# The First Session with Children and Adolescents

# THE FIRST SESSION
## with Children and Adolescents
### Conducting a Comprehensive Mental Health Evaluation

**Alvin E. House**

**The Guilford Press**
*New York   London*

© 2002 The Guilford Press
A Division of Guilford Publications, Inc.
72 Spring Street, New York, NY 10012
www.guilford.com

Printed in the United States of America

This book is printed on acid-free paper.

Last digit is print number:  9  8  7  6  5  4  3  2  1

**Library of Congress Cataloging-in-Publication Data**

House, Alvin E.
    The first session with children and adolescents : conducting
a comprehensive mental health evaluation / Alvin E. House.
        p. ; cm.
    Includes bibliographical references and index.
    ISBN 1-57230-750-1 (cloth)
    1. Mental illness—Diagnosis. 2. Adolescent psychopathology.
3. Child psychopathology. 4. Mental health services—
Evaluation. 5. Therapist and patient.    I. Title.
    [DNLM: 1. Mental Disorders—diagnosis—Adolescence.
2. Mental Disorders—diagnosis—Child.  WS 350 H842f 2002]
RJ503.5 .H683 2002
616.89′00835—dc21
                                                    2001055659

# About the Author

**Alvin E. House, PhD**, is a clinical psychologist whose professional practice has focused on psychological evaluation. For the past quarter of a century he has conducted assessments for medical, vocational, school, and forensic consultations. As an Associate Professor of Psychology at Illinois State University, he routinely teaches graduate-level courses in mental health diagnosis, psychological assessment, and psychopathology. He has coauthored a manual on observational assessment of children and has published articles and book chapters on intellectual, personality, and neuropsychological testing. His favorite consultative interests, in collaboration with his wife, Betty, are their children: Tiechera House Samuell and Brannan House.

# Preface

This book grew out of the two main professional activities of my life: clinical assessment and graduate education. While I do a certain amount of behavior modification and psychotherapy, and occasionally offer psychological consultation to agencies, most of my applied work revolves around psychological assessment and testing. From my interactions with child and adolescent clients, their families, and the other people in their lives, I have learned something about the process of evaluating the lives of children and the situations in which they function. In my other role as a university professor, I have a variety of assignments. I teach undergraduate classes, conduct research, write, and serve on university committees. Much of my work has focused on the professional education and training of graduate students in applied psychology. From my interactions with graduate students in clinical, counseling, and school psychology, I have learned about the process of passing on these lessons in evaluation to others. In this book I hope to convey to the reader my understanding of assessing youth, and to do so effectively, based on my other experiences in the professional training of students in helping professions.

The aim of this work is to help the reader conceptualize his or her initial contact with a new child or adolescent client. This is where all our future efforts to be of assistance to a child and her or his family begin: where we arrive at a preliminary understanding of what the problems are and what the situation in which these problems have developed is. This book is about the beginning, and how to make the most of it.

I have endeavored to make the focus and content of this book as easily applied as possible. I have made every effort to document the empirical basis for the opinions and recommendations I give here, but my primary goal is to improve the assessment skills of the reader, which cannot always come out of research and reports. In some of the text I discuss our attitudes toward youth or behavioral disorders because I believe that these attitudes often affect our actions as evaluators. By examining some of our own feelings and beliefs about those we serve and the process of the service, I believe we can become more effective and efficient in carrying out mental health assessments.

Most of the chapters in this book center on the problems most commonly seen in child and adolescent mental health evaluation. A number of relatively specific recommendations and suggestions are given for the reader to consider. When these guidelines for evaluation are common practice in the helping fields or have some documentation in the professional literature, I have tried to indicate this. For much of the day-to-day structuring of assessments, however, there is little specific direction to be found in the available literature. What I offer the reader when there is not an empirical basis for practice are the choices and procedures I have found helpful while working as a clinical psychologist over the past 26 years. Much professional education in the helping professions remains largely on the level of tutorial and mentorship, and many of my clinical skills were developed by modeling the actions of my professors and supervisors. Teaching by example, either personally or in a more abstract way through the medium of a book, will no doubt remain important in the education of psychologists, social workers, psychiatrists, criminal justice caseworkers, pastoral counselors, and other mental health specialists for years to come. Here I have striven to provide examples and illustrations of the principles of clinical assessment through segments of interviews carried out with youth.

Learning by emulation can be affected by the possible limits of generalization from the sample provided. If my experience is based on a representative sample of cases, then copying my behavior can be a very helpful strategy. If my experience is limited to a narrow range of cases, then applying even the most useful skills I have developed may not help with cases that significantly depart from the original sample. This is the great difficulty with teaching specific cases and clinical illustrations—how unique were the circumstances of this child's situation? How generally will the lessons of this case apply to other clients who are seen in the future? These questions always need to be on our mind as we try to learn from other people's examples and illustrations.

I have had the opportunity to evaluate a great many young people over the years, in a variety of professional settings. I hope that this large sample of cases includes examples that well represent the work most mental health professionals will be confronted with in their daily practice. The ultimate test will, of course, be when you, the reader, attempt to put my suggestions into practice in your own work. It is my sincere hope that you will find my lessons helpful to both you and your clients. My best wishes as you strive to serve your clients as faithfully as possible.

# Acknowledgments

I would like to express my thanks to wife, Betty House, who supported my effort to bring this work to completion and put up with many hours of my absence during its creation. I would also like to acknowledge the patience and encouragement of Christopher Jennison, my editor at The Guilford Press, who stuck with me through several slow periods.

Although I have been blessed with a number of extraordinary academic instructors and colleagues, some of the most important lessons I've learned have come from individuals far removed from classrooms. Among these teachers were my father, Frank L. House; my friend and brother, the Rev. Harold Hall; and the many young people who shared for a time my consultation office.

# Contents

# 1 The Mental Status Examination in Psychological Assessment

*A* child is waiting in your reception area. Usually he or she is accompanied by a parent or two; sometimes an older sister has brought him or her; occasionally a not-so-small group of parents, grandparents, aunts, and various siblings and cousins have taken over the waiting area. What are you to do with this child and the retinue? You are a psychologist, a counselor, a mental health therapist, juvenile probation officer, or psychiatric resident. Your years of training and study have brought you to this point—a child is waiting to speak to you. How do you begin learning about this other person, his or her life and difficulties, and what you might be able to offer?

All psychological, psychiatric, social work, and other human service interactions begin with an initial evaluation of the individual seeking services by the mental health professional. This evaluation can be informal, impressionistic, and unarticulated; it can also be formal, objective, and carefully recorded. In traditional discussions of assessment and evaluation, this initial evaluation was often referred to as the "mental status evaluation." It was based on your observations of the client's behavior, the client's report to you of what was going on, and on the data generated by asking your client to perform one or more tasks in the session. Some discussions of psychological assessment carefully differentiated between the mental status assessment, which was based on observations and actions in the session, and the client's mental health history, which was based on the client's self-report and content response to inquiry.

This differentiation between mental status examination and mental health history parallels the distinction drawn between a "sign" of mental illness (an observed characteristic) and a "symptom" of mental illness (the client's verbal report of a difficulty). Different health care professions have developed their own traditions and methodologies of initial assessment. Despite the various differences in approach, the fundamental nature of the initial contact with a client remains the same—understanding and formulation of the client's situation in a manner that allows assistance to be provided. The initial evaluation of a client, whether in a formal diagnostic process or as a first therapy contact, is the beginning of the process of providing that client with help. This basic core function remains the same whether the client is a child, adolescent, adult, couple, family, or other human system.

The purpose of this book is to consider the process of carrying out that initial mental health evaluation of children and adolescents with psychological and psychiatric problems. Whereas other books focus on the categorization of children's problems (House, 1999; Rapoport & Ismond, 1996), the emphasis here is on the methods used for obtaining data about youth. This information could lead to classification or treatment planning or could be put to several other purposes. Regardless of the particular diagnostic system being used in a mental health setting, certain basic information must be collected. You need to learn what is going on with that child who is waiting for you in the reception area, decide what needs to happen next for him or her, and get this plan put into action. You need to learn a great deal about your new client as quickly and efficiently as possible in order to achieve these various goals. This process is what I was trained to think of as a "mental status evaluation."

Mental status examinations typically seek to elicit signs and symptoms of psychological disturbance. These are the raw data that are organized into our understanding of a case, whether this organization is done by a diagnosis, a behavioral treatment plan, or any other kind of formulation. With the continuing effort to increase the reliability of psychiatric classification, a great emphasis has been placed on information that can be objectively assessed. As mentioned previously, a "sign" in this context usually refers to data that is directly assessed by the evaluator—observations of a child's actions in the office or on the playground, the child's responses to tasks presented to him or her, performance characteristics such as speed of responding. The characterization of this type of information as "objective" reveals the bias within most of the available literature on mental health evaluation—the belief that the evaluator is probably a more credible source of information than the available informants are. Behavior that is witnessed by the evaluator tends to be weighed as especially important, notwithstanding the many issues of observer reliability, drift, bias, and validity that must be addressed whenever human beings are used as measurement instruments.

Along with the observations and direct measurements taken by the examiner, the verbal report of the client must be considered. The conventional use of the term "symptoms" refers to the problems and experiences reported by the client. The child who tells us that she has been feeling "sad," has been crying a lot, and frequently thinks about killing herself is reporting symptoms. The parent who reports that the child has seemed "lost," is crying often, and has said she wishes she were dead is reporting symptoms.

Symptoms are critical to mental health assessment for a number of reasons. Many of the phenomena of interest to us do not occur in our offices and may not be able to be replicated within our offices—important aspects of a child's adjustment concern the events taking place on the playground, in the living room, and between peer group members. On some occasions the evaluator may journey to the classroom for an *in situ* observation; the clinician may role play the interaction with the friend that led up to the fight; but, however valuable these approximations are, the reality is that we must often depend on the verbal reports of our clients to open their world up to us.

A second aspect to our dependence on symptom report is that often the nature of the phenomena we are interested in is inherently private—the subjective experience of the child. To this we have access only by the child's grace and verbal report. There is not an "objective" measure of the frequency of suicidal thoughts or the intensity of anger; there is only what the child can report to us of these experiences. The challenge of collecting symptom data that are as reliable, valid, and useful as possible has been a major methodological consideration in the development of evaluation strategies.

The challenge of eliciting signs and symptoms of mental illness—cognitive, emotional, and behavioral responses that cause the client distress and interfere with his or her adjustment and achievement—in an efficient and effective manner is what makes mental health assessment the interesting and demanding activity it is. Initial assessment grew out of the general clinical tradition of diagnostic interviewing.

The initial clinical interview remains the basic activity for psychological evaluation, but increasing awareness of its limitations have opened the door for other approaches to assessment. One major development, especially for research, has been the development of structured interviews for children and for their caretakers. Structured interviews increase the reliability of results by standardizing the areas assessed, and they may further objectify the process by standardizing the wording of the questions and follow-up probes used to elicit interview data. Data can also be gained through having caretakers and children respond to printed stimuli—the behavior rating scales and self-report measures of psychological testing.

Increased standardization can also be seen in the tasks used to elicit performance data (signs) from clients during the evaluation. Cognitive aspects of adjustment especially can be measured by direct challenge. We can ask the child to speak, read, spell, draw, copy, and problem solve for us within the evaluation session. These requests can be informal, spontaneous, and original to this child in this situation, or they can be standardized and carefully planned. As with the interview questions, a series of tasks yields our formal assessment of mentation. Many of the ability tests of psychological assessment can be traced back in origin to the mental status items of traditional neurological evaluations.

The information obtained in the initial evaluation is used by the clinician to gain an understanding of the child and his or her situation and problems. In turn, based on this understanding, a clinician can build a case formulation, a psychiatric diagnosis, a therapeutic treatment plan, or a disposition recommendation. The initial evaluation may be guided by clinical and conceptual formulations, research needs, or legal mandates (Lifter, 1999) or by a combination of both professional and societal influences. The initial evaluation often leads to further assessment—formal intelligence and achievement testing for documentation of learning problems or mental retardation; medical evaluation of associated biological factors; further psychological evaluation of the child or important figures in her or his life. The final product may be a report with a codified DSM-IV (*Diagnostic and Statistical Manual of Mental Disorders,* 4th edition; American Psychiatric Association, 1994) or ICD-10 (*International Classification of Diseases,* 10th edition; World Health Organization, 1992) classification; an IDEA (Individuals with Disabilities Education Act, Public Law 94-142) qualifying categorization; an IEP (Individualized Education Plan) or treatment protocol to guide our interventions with the child over weeks or months; or simply a decision that no further action is indicated or necessary at this time. The beginning of all of these outcomes was an initial assessment of the child's abilities, emotions, and behavior—a formulation of his or her problems and general situation. I turn now to this first evaluation of children and teenagers. The child in your reception area is still waiting, but there is one bit of business that needs attention.

## THE INTERVIEW SEGMENTS

Many of the chapters in this book provide segments of interviews with children, adolescents, and occasionally their caretakers that are used to illustrate aspects of initial assessment and evaluation. In my courses such case material is usually popular; students enjoy "real-life" material. Case examples can often illustrate, quite meaningfully and in a brief manner, highly complex or subtle issues that can be difficult to adequately address in exposition alone. Clinical examples can put a human face on the abstract concepts of assessment, diagnosis, treatment planning, and intervention. Demonstrations drawn from actual practice can help convey the decision making and synthesis involved in applied clinical work. Moments from actual counseling sessions can also show us the difficulties and blind alleys visited by even the most experienced evaluator in a way that no purely conceptual discussion captures. For all these reasons, case illustrations have been used in much of this book. A reasonable question for the reader would be, "Are these examples real? Did any such children and teenagers ever walk this earth, or were they created solely for this work?"

As in much of our professional lives the answer is more complicated than the question would seem to call for; or, put another way, the answer is, "Yes and no." Yes, the youths are real; I knew all of them once upon a time over a career that has already spanned a quarter of a century. But many of them, perhaps most, would not recognize themselves in these pages; and few, if any, of their parents or other caretakers would have reason to believe they knew any of these children. Actually, those who might believe they did recognize a child would almost certainly be wrong. The case illustrations have been changed to protect the confidentiality of those involved. The changes went far beyond using different names, and that is where some of the complications come in. Different aspects of the clinical illustrations were altered to disguise the young people, in some cases to turn them almost entirely into someone else. In a few cases, a youth is really a composite of more than one actual child I encountered. In cases in which it didn't seem a pivotal point, some children have changed gender. Most have gained or lost a few months or years, symptoms have been substituted, many associated details (siblings, relatives, specific events) have been tampered with. The intent was to preserve the aspects of the case being used as an illustration while adjusting many other factors in order to provide the maximum protection of privacy and respect to the original real person. I ask you to trust my judgment that the changes were unimportant details to the particular point being made and that the information retained contains the essential and actual elements.

A further complication is that almost all the case illustrations are based on my memory of the interviews. My clinical records occasionally contain verbatim quotes, but never of extended exchanges. Most of my records contain the information gained, but not the exact route taken to obtain it. I have only a few tapes and transcripts of my actual sessions. The interviews presented here live in my mind because they were striking to me, because I had done something well (or very poorly), or because the youth had stepped out from behind his or her mask for a moment as a living, feeling, behaving individual. Unfortunately, we know that what we remember didn't necessarily happen that way. My confidence that I can actually recall a conversation with a 7-year-old in 1974 as I write this sentence in 2001 is real, but this confidence does not guarantee the accuracy of the recall. You and I are both at the mercy of my memories, and many things, of which the truth can be among the least, move memories. Fortunately, my part is really only of minor importance in these segments of conversation and interaction. What is really of significance are the lives of the youths presented here and how their lives were shared with another through question and discussion.

So my final answer to the question framed at the beginning of this disclaimer would be: Yes, the children are real; as real as any other person can be real to any of us. They once shared a time with me and now live in my mind and memory, and I have shared them with you as best I was able. I hope that they can teach you as they instructed me, for much of what I know of the practice of psychological evaluation was gained in the company of these children.

# 2 Evaluations of Infants, Children, and Adolescents

$W$hy should the assessment of the child scheduled for your next appointment require any special discussion? The problems appearing in youths are not usually essentially different in nature from those seen in adults. The diagnosis of mental disorders in children uses the same categories applied to the diagnosis of mature individuals. Treatment manuals are usually organized around the same problem topics. What is there about the developmental years that makes necessary a discussion focused on evaluation of adaptation difficulties during this period?

## DEVELOPMENTAL ASPECTS OF THE MENTAL HEALTH EVALUATIONS OF MINORS

In many respects the evaluation of infants, children, and adolescents is identical to the psychological assessment of adults and senior citizens: Circumstances are created in which information can be collected, and this information is used to guide further assessment, eventually leading to diagnoses, treatment plans, and the other dispositions arrived at in clinical work. Furthermore, many of the general heuristics of clinical investigation are identical: Interviewing remains the most commonly used assessment tool; the process in many ways depends on the goodwill of the client, so forming a positive working relationship is usually essential; and we are usually most interested in patterns of behavior, emotions, or cognitions. Given these important similarities, one might wonder, Why a book about the assessment of children? Despite many common features, there are several particular aspects of childhood and adolescence that influence the process of mental health assessment in unique ways. Consideration of these differences can lead to a better understanding of both the adjustment of minors and of the available empirical literature.

## The Impact of the Referral Source

A key feature in our available empirical literature on behavior problems in children versus adults concerns how the client came to our attention. Adults are usually self-referred. They have sought help; usually because something in their lives is causing them distress and unhappiness. The adult is miserable due to a serious depression or because his or her spouse will not stop nagging him or her about excessive drinking. In either case the adult has at least some degree of vested motivation in the process of the evaluation, sufficient at least to have spurred on the process of seeking help.

In contrast to this adult scenario, children, and to a lesser degree adolescents, almost never bring themselves into evaluation or therapy. They are typically in the consulting room because someone else in their world, usually a parent or teacher, has expressed concern about how the young person's life is going. This situation has several consequences. First, the child may not be distressed to the same degree by his or her actions, feelings, or thoughts as the adult who initiated evaluation is. All thoughtful readers will recognize that children and caretakers are not necessary upset about the same events and circumstances. Animal fears are quite common in young children but are almost never a reason for consultation; school phobia is a relatively rare extreme fear in childhood, but it is often a cause of referral for evaluation. *Children are evaluated for behavior that concerns the adults in their lives.* This basic difference in referral patterns affects, in turn, the available empirical literature on mental health phenomena in children. One can find many articles on school phobia or school refusal in children, a relatively rare extreme fear, but very few on animal phobias, a much more common extreme fear among young people.

A second important consequence of this difference in how children come to be in our waiting rooms has to do with their motivation to cooperate with the process. With adult clients, although circumstances vary and although there are enormous differences in the level of commitment and energy shown by adults undergoing assessment, they usually have a basic motivation to cooperate that grows out of the distress that initially brought them to us as clients. With children and adolescents this motivation cannot be automatically assumed. Children and teenagers may have little or no sense of personal urgency to cooperate so as to relieve their own suffering. Their actual motivation may often be exactly the opposite—they are exposed to a potentially threatening or actually aversive experience (the interview with you) without having a sense of how this might serve them in any way. Helping the young person understand how he or she can benefit from the planned evaluation can sometimes be critical in obtaining good data.

## Developmental Differences in Language Abilities

Another important difference between young clients and adults that affects mental health evaluations is skill and facility with language. As speech, language, and conceptual abilities increase over the first two decades of life, it becomes increasingly easier to obtain information from the juvenile client in the same efficient manner in which it is often obtained from adults—by asking questions and receiving answers. Despite all the well-documented limitations of interviewing, it remains a highly effective and efficient assessment tool. With young people, however, this tool is often constricted in application. The problem is not simply that children talk differently than adults do, more important is the reality that they may think differently, as well. As an illustration, consider feelings in children. Young children experience deep feelings, but attempting to carry out an abstract discussion of emotional states and symptoms with a preschool child is usually an exercise in futility. The emotional experiences are there, but the mental equipment to understand and the verbal experience to communicate these affective features of life is often lacking. Young children may be much more capable of expressing their feelings through art or play. Talking about feelings may be a skill still far off in their development.

Limited verbal skills affect not only our interviewing tools but also the various assessment devices we use—symptom checklists, adjustment inventories, and personality questionnaires. Examiners who wish to make use of these highly valuable tools must carefully consider reading levels, mental ages of standardization samples, and how concurrent validity was established in using even the simplest of psychological questionnaires with youths.

A positive outcome of the limited language abilities of the youthful client has been the early and consistent recognition by most examiners that other sources of data are essential in evaluating the mental health adjustment of children. Situational assessments, data obtained from collateral sources, observational measures, and the integration of multisource, multimethod data are all familiar topics within the literature on assessment of children. The impetus behind the development of these evaluation strategies has often been a recognition that interview techniques alone would not suffice. The benefit of the attention given to alternative approaches to assessment has been the appreciation of a much wider range of evaluation data than is often considered with adults.

## Developmental Perspectives in Data Comparison

A related development in approaches to the assessment of youth is the recognition of the need for developmentally appropriate comparison populations for nomothetic data. As attempts have been made to objectify and quantify measures of children's behaviors, emotions, and thoughts, attention has also been given to making sure that fair bases of comparison are used. Age- or education-level norm groups are usually employed for comparison with a given child's scores. In cases in which it has been shown to be of value, separate normative groups for males and females have been developed for some aspects of performance. Racial, ethnic, and subcultural normative comparison populations have been used in the development of some psychological measures of children. The use of age-graded norms has long been the standard in ability and achievement testing, and current evaluation approaches for emotional and behavioral adjustment tend to take a similar perspective.

## Developmental Differences in Presentation and Associated Characteristics of Mental Health Problems in Youths

The most obvious reason for differentiating the evaluation of mental health problems in children from the study of adult adjustment difficulties might be that the disorders themselves seem to be fundamentally different. If "depression" or "schizophrenia" in youths turn out to be quite different in symptom manifestation, etiology, or functional relationships than they are in adults, then it would make sense to speak of "childhood depression" and "childhood schizophrenia," and these topics would deserve their own study and consideration. As it has turned out, with our increasing knowledge of emotional, behavioral, and cognitive disturbances in youth, this is usually not the case. Depression, schizophrenia, phobias, and many other psychiatric disorders have been repeatedly found to be essentially similar in both adult and child cases. Although differences have certainly been noted, these developmental features often seem relatively minor, and the commonalities much more salient. So, although decreased libido is often a symptom of severe depression in adults but almost never mentioned in severe depression in prepubertal youth, the basic concept of a depressed state with multiple cognitive, behavioral, and physiological symptoms does seem to hold for children and adolescents, as well as adults. Overall, the available empirical literature does support major commonalities between the forms of behavioral disturbances in children and adults. This major conclusion, however, should not prevent us from recognizing that there can be important differences in the expression of disorders at different developmental points. As an illustration, the essential symptoms of posttraumatic stress disorder (PTSD) appear to be essentially the same in youth and adults: generalized hyperarousal, behavioral and cognitive avoidance, and intrusion of trauma-associated material. Children, however, appear to show a wider range of associated symptoms than do adults, symptoms that vary with a number of features of the trauma, the child, and the child's environment (Lipschitz, Rasmusson, & Southwick, 1998). Furthermore, traumatized children appear more likely than traumatized adults to develop PTSD as a chronic response to overwhelming stress (Lipschitz et al., 1998). Similar examples could be developed from a number of behavior disorders, even some that were initially conceptualized in terms of youth. Attention-deficit/hyperactivity disorder (ADHD) is increasingly being recognized as often continuing into adulthood, though it may show some change or attenuation of symptom presentation (Guyer, 2000). Appreciation of the developmental differences in symptom picture and associated characteristics of psychiatric disorders enhances our evaluations of children, adolescents, and adults.

## Stability/Instability of Behavior Patterns in Youths

A final difference that the examiner needs to consider in the mental health evaluation of youths is the relative stability of adjustment and maladjustment patterns in young people. The common perception is that the behavior of children may be more fluid when contrasted with that of adults. This is a general feature of the years of rapid developmental change, but it can also apply to many behavior problems. Measures of adjustment difficulty in children may be unreliable over time because the phenomenon itself may not be stable. A very basic and continuing challenge in research concerning both normal and abnormal behavior in children is determining how persistent, chronic, and generalized these manifestations are over time (see Lavigne et al., 1998a, 1998b). Some behavior problems (e.g., autism, mental retardation) are often quite stable over time, others are chronic but intermittent (many mood disorders), others have high rates of both stability and instability (e.g., ADHD, learning disorders), and still others tend often to disappear with the passage of time (e.g., enuresis, adjustment problems). The general nature of a problem (e.g., anxiety) may persist, but the specific symptoms manifested may change dramatically over time (cf. Craske, Poulton, Tsao, & Plotkin, 2001). This natural variability of behavior and behavior problems in children greatly complicates the process of learning about mental health challenges in youth. In some ways this represents a kind of "uncertainty principle" of psychological assessment. One can certainly assess the behavior, feelings, and thoughts of a child at this moment, but there is always a significant limitation in how safely these conclusions (even if accurate) can be generalized to future times. The longer the interval, the greater the uncertainty.

## BUILDING RAPPORT

Establishing a working relationship with the youths we are evaluating is usually a critical first step in assessment. In the absence of a cooperative exchange, the evaluator will be limited to observations and the reports of other informants, which is a very constricted base of data to work with. Social and verbal interaction provides a rich field of information for the mental health professional, if it can be accomplished.

### Rapport with the Young Child

Developing a productive working relationship with a young child depends on a variety of factors: the child's temperament, the manner of the caretakers accompanying him to the session, the historical relationship between child and caretaker, the circumstances leading to the evaluation, the child's history with health care providers, and your reactions to the child, parents, and situation, as well as other influences. Of these considerations, only your own behavior is subject to immediate and direct control. It is worth considering the other influences, insofar as the range of mediating events should make it clear that there is no "correct" set of actions you can take that will work with all young children on all occasions. As in many other clinical situations, you begin with assessment strategies that have worked well in the past and modify them based on reactions of the particular child currently being examined.

It is my usual custom to greet the parents and child in the waiting room or area. I introduce myself to the adults and clarify who everyone is. Typically the parent introduces the child; if this does not occur I introduce myself to the young person: "Hello, I am Dr. House. How about coming with me and talking a little; do you like games?" This greeting is accompanied by actions initiating a trip back to my office. I usually separate the child relatively quickly from the caretakers for at least a brief initial contact. This separation serves several purposes: First, I establish a precedent for the child going for a private conversation with me. Second, I observe how the child reacts to separation from his or her caretakers. Third, I establish my role as the one responsible for structuring the contacts with the family. Evaluation of the child's ease of separation from his familiar caretakers to go with an "approved but unknown" professional can provide important diagnostic and developmental data. The other two considerations are intended to increase the child's and parents' comfort, security, and rapport. I want to spend some time alone with the child. Demonstrating early in our relationship that this is a standard part of business appears to help put most children at ease. Similarly, most parents begin to feel more comfortable if the professional demonstrates evidence of confidence, prior planning, leadership, and organization.

If the child reacts very badly to an early attempt to separate him or her from his or her parents, I usually negotiate with the child and caretakers for one parent to accompany us briefly. Once again, my initial plan is to dismiss the parent relatively rapidly from the room, observing the reaction this precipitates in the client. I am very interested in the child's response if the parent objects to the child leaving with me. I usually simply inform the parent that this is my standard practice and that I would be most comfortable following it. If the parent persists, I offer to briefly discuss it with the caretaker(s) in private. This situation has occurred only a handful of times in many evaluations of young children.

Building rapport with the young child begins with the walk to my office. I comment on the child's clothing, possessions he or she is holding, the weather that day, where the child has come from, what plans the family has following the appointment, objects in the office that the child appears intrigued by, or any other topic that appears to have some potential interest to the young person. Children often respond verbally, but even in the absence of words, a range of reactions can be observed. Eye contact and facial expressions, body and defensive movements, cooperation or resistance to attempts to connect with him or her, all contribute to an initial impression of the child's current emotional state. Responding with words and actions to this emotional display begins building rapport between the child and the examiner. As the youth experiences the examiner as an adult who takes him seriously, listens to his words, notices how he feels, and tries to accommodate his situation, the child's sense of security and trust begins to build.

In the office the child is seated as comfortably as the furnishings allow. I offer a few words of explanation as to our plan of action: "I wanted a chance to talk to you about being here today, and what has been going on. Your mother called me and said. . . . Let me ask you a few questions. . . . " From this basis mental status inquiries proceed. If the child has difficulty responding to these questions, I make a transition into more overt activity: "Would you like to draw something? Here is some paper and markers, show me what you can draw"; or "Have you ever played 'Simon Says'? Lets try a game."

## Rapport with the School-Age Child

With the school- or "latency"-age child, the most consistently effective path to rapport building for me has been movement into discussion of the child's favorite activities. School-age children in a professional's office are often most comfortable and least defensive discussing external events and activities—hobbies, sports, part-time jobs, school activities, youth groups, and so forth. Elicitation of this information begins both to build up a database about this child's life and to establish a pattern of communication between child and examiner. This can serve as a foundation for movement into topics less easy or comfortable to explore aloud in front of a stranger—peer relationships, conflicts with friends and rivals, personal or family failures, losses, and so forth. Sensitive discussion of these more emotionally charged subjects helps demonstrate the safety of some initial sharing with the interviewer of highly threatening issues—conflicts with parents, perceptions of family stress, fears, perceived weaknesses, and so forth. With certain exceptions (e.g., suicide, which needs to be addressed directly at the appropriate time), the general strategy of fading or successive approximations is a highly valuable one for organizing interview content—beginning with topics easy for the child to discuss and moving into more difficult areas as initial respect and trust is established.

The issues of the child's loyalty to his or her parents and family members and respect for the family's privacy or "secrets" becomes an issue for many children during the elementary school years. Some children may experience great distress or guilt on realizing that they have criticized a parent or revealed a sensitive family event in front of an outsider. Reiteration, in appropriate language, of the rules of the therapeutic relationship and sensitivity to the possibility that the child may be saying things about which he or she will feel bad later are both essential features of interviewing school-age children. Respect for the multiple demands on the child's loyalties helps build rapport. Cognitive reframing of both the events reported (in at least potentially neutral terms) and of the child's participation in the evaluation as a clearly positive action for the long-term benefit of his or her family can help reduce the conflict potentially engendered by the child's responsiveness in the interview.

## Rapport with the Adolescent Still Attending School

The prospect of interviewing adolescents tends to terrify many mental health professionals. A significant proportion of the underground humor of clinicians' subculture revolves around the intractability, haughtiness, and evil of the typical teenager. How many times do we hear in the staff lounge glib comments such as, "Adolescence is a mental illness." Teenagers often seem a challenge to us, no less than to their parents, not so much by what they do but by their very existence. At the same time, most of us know some colleagues who enjoy working with adolescents and seem highly skilled at it. I would suggest that a careful consideration of "teen effective" counselors would reveal very little difference in their interviewing, therapeutic, or diagnostic skills from those of the more typical "teen phobic" counselor. I believe that the effective differences have to do with the attitudes, beliefs, and values of the counselors who work more effectively with adolescents. Specifically, I believe the essential elements of success in forming working relationships with adolescents are our tolerance of differences in motives, our own and the clients' honesty, and our respect for those in a weaker position than ourselves. Although these may be valuable or important clinician attributes for work with many or all clients, for work with teens I believe they are vital.

Most of us recognize and accept to some degree individual differences. We look about us and see that people are different in many ways. Some of our friends are taller than we are and some are shorter; some are physically stronger and some weaker; some learn more rapidly than we do and some struggle more than we do. Through our lives, our upbringing, the people who influence us, and our training we come to some position about these differences. Most individuals in mental health fields see themselves, and hope to be perceived by most others, as "tolerant" of differences. But most forms of tolerance have limitations, especially if the difference is often not openly articulated. I would suggest that an aspect of human difference that is especially difficult to appreciate is that in basic motivations. The possibility that not all people really want what we want can be easily said but can be very hard to accept emotionally. For the typical mental health professional, no less than for many parents, the inner certainties that everyone would really like to do well in school if they could, that we all do want to get along with others, and that everyone would feel better about doing their fair share of the work may have never been questioned. Adolescents often question these assumptions by their every action and inaction. They resist the imposition of values from without. Unless the counselor can tolerate the adolescent's ambivalence toward standard values and beliefs, can actively work at helping the youth to learn what he or she is beginning to think, and can help articulate "common cause" between adolescent, family, and counselor, it will be very difficult to work effectively with the youth. This is a imposing task that at times exceeds our achievement, but it is a necessary first step in my experience.

Most mental health professionals value honesty in human relationships and profess the functional strength of honesty within the professional relationship. At the same time, we often avoid certain topics with many clients because we would rather not be fully open and honest with them, possibly for very good reasons that are in the clients' best interests. With certain clients this conflict becomes central to establishing effective rapport, in particular, clients with borderline personality disorder and clients (regardless of the nature of their problems) who are teenagers. Much like the individual with borderline features, an adolescent is often exquisitely sensitive to mendacity. They hear the reverberation of the half-truth, the slight evasion, the less than total candor in our voices; see the shift of our eyes; feel the change in our body language. Many adolescents expect to be lied to by adults, they are ever alert for it, and it seldom escapes their attention—unless they want to be lied to. It is a paradoxical truth that teenagers are both the most difficult and the easiest group of people in the world to successfully deceive. The difference is, of course, whether the lie is congruent with what the youth would like to believe. The car salesperson suggesting that the teenager could easily come up with the payments through his or her part-time job may be experienced as a "solid" and unbiased source; whereas the parent's remark that "we just can't afford it" is easily recognized as a half-truth. This example was chosen to illustrate an important point—that the parent may be stating the facts to a certain extent: The family cannot easily afford another vehicle. But this is not the whole truth. The parents may be unwilling to commit the family's money to this venture because they don't believe that the teen will be responsible about his or her side of the contract. Perhaps the parent isn't convinced that the young person deserves this possession or thinks that other members of the family have a greater claim on the division of resources. Perhaps all of these and other thoughts and feelings go through the parent's mind. All that is said is, "We can't afford it," and the teenager hears the omissions and feels deceived.

I have found that working with adolescents living at home (in a dependent state) tends to require a demanding commitment to honesty. Full and complete disclosure has to be the rule for there to be any hope of gaining the young person's cooperation. This commitment can require a great deal of effort from the examiner because it causes us to carefully inspect our actions and words with the adolescent and with the family for their consistency and openness. It also requires humility and the capacity to admit our errors when we discover the times we have not been fully honest with the adolescent. This may not occur during an initial evaluation, but I suggest that it almost inevitably occurs in ongoing relationships. How we handle lapses of communication is much more critical than their occurrence. Most teenagers recognize a truth that many adults may have forgotten: Everyone does lie at times.

This does not make lying right, nor does it mean everyone is untrust-worthy. The people who don't have to lie about their lies can usually be believed (about most things). In at least this respect it is good for coun-selors to be like adolescents.

### Rapport with the Independent Adolescent or College Student

In my experience, work with emancipated adolescents, high school graduates, or college student proceeds best if they are treated as adults. Legally they may well be so, but even if not, it is almost always most productive to treat them as adults to the degree possible. Special cir-cumstances (e.g., guardianship by the state office of child and family protective services, probation status, etc.) may prevent according the young person the full privileges of adult status. If this is the case, im-mediately bring it up for discussion, clarify how this special circum-stance may affect our relationship and work, and negotiate the best possible working relationship under the circumstances. Approaching the problem in this direct and respectful manner usually helps initiate good rapport with the youth. The key psychological variable is that I re-ally do consider these clients to be functionally adults, even if they are not accorded this status by society. Their perception of this attitude on my part helps establish a working relationship.

## SPECIAL PROBLEMS AND POPULATIONS

Several subgroups within the general population of children and ado-lescents present special challenges for accurate and comprehensive evaluation. These youths have particular characteristics that complicate the evaluation by affecting the confidence that can be placed in our usual tools of assessment. In some cases these limitations can be com-pensated for, and in all cases the possible impact of atypical features should be borne in mind. Both the conclusions reached and the confi-dence we can place in our interpretations can be touched by these fea-tures.

### Evaluation of the Severely Compromised Infant and Child

The assessment of children with severe physical or cognitive disability or both presents a great challenge for the mental health practitioner.

Careful observation and description of functional competencies can be valuable in the evaluation of grossly impaired children. The emerging literature on neuropsychological assessment of infants and young children can be a useful reference for this work (Aylward, 1997). Bucy, Smith, and Landau (1999) present a very practical discussion of evaluating preschool children with significant developmental disabilities.

Evaluation of very young children presents challenges similar to those of assessing severely compromised youth, and the literature on behavior observations and evaluation of young children can be drawn on to aid our work with developmentally delayed children. Dunn (1999), for example, reviews the assessment of sensorimotor and perceptual development in preschool children and shows how careful attention to observational data can guide the evaluation of very young children. She illustrates, for example, the progression of grasping patterns used in drawing or writing as the child's fine motor development progresses. It is relatively easy for the examiner to note whether the child uses an immature fisted grasp, a palmer or lateral grasp, or a more mature pincer or tripod grasp. Attention to such behavior during the session increases the detail and depth of our evaluations. Similar approaches have extended neurological evaluation to infants (Majnemer & Mazer, 1998)

Observations of children in structured situations have a long history of application in clinical assessment. W. H. Miller (1975) used structured situations in a therapy playroom to observe the interaction between children with behavior problems and their parents. Such techniques have continued to be utilized with a wide variety of problems. Handen, McAuliffe, Janosky, Feldman, and Breaus (1998) demonstrated the usefulness of controlled observations in evaluating children who showed both cognitive impairment and ADHD.

## Sensory Limitations

Sensory limitations and handicaps bring both a direct and a less obvious set of problems to our evaluations. The overt and immediate consequence of significant problems with either visual or auditory senses is that assessment approaches that rely on these information channels are compromised for evaluation purposes. Even in informal mental status evaluation, we typically rely on a variety of stimulus events. We ask questions that rely for their validity on the assumption of normal auditory registration. We ask the child to read text, copy a drawing, assemble a puzzle, model our movements—all depend on visual acuity. Developers of psychological, developmental, and educational tests have worked to create alternatives to standard measures that are not dependent on all the sensory channels usually invoked by common instruments. Nonverbal intelligence tests for deaf and hard of hearing clients and hepatic intelligence tests for the blind and visually impaired have been available for many years. To what degree the alternative measures are truly compatible with standard measures remains an ongoing question for researchers.

The less obvious and possibly more important complication brought about by sensory and motor difficulties (see the following section) has to do with the question of what constitutes normal development for a child with a major sensory handicap. Our formal, empirical, quantitative expectations of child and adolescent development and our informal, subjective, qualitative impressions of normal progress through life's challenges are based almost entirely on experience and research with physiologically intact human beings. Major sensory and motor handicaps affect a relatively small fraction of our population, and the lives of these children have had relatively little impact on the development of mental and psychological tests and measures. Articles may report that the mean tested IQ of a group of congenitally deaf children differs from that of a chronologically matched set of control children. Does this difference mean the same thing that it would if a group of children with normal hearing received comparably low scores? My clinical impression is that it often does not. Our ability to generalize from the limited set of test behaviors available to us in an evaluation to the broader and more important domain of the child's performance and adjustment outside the evaluation circumstances seems more limited for children with important sensory (and motor) handicaps than for the general population of children.

I am not suggesting that we abandon our tools and procedures of evaluation but that using a great deal of caution in our interpretation of results is very prudent with children who have sensory limitations. The evaluator should be very alert for evidence that is discrepant from formal results and should interpret this evidence as fully as they do the quantitative data from this testing. Roberts and Hindley (1999) provide an excellent review of the issues involved in assessing psychiatric disorders in deaf children. More work of this kind, considering other sensory handicaps and how they interact with our assessment of the child's emotional, behavioral, and cognitive adjustment and development, would greatly add to the literature on mental health assessment of young people.

## Motor Limitations

Many of the preceding comments about sensory limitations apply equally to motor problems. Motor control problems, however, do provide an opportunity to discuss another aspect of the evaluation of special children—the impact of different degrees of impairment. When a child is missing his or her right arm, due either to a congenital medical condition or to an accident at a later age, this difference is very obvious. The child, the child's family, peers, and teachers are all aware of this difference—it cannot be escaped and can barely be denied. This difference becomes part of the perception of the child—her image of herself and the image held of her by others.

More subtle motor problems, however, can be invisible to others. The child with mild cerebral palsy, for example, may not appear obviously handicapped to others. Although this may be a relief to the child's parents and often to the child himself, it is not without consequence or cost. The motor control problem is still there; it is just relatively invisible. When the child has problems with motor control, the adults and peers with whom the child interacts will reach other conclusions about the nature of these problems. Other children may decide these youngsters are "clumsy" or "slow" or "stupid" for dropping the ball all the time in games. Teachers may see in the child's poor handwriting evidence of deliberate oppositional tendencies or laziness: "If he would just try a little more I'm sure his printing could be neater." These reactions from others begin to

---

### Case Illustration 2.1. Tiechera's Helper Arm

A bright and active 5-year-old girl, Tiechera, lacked a lower left forearm and left hand due to a congenital malformation. She was learning to use a mechanical grasping device, which her parents thought would be more valuable to her than a cosmetically more circumspect but functionally less useful molded prosthetic arm. The physicians and physical therapists involved referred to the mechanical device as "Tiechera's helper arm," and this language was adopted by the family and school. Tiechera brought her helper arm to school and demonstrated what she was beginning to be able to do with it. The other children were very fascinated by the device, all wanted to see it work, some wanted to hold it, and a few wanted to try it as much as they could. Very quickly it became an accustomed sight, and little attention was paid to whether Tiechera was holding something in her flesh-and-blood hand or in her helper hand.

shape the child's self-perception and self-esteem. Careful review of medical and developmental records, interviewing of caretakers, and observation of movement, posture, and constructional behavior can contribute to the accurate evaluation of the child with motor problems. This assessment, in turn, can be used to begin addressing the child's needs, both instructional, psychological, and social.

Another aspect of atypical motor (or sensory) functioning concerns whether the limitations are congenital or acquired. In general, if a child has enjoyed normal sensory or motor function for a period, typical development has been supported for that time. When the sensory channel or the motor system is lost or compromised to some degree, the specific performances served by that system are limited in the future. However, the child has still had the advantage of a history of full development up to the time of the injury or illness. A simple example pertains to speech and language development in children with hearing impairment. Even total loss of hearing after a few years of normal auditory input often yields a child with fairly good speech and English language abilities. Congenital hearing loss is almost inevitably associated with severe speech problems, as well as language limitations, for standard English (the child's facility with non-auditory based language— e.g., American Sign Language (ASL)—is an independent issue). It is less obvious, but a similar developmental process appears to occur with loss of motor ability. The total picture of developmental competence appears significantly different in a child who has experienced typical motor ability up to a point of illness or injury than in a child with congenital limitations. You will find it useful to note in evaluations the history, as well as the degree, of motor (or sensory) difficulty.

## The Nonverbal Client

The child or adolescent who does not speak is among the most challenging clients seen for evaluation. Meaningful evaluation of the young person who does not participate in the almost universal symbolic exchange of ideas calls for ingenuity, patience, and perseverance.

### Hearing Impairments

Hearing impairment is the most common causal factor of speech and language problems. Hearing limitations bring difficulty to the assessment contact from two directions.

First, our capacity to communicate with these children is compromised—they do not understand what we wish to communicate to them because they cannot clearly hear us. The evaluator needs to utilize pantomime, gestures, written or signed instructions, pictorial directions, and whatever other devices or aids may assist their ability to effectively communicate with the young person. The evaluator may need to enlist the aid of a translator with competency in signing. All of these modifications of standard assessment procedures have potential, often unknown, implications for our results and interpretations. Although the frustration of this situation can perhaps begin to give us an appreciation of what the child may go through almost daily, it does nothing to help us communicate adequately to secure useful and reliable data from the evaluation.

Second, the child's ability to communicate with the examiner is compromised. The young person may also need to rely on alternative modes of communication, which may be more or less satisfactory for the needs of the evaluation. American Sign Language (ASL), for instance, is a complex system of symbolic communication, as are oral languages such as English or Japanese. Just as hearing children vary in their rates of acquisition of standard English and in their abilities to express complex messages, such as their perceptions or feelings, children who are developing a manual language vary in their facilities with their coding mechanisms. The introduction of a third party to serve as a translator and often to offer at least an informal assessment of the child's skills with ASL may be unavoidable—few mental health counselors are fluent in manual communication. A third party in the evaluation room, however, introduces a number of potential complications. The most likely possibility would be someone from the child's family. His or her parents may have gained some skills with ASL, and they are readily available, but how skilled are they? Furthermore, how comfortable is the child at passing private messages through a parent? Professional translators bring an established degree of technical competence but represent yet another stranger for the child to grow accustomed to.

## Language Impairments

The child with an expressive or a receptive–expressive language disorder is at distinct disadvantage in dealing with his or her world. We rely every day on our ability to use symbolic communication with others.

Individuals with severe language disorders have at times been misidentified as psychotic (Strub & Black, 1988). Psychological evaluation of the child or adolescent with severe language dysfunction can be very difficult because of the pervasive effects of this domain of functioning. It becomes especially important to attempt to isolate the point of dysfunction in the child's performance: Did he understand the question or direction? Can she process a solution? Can he communicate the solution or response? Can she demonstrate in some alternative manner her solution or response? The more clearly we can understand at what level the child's performance breaks down, the more clearly we can communicate his or her difficulties to others and plan remediation and treatment.

## Autism

The behavioral syndrome of autism is in part defined by language disorder and is frequently associated with mutism. Further, the child's behavior is often oppositional and, by definition, his or her response to social stimulation is inevitably atypical. One important challenge of assessing children with autism and other severe behavioral disorders is attempting to determine what the child *cannot* do and what he or she *will not* do at this time. Although the immediate practical differences are small, the longer term implications for education and habilitation can be of some significance. Higher tested intelligence and other indications of higher general cognitive ability have consistently been found to be an important positive prognostic variable with autism (Klinger & Dawson, 1996; Rapin, 1997; Wing, 1997).

## Selective Mutism

A special case of nonverbal behavior in childhood is selective mutism, in which evidence exists that the child can speak but does not. Children manifesting selective mutism often have normal mental abilities and usually cooperate with nonverbal intelligence tests and other ability measures, which helps in establishing these aspects of the child's condition. It is more difficult to effectively evaluate other areas of the child's personal and social adjustment, as one important source of data is not available. The possibility of other anxiety or social adjustment problems or both should be carefully evaluated. Overall, the empirical literature supports conceptualizing selective mutism as a social anxiety syndrome (Dummit et al., 1997; Kopp & Gillberg, 1997; Steinhausen & Juzi, 1996). A small subgroup of children with selective mutism also have a history or comorbid occurrence of speech and language problems. Finally, at least some case reports have described the concurrence of selective mutism with serious behavioral or emotional disturbance. Whether these cases represent merely statistical coincidence or a small subgroup with functional comorbidity is not clear.

## Mental Retardation

The nonverbal child with putative mental retardation presents the obvious challenge of establishing whether the child does in fact have any significant cognitive limitation or is only nonverbal for some reason. Our everyday and many formal conceptualizations of intelligence are so intimately associated with oral and written language use that it is difficult to separate the two. The child who is talkative, quick to question and answer, and seems to read voraciously is commonly perceived as bright, intelligent, possibly gifted. My observation is that adults may systematically overestimate the intelligence of highly verbal children. Conversely, the child who does not speak is just as universally regarded as mentally slow, and once the attribution of retardation is made, it can become the explanation for the child not speaking. We realize that a child is mentally retarded because he does not speak and understand that he does not talk because he is retarded. The circularity of this dance of illogic has been missed even by professionals.

Nothing in the concept of mental retardation implies muteness. Language use is a learned behavior, and this learning is affected by mental retardation. Mentally retarded children learn more slowly; this is explicit in our concept of mental retardation. But the absence of language is not consistent with any but the most profound cases of mental retardation alone. The condition of a completely nonverbal child or adolescent with mild mental retardation, for example, would require explanation. It is not adequate to say that the child is not talking because he or she is mentally retarded. In a mildly retarded child, we would expect possibly mild speech problems and mild language limitations. Severe language compromise or the absence of speech would suggest comorbid disorders, in addition to the mental retardation. Probably one of the more historically common evaluation errors with mentally retarded children has been the failure to identify comorbid diagnoses, some of which could be treated.

## SENSITIVITY TO DIVERSITY AND CULTURAL ISSUES IN ASSESSMENT

Increased discussion and consideration of possible roles played by cultural and ethnic background features in children's presentations, both normal and deviant, has become a positive trend in mental health evaluation. The consideration of cultural issues in DSM-IV represents a clear advance over previous diagnostic formulations (Smart & Smart, 1997), although issues of concern remain (Cervantes & Arroyo, 1994; Novins et al., 1997). This is to be expected; the role of cultural and ethnic background in shaping behavior is tremendous and can hardly be neatly dealt with by simple formulations. The related topic of how cultural differences may interact with the use of evaluation instruments, such as behavior rating scales, is just beginning to be addressed (DuPaul et al., 1998; Ramirez & Shapiro, 1998; Reid, 1995). The real significance of these and related publications is that cultural variables have become part of the ongoing dialogue regarding children and adolescent behavior and adjustment. The fundamental goal of all mental health evaluations is to understand the youth's actions as fully as possible in light of all the unique and shared circumstances of the young person's life. Formal consideration of how the multicultural diversity of present life contributes to a particular child's situation can only enrich our understanding.

Our increased sensitivity to cultural influences in the presentation and course of mental health problems also reflects a greater sensitivity to the range of variables that interact to shape behavior. Although most psychologists view behavior as a product of the individual and the environment, the conceptual and methodological sophistication to begin to understand this interaction has only begun to emerge in the social sciences. Family violence, for example, would probably be viewed by almost all therapists as a risk factor for adjustment problems, but gender differences affect the impact of this risk (Cummings, Pepler, & Moore, 1999; Jankowski, Leitenberg, Henning, & Coffey, 1999). The forces of poverty, another well-acknowledged risk factor, appear to be moderated by both personal (Ripple & Luthar, 2000) and ethnic (McLeod & Nonnemaker, 2000) characteristics. Even the influences of dire circumstances such as homelessness interact with other variables of the child's case (Cummings et al., 1999; Schteingart, Molnar, Klein, Lowe, & Hartmann, 1995). In order to best serve our clients we must continue striving to appreciate their individual lives in all the historical, cultural, socioeconomic, biological, and personal frameworks in which these lives are embedded. It is from this understanding that the maximum opportunities to provide service develop.

# 3    Sources of Data

*W*hat do you need to learn about the child waiting to see you? To make full use of the time available for the initial evaluation, an examiner must take efficient advantage of the variety of data available about the child or adolescent. In the initial contact, the primary data are our observations of the client, what he or she can tell us, his or her responses to tasks, and the reports of the caretakers who have accompanied the young person to the session. As the case develops, other information can be gained through formal psychological testing, interviewing a wide range of collateral sources, and accessing prior medical and educational records. Consideration of how to most effectively use the various data, even prior to their availability, allows for a well-organized process of assessment.

## OBSERVATIONAL ASSESSMENT

One of the most valuable sources of information available to the examiner is his or her own observations of the youth's presentation and behavior within the session. These things provide a direct sample of the young person's approach to the world, to novel situations, and to challenges. It also represents the outcome of a significant interaction between the youth and his or her caretakers: the decision that the young person should come for a mental health appointment. The presentation and actions of the child or adolescent offer valuable hypotheses about how the path to your door has been traveled.

Your initial view of the child offers one of the few pictures of that individual that is unaffected by any interaction with you. Beginning with your first few transactions with the youth, the behavior you see will inevitably represent an interplay between the child and yourself, shaped in part by forces neither party may be totally cognizant of. Here, in the first few seconds of contact, is a view of another person not yet influenced by your contributions.

## First Impression

How do you initially find the youth? Turned to the wall while waiting alone in your reception area? Politely sitting between two caretakers with hands folded in lap? Scattering your magazines, brochures, and the secretary's belongings about while parents shout orders and threats? Unknown events and discussions have led to this event: A child or adolescent waits for contact with you for a mental health evaluation. Depending on the procedures of your setting or organization, as well as on your own standard practice, you will often have some preliminary information regarding the case; you may have had discussions with the caretakers or on rare occasions may even have spoken with the youth on the telephone. Here, usually for the first time, you come into the personal presence of the young person you are going to attempt to help. What initial impression does he or she make on you? This first contact offers a sample of how the child deals with novel and potentially threatening situations. His or her opening stance may be rebellious, assertive, passive, anxious, or fearful.

How do the caretakers present themselves in this initial physical contact? Is the family deferential, hostile, withdrawn, and passive? Is the child here with a caseworker he or she met only minutes ago? Often one caretaker has accompanied the child, usually a mother. Is this the person whose concerns led to the evaluation or the parent whose work schedule coincided with the available appointment time? It would be foolish to place too much importance on the initial impressionistic pictures formed of the youth and those who accompany him or her, but it would be equally foolish to completely ignore this experience and the potential data contained within it. Initial impressions shape many social transactions and experiences, and this child and family has created an initial impression on you. This impression may or may not represent how they come across to other professionals (teachers, pediatricians, etc.) or to other people in general; only further data will answer that important question. Your initial impressions begin to present you with hypotheses to be further evaluated; this is its potential value.

The caretakers have usually had the task of bringing the young person to the appointment. Here is an opportunity to sample their organization and follow-through. Did the family arrive early, on time, or late? Did they remember to bring in materials you might have requested in preliminary contacts (school or health records, questionnaires mailed to the family before contact, samples of satanic artwork)? The practical demands of current psychological practice require most of us to make maximum use of all available contacts with clients. Rapidly forming an accurate and realistic view of how much effort and responsibility can be expected from parents outside of the session is very important for efficient treatment planning. Concrete illustrations and examples of how the family effectively carried through (or failed to do so) can form the most meaningful basis to give the family feedback to effectively set up future assignments. Carefully noting and recording such behavior from the time of first contact helps facilitate the process.

## Separation from Parents

My standard practice for the first interaction is often to seek at least a few minutes of time alone with the young person I am seeing. I am interested in how the youth handles separation from the parent(s) or other caretakers who have transported her or him. It is a strange situation, and typically I am unknown to the child; but usually we are in a legitimate setting (clinic, hospital, doctor's office), and I have at least the tacit approval of the child's parents. How does this emotional calculus play out in the responses of this particular youth? The majority of young children, early school-age and middle school-age children, adolescents, and young adults I have interacted with over the years separate and come to my office easily and without undue distress. Variations from this expectation offer potential information—how does the parent react? What is the nature of the child's reaction to separation? Does he or she show apparent fear and cling to a caretaker? Is he or she rebellious and oppositional? Is his or her behavior totally disorganized, requiring physical management? I almost never physically prompt a child to accompany me, relying totally on verbal requests (and the encouragement of the parents). Neither do I attempt to physically restrain a child who leaves my office. I ask her to sit back down and usually accompany her if she does leave. It has been my experience that physical intervention has almost never been necessary across many years of practice. Important exceptions have included children who showed autism and other pervasive disorders, children who showed schizophrenia and other psychotic disorders, children with profound and severe cognitive or neurological impairment, and physically aggressive and violent children.

Along with observing of how the child handles separation from the parents, watch his or her initial response to your office. Some children wait for you to indicate a chair; others hop up into the most interesting chair available (often yours). How does the child adapt to this new environment? Is there inquisitive behavior—visually scanning the room, manipulation of chair controls or pillows on a couch, questions about the room and its uses? Children show a great range of initial behavior on entering an examiner's office—from helpful participation in your planned agenda to abruptly switching off the lights and plunging the room into total darkness to simply getting up and leaving the session prematurely. Sometimes these actions are consistent with what you have been told are the caretaker's presenting concerns and some-

---

**Practice Note 3.1. Disruptive and Intolerable Behavior**

It is important for the child mental health specialist to be prepared for the rare event of violent or other unacceptable behavior within a session that cannot be verbally controlled. As a starting point it is wise to periodically review the written policies of your agency regarding the handling of unacceptable behavior within a client session. If you that discover your agency does not have written policies, it would be prudent to strongly encourage that such policies be developed. Even, or perhaps especially, independent practitioners would be well advised to develop written policies for their own practice with respect to these and other matters. It is especially important to note what the expectations of your agency are with respect to how you should immediately deal with aggression, destruction of property, elopement, and so forth—who should be immediately and eventually informed and what records should be made concerning the event. In some situations it may be necessary that persons or agencies (juvenile court officers, state child protective departments, custodial parent) outside of your clinic be notified of the event. There should be policies for how this nonfiction is conducted and documented. The foremost consideration in all actions should be the protection of the child for whom you have taken temporary responsibility, as well as the protection of yourself and other personnel and the protection of the property and resources of the agency for which you work.

---

times such behaviors are unexpected, idiosyncratic responses. Most children, at an initial appointment, are well behaved and compliant with the examiner. Variation from such behavior is notable. Most oppositional behavior during an initial appointment appears to be primarily motivated by attention seeking, usually from the caretakers. Resistant behavior typically reflects anger or fear. Disorganized behavior may result from extremely high anxiety (a benign possibility) or serious psychiatric disturbance.

When the child refuses to accompany you to the examination room or leaves your office prematurely, the question arises of how the parents will handle this behavior. Most parents will side with your expectations if you have made it clear that you want some time alone with their child and will communicate their position clearly to the child. This may resolve the difficulty. If it does not, you may have to consider varying your standard practice. Possibly more noteworthy is an inconsistent or contradictory response from the caretakers. An apparent inability to deal unambiguously with your simple expectations may be an initial indication that this family will be difficult to work with. This is not necessarily pejorative—in my experience some families who have been difficult to work with at first have eventually been successful cases—but it does begin to inform your expectations, especially with respect to how quickly things will be accomplished.

In some cases, the caretaker may have more difficulty separating than the child does. Occasionally I have had caretakers request (or insist) that they be present during my initial interaction with their child. If the child has a history of adverse reactions to separation or has suffered a trauma, this may be understandable, but your response should be carefully considered. If I perceive little or no anxiety on the part of the child at the impending relocation, I tend to be firm in my expectations and am curious about any difficulty the parent has in accepting this fairly common practice. I may leave the child in the waiting area (appropriately supervised if necessary) and meet alone with the parent(s) to discuss my practice and their concerns. On literally a handful of occasions over the years, this conversation has led to the parents deciding to withdraw from further participation. Several cases in this very small sample involved forensic issues, and I had suspicions regarding the motivation of the caretakers, but in reality you may never know what led to the decision to withdraw. Although you as examiner need to be flexible and to accommodate individual differences in clients, your standard practice should reflect the procedures that you have found most helpful for the majority of your clients. It is not a casual or trivial thing to deviate from your standard practice, especially because it may affect your evaluation results in unknown ways that are impossible to fully analyze. Although I often tolerate variation in my preferred practice to increase the sense of security or comfort of a child, I usually do not do so just to humor a parent.

## Gait and Posture

The child's natural gait and posture provide an initial sample of his or her gross motor repertoire. The mental health evaluator lacks the training or conceptual vocabulary of the physical therapist or physician, but he or she can make a basic discrimination regarding these samples of gross motor behavior. The child's standing posture and gait is typically unremarkable. Gross variation from this base-rate expectation should be noted and explored further when the parents are interviewed. The child's posture in a chair is similarly expected to be typically erect and relaxed. Variation from this may reflect fatigue and withdrawal (child lies down or slumps in the chair), limitations of attention and concentration (child fidgets in the chair, or rapidly changes posture), anxiety (child displays rigid, withdrawn postures or startle responses), or other emotional states or behavioral reactions of the child. I find it helpful to record behavioral descriptions of the child's standing and sitting posture and gait or to note if these are different from the expectations.

## Dress and Grooming

The child's presentation includes his or her clothing and physical hygiene. My expectation is that children are usually prepared to be brought to a doctor's appointment. For the child to arrive dirty, smelly, or soiled may reflect either serious disorganization on the part of the caretaker or a serious deviation from typical standards of acceptable care. Either variation has important implications for how the child may be sent to school, to friends' homes, or out into the community. Such a presentation may affect the reception the child receives outside the home. Alternatively, it may mean that the child left home properly groomed but that this state could not be maintained for the trip to your office. One very hyperactive child I saw once had dug up a plant in the yard outside the building while his mother was getting his younger sibling out of a car seat. The family arrived in my office with the client's fingernails encrusted with dirt, his clothing soiled and disheveled, and a tearful mother holding her youngest child by one hand and "my" flower in her other hand. This initial presentation was both informative and diagnostic of the family's difficulties.

The issue of clothing takes on another significance when the youth is of an age at which he or she begins to chose his or her own dress. My expectation is that most parents wish their child to move in the community and to your office attired somewhere within the range from "clean and casual" to "dressed for church or synagogue." Most preadolescents and teenagers prefer the range from "casual (clean optional)" to "making a statement." The content of "making a statement" may vary tremendously—the carefully considered, currently fashionable, name-brand look that costs several hundred dollars; the current fashion statement designed to make any adult cringe; the specialty niche look (gang colors, for instance). Parents may often comment on the young person's appearance in or out of the youth's presence: "You can see how he dresses; we had a fight just to get him to put on clean clothes before coming here." In my own notes the phrase "adol standard" refers to dress that might be unacceptable from adult or child clients but that is within the typical range for teenagers from the youth's socioeconomic background. Such judgments are subjective and require some familiarity with the clothing usually worn in the hallways of public schools in your area, as well as the dress affected by different cliques within the youth community ("preppies," "hoods," "sluts," "jocks," "skaters," etc.).

## Actions within Your Office

Much of the behavior we are interested in as mental health evaluators occurs outside our offices in other settings. A small range, however, can be directly sampled within our environments. The behavior of our client within the session provides one sample of his or her behavior against relatively known stimulus features: an unfamiliar setting, a "professional" context, an authority figure, a time-limited and structured relationship. The child's temperament, abilities, and coping skills are reflected in his or her spontaneous interaction and behavior and response to our questions and tasks.

The child's spontaneous speech and language, oral comprehension, and other communication responses provide a rich sample of his or her verbal strengths and weaknesses, as well as one facet of his or her social skills. Human beings interact with both their world and themselves through their language. Children seek knowledge through questions, comprehend the messages of others to varying degrees, and self-direct their own actions. Their speech provides an opportunity to assess their articulation, expressive language, and pragmatic communication. Simple rating scales such as the Multilingual Aphasia Examination (MAE) Speech Articulation Rating Scale (Benton et al., 1983) can help quantify our assessments for comparisons over time. Clinical impressions of the level of working vocabulary, observations of word-finding difficulty, and any apparent lapse in oral comprehension can be noted and followed up for more formal assessment. Spontaneous conversation also allows for initial impressions of the child's level of social awareness and functional communication. If the child has a speech disability, we can also observe his or her frustration tolerance and adaptation to communication difficulties.

The child's ability to attend and stay mentally focused during the evaluation provides a sample of his or her concentration abilities. This is a one-on-one situation with novel participants and events—optimal circumstances for maintenance of attention and concentration. Evidence of distractibility and poor concentration can be very meaningful within this context. Even children with attention-deficit/hyperactivity disorder can usually maintain their focus within brief, individual evaluations; lapses of mental focus are usually significant. The list of potential alternative explanations is relatively short (high anxiety, thought disorder, chemical effects), and a hypothesis of a delay or impairment in cognitive functioning may add to the list of factors to evaluate.

The child's compliance, cooperation, and task motivation provide another important set of initial observations of in-session behavior. My baseline expectation is that most children (even those with behavior disorders) will be relatively well behaved in an initial evaluation. This behavior is often a source of great frustration and confusion to their parents, who proclaim that the child is "different" at home. They are correct, of course. Task performance behavior, including instructional compliance, is highly situationally specific in most children. The same features that tend to maximize the child's attention and concentration during an initial evaluation work to enhance his or her cooperation. Against this background, difficulties with child management in an evaluation setting also tend to be very informative and usually suggest severe clinical disorders in children. In adolescents the same pattern may also reflect a marked power struggle between the teenager and caretaker.

Anxious and fearful behavior is seen with some regularity in children during evaluations and lacks the information value of externalizing or acting out problems. The anxiety reactions may be too specific to the context of a "doctor's office" to be diagnostically useful. More potential value lies in observations of how the adults cope with and handle the child's distress and of the child's response to soothing efforts by others. It is valuable to note any indications of the child's own ability to self-soothe—his or her own coping responses to tension and fear.

Highly agitated and disorganized behavior within your office can also be of important clinical significance. The absence or loss of self-control and other control in youth is rare in the absence of severe neurological or psychiatric disorder. Maintaining calm detachment is not a normal reaction to having your office completely disrupted, but it is useful to try to note whether the child's actions appear random and undirected or show purposeful destructiveness. Evidence of differential reaction to the intervention by others (familiar vs. unfamiliar agents) has practical importance. Finally, note whether the behavior is accompanied by signs of high emotional arousal (crying, dilated pupils, rapid breathing, facial expressions of fear, anger, distress) or whether the frenzy is carried out in an emotionally absent and detached manner. These observations can be useful afterward in discussing the events with the child's caretakers, in part to begin establishing how typical or novel the disruptive behavior you observed is for the child.

## Behavior within the Larger Office

A second "setting" that should not be overlooked within the office environment is the reception room or larger office area. The child usually spends some time here waiting with one or more caretakers or perhaps alone or with the minimal supervision of a secretary or receptionist. These seemingly slight changes from the situation in your office often provide interesting and informative behavioral contrasts. For instance, children with clinical ADHD, as noted previously, can often maintain reasonable cognitive focus during your evaluation of them. In the less structured and less directed setting of the reception area, however, the behavior their parents and teachers have complained of may be more readily observed. The books and magazines or toys provided for the occupation of young visitors may be heaped into piles or scattered about. Your rack of brochures on parenting tips or social service agencies may have been emptied, each marked with a bright crayon streak, and discarded. Office plants, any apparatus with moving parts, and antique furniture or fixtures are at risk. Tables, chairs on casters, and cabinets with interesting objects on top may provide significant physical risks for the child, who will discover a variety of inappropriate responses to these stimuli. You need to carefully inspect your outer office area to ensure the safety of both your young clients and your belongings. You can also gain additional information by observing the child's behavior in a situation different from the formal evaluation contact.

### *In Situ* Observations

Before leaving the topic of observations, I should say a few words regarding data gained by observing the child in other settings, especially settings natural to the child's life. Observational assessment of behavior is a tremendously valuable evaluation approach that has been harnessed to great effect by both ethnologists (McGrew, 1972) and social learning theorists (Patterson, 1982; Wahler, House, & Stambaugh, 1976). Unfortunately, the pressures of typical clinical practice seldom make *in situ* observations feasible. School psychologists make observational assessments in classroom settings and sometimes in other situations within schools. Social workers make home visits and conduct observations of parent–child interaction in home-like settings. Observational assessment in natural environments by psychologists and psychiatrists is usually restricted to research projects. The practical difficulties notwithstanding, direct observation of behavior has tremendous potential to clarify questions about the most accurate diagnosis and functional analysis of behavior and should be considered as an adjunct evaluation tool in complex or difficult-to-resolve cases.

## INTERVIEW DATA

Despite all its potential limitations, the exploratory and hypothesis-testing clinical interview remains a highly effective and efficient tool for learning about and understanding the difficulties of another person. The utility of the interview is enhanced if we recognize its limitations. Through verbal exchange clients can share with us perceptions (1) of events, experiences, and relationships that they are aware of, (2) that they are able to express in language, (3) that we have made them feel willing to share with us, and (4) that we have let them know are important or of interest to us. The first two considerations concern ability, the third concerns willingness, and the final consideration concerns the interviewer's communication with the client.

In general, clients can only tell us about knowledge they are cognizant of. There are exceptions to this generalization, but for the most part people can only share what they know. Interviewing clients about nonverbal aspects of their interpersonal presentation, for example, is often of little use because clients are not usually in a position to observe and gain feedback regarding their nonverbal behavior. As another example, in the absence of instrumentation, most clients cannot accurately report to us their blood pressure. They don't really know the answers to the important questions we might have. Other methods of inquiry (role playing, for instance) are necessary to illustrate the qualities of interest. Some assessment techniques (e.g., self-monitoring) can lead to greater recognition of one's own actions and reactions, increasing the client's awareness and possibly facilitating a more meaningful exchange with the clinician. With children and adolescents, as with adults, there is little to be gained in inquiries about events or knowledge that lie outside the youth's understanding.

Awareness alone, however, does not ensure that interview inquiries will elicit useful data. The client not only has to have had the experience about which we ask but also has to be able to express this experience in a language we mutually comprehend. A client may "not have the words" to give communication to the idea they wish to share with us. Emotions may be especially difficult to capture with language. Children may have as wide a range of affective experience as adults do, but their verbal expression of feelings is not as differentiated. Certain interview techniques have been developed to address this type of difficulty with respect to particular experiences. Pain rating scales, for instance, ask clients to quantify the qualitative experience of discomfort by using a digital range ("On a scale that goes from '0' for no pain to '10' for intense, unbearable pain, tell me how you're feeling now"). Similar devices have been used to facilitate client's communication about fear, anxiety, and anger. Analog devices such as a "fear thermometer" have been used with children for the same purpose.

Many of the data we seek in evaluating the mental health problems of clients are potentially embarrassing, confusing, or conflictual for the individuals speaking with us. Our inquiries increase the client's temporary discomfort, and he or she experiences mixed motivations regarding cooperation and full disclosure. Children may experience a sense of conflict over being asked about "family business," even when the points of concern are well within the normal range of family experience. Older children may be reluctant to incriminate themselves with open accounts of acting out, instigating problems for their siblings, or manipulating adults. Teenagers often have an intense desire for privacy regarding their personal lives and are hesitant to trust any adult and any outsider. All must be helped to believe that cooperation is in their and their family's best interests. We can do this by clearly communicating the purpose of the inquiry, how the information obtained will and will not be used, the degree of confidentiality that exists for the client, and the rules that govern the actions of the examiner. Providing clear, direct, and usually unambiguous questions further assists the youth in giving us clear, direct, and unambiguous answers.

Much of the literature dealing specifically with interviewing children and adolescents is based on clinical experience, and relatively empirical evaluations of these useful hypotheses are available. Nevertheless, until more data becomes available, this "conventional wisdom" represents our best basis for practice. Logan (1989) discusses adjustments in interview style and techniques to accommodate the developmental status of children. I found especially cogent his observation about the limits of changing our behavior when interacting with youths: "Some people change their tone of voice when talking to a very young child. This is not necessary and may sound patronizing or condescending to a child. Therapists must respect children in the same manner as they respect peers and convey this respect in the same way" (p. 312).

Finally, it is a truism that "you get what you ask for." Clients tend usually to answer the question we ask. If we don't ask about something, they may or may not volunteer the information. The task of the examiner is to systematically elicit the data that will help clarify the client's problems; the development, course, and response to self-help and prior treatment efforts; and any related information. Examiners may be guided by general topics, informal outlines, detailed protocols, or structured interviews. Their level of inquiry may be for informal screening purposes, guided by outcome criteria (DSM-IV or ICD-10), or a full, comprehensive examination. The January 2000 issue of the

*Journal of the American Academy of Child and Adolescent Psychiatry* devoted a special section to structured interviews developed for diagnostic assessment of children and adolescents (McClellan & Werry, 2000) and reviewed the major instruments available (Ambrosini, 2000; Angold & Costello, 2000; Ernst, Cookus, & Moravec, 2000; Reich, 2000; Shaffer et al., 2000; Sherrill & Kovacs, 2000; Valla, Bergeron, & Smolla, 2000; Weller, Weller, Fristad, Rooney, & Schecter, 2000). We need to keep in mind, however, that even structured interviews are not immune from unsought subject effects and distortion (Perez, Ascaso, Massons, & de la Osa Chaparro, 1998). There is no perfect solution to the challenging process of learning about another person's life.

A challenging and complex aspect of interviewing youths is the concern of how much, if any, confidentiality the young person is entitled to, especially with respect to communications he or she would rather were not shared with parents or other guardians. Beyond the clinical and ethical issues involved, there are legal constraints on the right of privileged communication, and these partly depend on the age of the youth. A variety of positions have been taken by clinicians, and it is worthwhile to review different discussions (cf. Bartlett, 1996; Logan, 1989). My experience has been that, as long as your position is consistent with state statutes, the most critical aspect of settling this potential difficulty is to have a clearly understood policy in place before interviewing begins. My typical position with youth (which I discuss in the presence of the child and the parents) is that they can tell me things with some expectation of privacy but that there are limits to this privacy. Their parents, for instance, usually want to know my conclusions and recommendations in the case—this expectation on the parents' part is completely reasonable and appropriate. Although the youth and I will discuss revelations regarding my impressions and recommendations before these formulations are shared with the parents, there is no real question regarding the sharing. In contrast, specific details of past actions or events that the child relates to me are not usually shared without the child's consent unless I have concerns regarding the child's safety. I use multiple examples with the family to illustrate this point and to ensure that we all have an understanding of the "ground rules." This explanation requires some amount of time but tends to be well worth the investment in the long term. Release of any information to anyone other than the child's legal guardians (or even to the guardians in some states and with older adolescents) requires the written consent of the guardian (and possibly the youth, depending on age and state

## Interview Segment 3.1. Position on Child/Adolescent Privacy

Most mental health examiners are quite familiar with and comfortable dealing with privileged communication, confidentiality, and the ethical and legal issues surrounding these areas as they pertain to communications with other parties "outside" the therapy. There may be less familiarity and more difficulty regarding how to handle issues of privacy between the therapist and different members of the client's family, especially when the child or adolescent client wishes information withheld from his or her parents. My experience has been that the most crucial aspect of resolving this dilemma is to deal with it openly at the beginning of the counseling and to secure joint agreement on a working policy. The details of this policy are probably less important than having a frank discussion in which all parties can voice their concerns and obtaining informed consent from all members of the family as to the working policy that will be followed. The subsequent dialogue is an example of such a discussion involving myself, Fred Z (a 12-year-old boy with mild behavior problems), and Fred's parents (Mr. and Ms. Z). The examiner, client, and both parents are all present at the time of this interaction.

EXAMINER: OK, we've talked about confidentiality, your right to have privacy about whatever goes on here, unless you and your parents give written consent for me to release information. Now we need to discuss something else—how much privacy you have about anything you might tell me that you wouldn't want your parents to know. Working with a counselor tends to go best when people feel free to say whatever is on their minds without worry about that getting repeated to other folks. On the other hand, your parents care about you and have a duty to stay informed about what is going on with you. This creates a problem for all of us sometimes. Can you tell me what the problem might be?

FRED: I tell you something and then get mad when you tell my parents.

EXAMINER: Exactly. Or your parents get mad because I won't tell them. Either way someone is really upset and that might spoil any good that could get done for you and your family. What we need to do is agree on some rules so everyone will know what to expect, and there will be less chance of things going badly.

Here are my usual rules. First of all, parents are not usually interested in the particular details of what you tell me. They want to know about what I think is going on, what I propose to do about it, and how this is working out. Sometimes they would like some advice about how your family could work better together. These are all very worthwhile questions for your parents to have, and I need to be able to talk with them about these things. You will always know what I am going to tell your parents, because we will have talked about that first. Most of the time you will probably be with us while I am talking to your parents, so you will know exactly what I have said. How does that part sound?

FRED: OK, I guess.

EXAMINER: Fine. Now, here is the other part. Suppose you tell me something and don't want me to share this information with your parents. Maybe you did something you don't want them to know, or say one of your friends did something but, again, you don't really want your parents to know about this. You tell me that you want this kept private between you and me. What will we do then?

FRED: I don't know.

EXAMINER: I do. I won't tell them.

FRED: You won't?

EXAMINER: Nope. I might want to, but it just doesn't work out very well if I do. I've tried it different ways. You really need to believe that you can trust me to keep your confidences if this is going to do your family any good. There is an exception.

FRED: Yeah, I figured.

EXAMINER: It's the same as the one on your overall confidentiality—if I am worried about your safety, or anyone else's physical safety, then I do whatever is necessary to keep you safe. Even if I have to violate your privacy. Let me give you some examples, so we are all very clear as to how I would act.

If you told me you had shoplifted a record from a store but didn't want me to discuss this with your parents, I wouldn't, even though I would be very concerned about how much trouble this could cause for you and your family.

If you told me you were smoking cigarettes and you didn't want your parents to know, I wouldn't tell them. I think smoking is very dangerous and a very bad habit, but the danger is usually long term. I wouldn't tell.

Suppose you told me you had been using some pills that a friend gave you at a party but you didn't want your parents to find out. Your parents are going to know about this. I would prefer that you told them, we could talk to them together, but they are going to know. If you won't tell them, I will. There are too many physical dangers involved in using drugs you get from other people for this to stay private, no matter how upset you get about me talking to your parents.

FRED: What about drinking?

EXAMINER: Good question, and harder to answer. In someone your age I would probably treat drinking like other drug use, and insist that your parents be informed. In you were 10, I would report any alcohol use to them. If you were 18, it would depend on what you told me about your drinking. Any suggestion of drinking while driving or other irresponsible behavior while drinking, and your parents are going to need to know about it.

Here's another example. Suppose you were the one who broke the television, and your parents have blamed it on your older brother. He's in major trouble about this and you tell me what really happened. I'm not going to tell your parents, even though this is causing lots of unhappiness between them and your brother.

FRED: Yeah!

EXAMINER: I would be talking with you about needing to put things right with your family.

FRED: Oh.

EXAMINER: But I wouldn't do that for you.

FRED: OK.

EXAMINER: If you told me about having a gun in your locker?

FRED: I'd never do that. But if I did you'd tell.

EXAMINER: Right. And if you told me you were going to run away from home and head for Chicago?

FRED: I don't know. You wouldn't tell.

EXAMINER: I would! There are a lot of dangers for kids who are on the streets. You might not realize how dangerous running off to the city was, but I would consider that a real risk to you and would inform your parents.

FRED: So you're going to tell if you think I'm in danger, or somebody is.

EXAMINER: That's right. Otherwise we would talk about it, I might really push you to talk to your parents, but I wouldn't without your agreement. How does that sound to everyone?

MR. Z: If we asked you about something Fred did not want us to know, would you lie to us?

EXAMINER: That's an important question. The answer is, "No." I'm not going to lie to you about your son or anything else. For one thing, I'm not very good at it. For another, I don't believe lying is usually a helpful way of dealing with problems, either for you or for me. I am pretty good at not answering questions I don't want to, but if you kept at it—you could probably figure out there was something I was not saying. Since there are only a few situations in which you would find me evasive, that would tell you a lot. For this to work it is important that you agree not only to the rules, but to the idea behind those rules. You can't use me as a lie detector for your family. It won't work if you do try, and it will almost certainly spoil any real good that I can do for you. I want to try and help your family, and I certainly don't want to withhold any information that would help you. But, unless Fred is in some real danger, he needs to be in control of who he shares information with. Otherwise he is not going to feel free to talk openly with me. Any other questions?

This approach was originally suggested to me by a colleague, Dr. Daniel Graybill, at Illinois State University. I have used it for over a decade as my preferred position regarding intrafamily confidentiality. This protocol is not without difficulties, and I offer it only as one possible solution to the challenge of privacy and disclosure with juvenile clients. The most important aspect of this example is that the topic is brought up early and straightforwardly in the counseling process. As mental health professionals we have a responsibility to our clients and their families to educate them regarding the choices that will govern our relationship during counseling and the impact of these choices on that process.

---

statute). It is interesting to note that issues of confidentiality as they pertain to the delivery of services to adolescents has become a important topic within the broad field of primary medical care (Alderman, 2000).

## QUESTIONNAIRES AND SYMPTOM SCALES

A large number of general and specific symptom questionnaires have been developed for use with children to help assess behavioral and emotional difficulties. Some instruments are analogues of self-report behavioral screening questionnaires designed to be completed by caretakers (e.g., Achenbach, 1991; Goodman, Meltzer, & Bailey, 1998). Some have been extensively investigated with respect to psychometric properties, reliability, and validity (e.g., Dadds, Perrin, & Yule, 1998; Finch, Saylor, & Edward, 1985). I make no attempt here to offer any comprehensive review of specific instruments; I have found some to be quite useful and many others to be less so. In the clinical application of such instruments we need to take into account the attitude of the child, as well as his or her reading skills. When I make use of symptom report scales with young people, it has become my practice to remain in the room with them as they complete the instruments. This allows an opportunity for unobtrusive observation of their test-taking manner, as well as the time and apparent care they take in responding to different tasks. Self-report questionnaires can offer the evaluator quantitative data that can be evaluated with age-based and (if indicated) gender-based norms. This can be a tremendous contribution, but only if care is taken to ensure that high-quality data are obtained. It is critical to ensure that the young person understands the task and the instructions and that his or her cooperation has been secured to the fullest extent possible.

It is also necessary for evaluators to realize that using questionnaires to screen for low-frequency problems has certain psychometric limitations. Even instruments with good sensitivity and specificity will misidentify many cases when the disorder in question has a low base rate (Clark & Harrington, 1999). Self-report questionnaires have a valuable role in mental health assessment, but they are ultimately only another tool, useful as long as their limitations are appreciated (Kresanov, Tuominen, Piha, & Almqvist, 1998).

## BRIEF TESTING

Traditional mental status examinations used a combination of interview and brief performance tasks to assess the symptoms and signs of mental or neurological disorder (Sarma, 1994). Many of the performance tasks were verbal and focused on evaluation of the sensorium or higher mental functions: orientation, attention, verbal fluency, oral comprehension, mental calculations, abstract reasoning, judgment, and memory. Other performance tasks might involve the apperception or manipulation of materials and assessed constructional abilities (drawing, copying), spatial relationship skills, writing skills, comprehension and memory, written arithmetic skills, and confrontational naming abilities. Derived in large part from clinical neurology and psychiatry, analysis tended to be qualitative rather than quantitative and was highly dependent on the clinical experience of the examiner. The qualitative neuropsychological investigations of Alexander Luria represented one extension and elaboration of this approach. The more quantified and standardized approaches of the modern mental status examination (Strub & Black, 1993) and of "behavioral neurology" represent another. Finally, several important similarities between the brief testing of the mental status examination and the more extensive and formal evaluations of psychological ability testing can be seen. Both mental status and intelligence testing attempt to assess a number of important domains of cognitive ability. Both present the client with problems or challenges to be solved. Both tend to comprise a number of specific items that are either passed or failed. Important differences are (1) the depth of testing—intelligence tests tend to be longer, with more items, and are hence more reliable; (2) the normative (nomothetic) versus individual (idiographic) basis of scoring and interpretation; (3) the standardization of instrument and procedure—individual practitioners may be very consistent in items and methodology with mental status assessment, but only a few protocols are standardized to be point of being an identified instrument (e.g., Mini-Mental State Evaluation; Folstein, Folstein, & McHugh, 1975) that has an accepted form and sequence. The brevity of mental status performance items contributes to both their efficiency in identifying severe and persistent mental disorders and their frequent relative insensitivity to mild or fluctuating difficulties. The length and rigid structure of intelligence tests contributes to the reliability and sensitivity to mild and borderline limitations of mental functioning and also to their cost, both in financial resources and professional time. Brief testing can make use of tasks that allow for quantitative scoring and interpretation, providing for more objective assessments. Brief testing can provide reasonably reliable baselines against which change can be assessed and can provide a solid basis on which to reach decisions regarding more expensive evaluation. The empirical literature on mental status examination has grown increasingly sophisticated, and a growing body of data exists on the sensitivity and specificity of many traditional brief testing tasks, such as serial seven subtraction, orientation, or figure copying (see Franzen & Berg,

1989). In addition, continuing research illustrates new and creative ways to evaluate the performance of youths (see, e.g., Bishop, 1998).

## COLLATERAL SOURCES OF DATA

The collection of data from others who know the youth is crucially important to the full and accurate assessment of young people. Children may lack the cognitive development to understand or be able to report relevant information; adolescents may have difficulty understanding or appreciating the relevance of the attitudes and perceptions of others. Across the range of the developmental years, children and adolescents may intentionally withhold or distort information. Children may act to protect family or sibling secrets (mother and father argue at times; little brother torments the family pet). Teenagers often have an exquisitely developed sense of privacy and frequently have learned that controlling information is a powerful technique for interpersonal influence. Gaining the perspective of multiple informants seems indispensable for the best evaluation of youths. The issue of who can provide the most useful information varies with the problem being assessed, with the age of the child, and with the available pool of informants. La Greca and Lemanek (1996) discuss the question of the "best" informant as a function of the child's developmental level and the focus of assessment (see Table 3.1). Whenever practical, collecting data from multiple informants is valuable. The usefulness of considering several sources of data can be demonstrated across a wide range of behavioral questions (see, e.g., Holmbeck et al., 1998; Rubio-Stipec et al., 1996; Webster-Stratton & Lindsay, 1999).

The basic tools for gathering data from collateral sources are interviews, printed surveys or questionnaires, behavior checklist and rating scales, and behavior diaries or event-sampling observations by caretakers.

### Interviews of Significant Others

Interviewing informants parallels the process of interviewing clients. The validity of caretaker reports is limited by (1) their knowledge and awareness of the child's behavior and adjustment, (2) their motivation to honestly and fully disclose what they know, (3) their global beliefs and attitudes about child development and child rearing, and (4) the

**TABLE 3.1** "Best" Informant as a Function of Both Developmental Level and Construct of Interest

| Construct | Infancy/ preschool years | Elementary school years | Adolescence |
|---|---|---|---|
| Behavior problems | | | |
| Externalizing behaviors | Parent, teacher | Parent, teacher | Teenager, parent |
| Internalizing behaviors | Parent | Child, parent | Teenager |
| Family functioning | Parent | Parent, child | Teenager, parent |
| Health-related areas | | | |
| Behavioral distress | Parent, observer | Parent, observer | Teenager, observer |
| Conceptions of illness (e.g., AIDS) | Preschooler | Child | Teenager |
| Disease management (e.g., adherence) | Parent | Parent, child | Teenager, parent |
| Health beliefs and attitudes | Parent | Parent, child | Teenager |
| Illness perceptions (e.g., symptoms) | Parent | Parent, child | Teenager, parent |
| Quality of life | Parent | Parent, child | Teenager, parent |
| Subjective distress (e.g., pain) | Preschooler | Child | Teenager |
| Peer relations/social competence | Teacher, peers | Peers, child | Teenager |
| School functioning/ academic behavior | Teacher | Teacher | Teenager |
| Self-perceptions (e.g., self-concept) | Preschooler | Child | Teenager |

*Note.* From La Greca and Lemanek (1996). Copyright 1996 by Kluwer Academic/Plenum Publishers. Reprinted by permission of the author and publisher.

skill of the examiner in facilitating their open and complete report. As with youths, the reliability and accuracy of the information produced by caretakers is usually enhanced by initial general inquiry followed up with specific, objective, and behavioral inquiry, along with numerous requests for examples, contrasts, illustrations, and comparisons with siblings and peers. There is room for some cautious optimism. Empirical evidence supports the common working belief that caretakers can provide a reliable history of their children's emotional and behavioral problems (Kentgen, Klein, Mannuzza, & Davies, 1997) and general mental ability (Waschbusch, Daleiden, & Drabman, 2000).

This optimism, however, must be qualified by awareness that a number of variables other than child characteristics can influence the report of parents. Emotional distress in mothers can bias their reports toward more negative perceptions (Garber, Van Slyke, & Walker, 1998). The cognitive distortions of depression may readily affect the view of parents toward their children—affecting the caretaker's perception of the child's level of functioning, the seriousness of any difficulties, and how likely positive change would be. There may be general halo effects (Kendziora & O'Leary, 1998), as well as specific areas of over- or underappreciation of a youth's difficulties. This topic is complex, and it is difficult to evaluate how much distortion may enter into the impressions of depressed parents—there is evidence, for instance, that maternal depression not only distorts mothers' ratings of their children's behavior but also interacts independently with childhood behavior to exacerbate problems (Boyle & Pickles, 1997). Ultimately, the use of multiple informants and repeated samples gives us the most secure basis on which to formulate conceptualizations.

The reports of parents and other adults on externalizing behavior problems, such as fighting or disobedience, are usually in greater agreement with other external measures than are reports of internalizing problems such as depression that require inference regarding private states. However, low-frequency acting out, such as stealing, may be missed by caretakers, and these reports may show poor reliability against other measures. Parents' reports regarding their child's cognitive abilities may have some general validity but show a great deal of variation in accuracy across different domains of cognitive performance (Waschbusch et al., 2000). The general conclusion to be drawn here is clear—single sources of data are suspect.

Actively engaging the parents or other informants in the assessment process and helping them understand their vital role in the evaluation may help improve the quality of the data they provide. Research by Edelbrock, Crnic, and Bohnert (1999) with the Diagnostic Interview Schedule for Children (DISC), a structured interview for diagnostic classification of child problems, found improved reliability in the DSM diagnoses generated over a 1-week interval when parents were given an overview of the assessment areas and examples of criteria in everyday language. Rather than viewing parents, teachers, and other informants as passive and flawed sources of data, we can approach informants as concerned adults who are trying to serve the children in their care. Helping them understand how they can assist our similarly motivated efforts by working toward a joint understanding of the behaviors and problems of the young person generates not only a more comprehensive data set but also a more reliable one. A similar active engagement approach to interviewing children has also been shown to be productive (Saywitz & Snyder, 1996).

The data gained from interviews with parents, teachers, and other informants can be used in a variety of ways to further our understanding of adjustment problems in youth. Rubio-Stipec and colleagues (1996) used the structured interview data generated by the Revised Diagnostic Interview Schedule for Children (DISC 2.3) to generate continuous scale measures of four broad symptom scales (depressive disorders, conduct disorder, oppositional defiant disorder [ODD], and ADHD). The obtained measures were shown to be reliable and sensitive to the targeted psychopathology. Although most clinical assessments do not utilize such a sophisticated methodology, continuing research may well yield practical and efficient measures that make more efficient use of collateral report data.

## Surveys and Questionnaires

The judicious use of printed surveys and questionnaires can greatly increase the efficiency of the clinical evaluation by gathering a great deal of information in a systematic fashion while the examiner is otherwise engaged. Probably most clinics make use of some preliminary data sheet completed prior to contact. Such face sheets usually include, at a minimum, demographic, residence, employment/insurance, and family data information on the client, parents, or other caretakers. Many initial forms include inquiries as to presenting concerns, problems to be addressed in counseling, referral questions, and so forth. The availability of word processing resources in almost all settings creates excellent opportunities to augment this basic information with a great deal of easily obtained clinical data. Some care should be given to the reading level required by any such inquiry, the size of the font used, and the amount of space provided for a response. At some point the informant's prior education and expected reading skills need to be considered relative to this manner of gaining information. Melchert (1998) reviews a number of instruments that have been used in assessing family history.

## Behavior Checklists and Behavior Rating Scales

Behavior rating scales, completed by an informant regarding the identified client, have become standard practice for the evaluation of a number of behavior problems of youth. Barkley (1998a), for example, has come to describe the use of such instruments as essential for good practice evaluations of children suspected of manifesting ADHD. These tools allow parental and other caretaker perceptions to be systematically sampled in a consistent manner. This, in turn, opens the possibility of normative analysis—the quantified results of a caretaker's ratings can be contrasted with comparable comparison groups. Demographically adjusted norms (age and gender or age and grade level) exist for the evaluation of a number of behavior report scales. Good convergent validity has been demonstrated between behavior rating scales and structured interviews (Biederman et al., 1993) and between behavior rating scales and direct observations (Skansgaard & Burns, 1998) for high-prevalence disorders such as ADHD.

Behavior rating scales can also help to control to a degree the effects of negative bias that difficult child behavior can produce in caretakers. Teachers, for instance, have been shown to be less influenced by negative halo effects due to oppositional behavior in their evaluations of overactivity and inattention when their behavior ratings are based on operationalized criteria (Stevens, Quittner, & Abilcoff, 1998). Troublesome child behavior can elicit strong emotional reactions from parents and teachers, reactions that may shade their other perceptions of the child, especially global perceptions that are not anchored by specific behavioral criteria. Rating scales can help focus the attention of the informant on the relevant domain to be considered and reduce the potential influence of generalized evaluations.

The use of behavior rating scales does not solve all assessment difficulties. There tend to be systematic differences in how adults and youths perceive the emotional and behavioral problems of young people. Adults, for instance, tend to rate children's adjustment problems as being more severe than do the youths in question (Handwerk, Larzelere, Friman, & Soper, 1999). Data have been reported that raise concern regarding possible subject bias in teachers' behavior ratings of ADHD characteristics in children (Reid, 1995; Reid et al., 1998; Sonuga-Barke, Minocha, Taylor, & Sandberg, 1993). Unrelated physical problems of the child can influence scales intended to reflect behavioral adjustment (Holmes, Respess, Greer, & Frentz, 1998). Additionally, the validity of adult behavior ratings obviously vary with the adequacy of the caretaker's sample of the youth's behavior. In the common event of a discrepancy between behavior ratings by adults and the youth, it is by no means clear which perception forms a better basis for clinical decision making. Identical issues are involved in comparing behavior ratings from different adult sources—mothers with fathers, parents with teachers. The use of multiple informants in making evaluations is usually recommended (Mitsis, McKay, Schulz, Newcorn, & Haperin, 2000; Power et al., 1998).

The context in which behavior ratings are obtained is another consideration that affects their reliability and validity. Epidemiological studies of community samples may not directly translate into valid conclusions applicable to clinical populations (MacLeod, McNamee, Boyle, Offord, & Friedrich, 1999). Carefully considering independent indications of the severity of behavior problems in children and adolescents (Leon, Lyons, & Uziel-Miller, 2000) may be very helpful in studying the data from behavior rating scales. In my practice I have found behavior rating scales very valuable, but they are only one source of information and need to be balanced against other sources of data. A conceptualization or diagnosis is not made on the basis of behavior report scales but as a considered professional judgment based on all available data. Viewed from this perspective, behavior rating scales are useful indeed. A variety of specific instruments have been developed, and more are sure to appear. I draw the reader's attention to the efforts of Robert Goodman in England, who has produced a fine instrument both broad areas of behavioral disturbance, as well as some aspects of successful adaptation (Goodman, 1997; Goodman & Scott, 1999).

Evaluation conclusions are further complicated by the reality that different assessment methods yield different results. Behavior rating scales and interview methods may have different sensitivity and specificity for various emotional and behavioral problems in child clinical populations (see Green, Foster, Morris, Muir, & Morris, 1998). It is the task of the mental health evaluator to carefully weight all the available data in arriving at her or his final diagnostic impression and clinical plan.

## Behavior Diaries and Event-Sampling Observations

One methodological approach to getting around the prohibitive cost of using the examiner or professional external observers in naturalistic settings is to employ natural agents within the situation to gather data. Parents and other caretakers can be asked to record instances of behavior (compliance with adult instructions; arguments with siblings; hitting another child), duration of action (how long the child can occupy herself while father prepares dinner; latency to "lights out" at bedtime;

length of piano practice), behavior ratings (global rating of good behavior on a 5-point scale three times a day; child's apparent unhappiness several times a day). Behavior therapists have made extensive use of these forms of assessment to augment other sources of data. Such data would not usually be available at an initial evaluation unless some instructions had been communicated to the family prior to their initial visit, but one outcome of the initial evaluation might be the formulation of such homework assignments that would add to the data at follow-up sessions to clarify diagnostic and functional analysis.

## PSYCHOLOGICAL TESTING

Formal psychological testing may be an established element of a child's initial mental health evaluation, or a decision to seek or not seek psychological assessment might be one of the outcomes of the initial evaluation. Standards of practice will vary with philosophy of the agency, the youth population served, the available personnel and their expertise, and the historical patterns of practice. A full discussion of this topic is well beyond the bounds of this book, and an extensive literature exists that deals with the psychological assessment of children and adolescents. An initial starting point for the reader interested in this topic would be the discussion in Kronenberger and Meyer (1996). For our purposes, it may be helpful to consider briefly some of the potential indications for psychological testing.

### Mandated Psychological Testing

A variety of child care or social service agencies operate under guidelines that require psychological testing of certain populations of youth. A psychological evaluation may be mandated by a school system in order to qualify children with learning problems for special education services. Programs for children with disabilities or for an adjudicated delinquent may require a psychological battery to establish eligibility for service or to gain admission to various treatment facilities. Courts may require psychological assessments as a part of adjudication procedures. Common across all these examples is the fact that the decision to test the child has not been made by the examiner but by external considerations. The examiner's only job is to assess the youth and communicate the results of this evaluation.

## Elective Psychological Testing

The key feature in elective testing is that, based on data available (previous records, brief task performances, observations, etc.), the examiner has decided that formal psychological evaluation is indicated. The primary consideration should be formulating as clearly as possible the question(s) for which answers are being sought. As in treatment planning, the professional training, knowledge, and skills of the professional evaluator come into most play in the planning of meaningful and efficient psychological assessment. Many, possibly most, psychological instruments can be administered and scored by paraprofessionals or computers. It is the selection of the most appropriate measures and the integrative interpretation of results that require training, experience, and creativity.

## PREVIOUS RECORDS

The effective use of previous records can greatly improve our evaluations of the cognitive, emotional, and behavioral problems of children and adolescents. The challenge is to obtain these records efficaciously so that data become available in a timely manner. Whenever possible, I ask the youth's primary caretaker(s) to assume responsibility for acquiring records for review, if possible prior to my initial contact with the young person and his or her family. The typical initial telephone contact can be used to instruct the caretaker regarding desired records and to provide guidance, if necessary, in obtaining these. If at all possible, prior records are reviewed before the family is seen. The need to have as much information as possible is one reason to give the caretakers the task of assembling prior records. Another reason is that caretakers can access some records more easily than the professional can, either in person or by having the relevant professional or agency send records directly to the evaluator. A final consideration is that this task also provides a sample of the caretakers' behavior. Their responsibility and success in carrying out this initial assignment may foreshadow the follow-through and success seen on subsequent homework. This simple beginning provides an opportunity to begin establishing the active role of the caretakers as partners in any services provided to their children.

Even when background records are obtained by the caretakers, it is prudent clinical practice to obtain releases of information from all involved professionals. Having releases on file facilitates communication with the other professionals if follow-up inquiries are indicated or if consultation is needed for treatment coordination or planning. Reluctance of parents to sign releases of information is unusual, and if this happens, the reasons should be carefully explored. On very rare occasions parents may have legal or personal agenda independent of their concerns for their child; for instance, protecting a family secret or trying to bolster a change-of-custody suit. In these cases, it is especially important that the role and responsibilities of all parties be carefully clarified. Such clarification is the best foundation for avoiding frustration on the part of any of the involved parties.

## School and Academic Records

I am usually interested in seeing elementary school, middle or junior high school, and high school transcripts; records of any achievement testing; and any psychological, social work, speech, or special education reports within the school files. If parents have kept report cards, especially from the first few grades, it is often useful to review them. Samples of written work in English, spelling, and arithmetic, as well as artwork, from different years of school or different ages are worth at least a quick review, if they are available. These records provide documentation of the child's prior level of academic achievement, as well as teacher's perceptions of work habits, social adjustment, and general adaptation to the school environment. The pattern of school achievement can suggest hypotheses to be further evaluated. For example, a child's grades may be relatively stable and unremarkable (mostly S for "satisfactory," very few S+'s, an occasional N for "needs improvement") for the first 3 years of school (kindergarten through second grade). Then there is a distinct drop in achievement, from mostly D's to mostly F's across the next three grades. There are several possibilities that need consideration. Possibly the child's level of general intelligence is borderline, and he or she has begun to "top out" in his or her response to the standard curriculum. Perhaps there has been an environmental change that contributed to this decline in schoolwork: parental divorce, shifting placement, or insufficient parental support of school work. Perhaps these grades are recording the premorbid decline seen in some children prior to an initial schizophrenic episode. What is present in these records is evidence that the child's academic performance had been adequate for several years and that something then changed.

An important task for the evaluator is to learn what accounted for this shift in achievement.

Other information that may be available through school records could include data on absences, tardiness, and contacts with the school nurse. Patterns of absences in the spring and fall are sometimes associated with allergies. Frequent late arrivals at school can be a consequence of family disorganization, attention or behavior problems on the way to school, or inadequate family resources. The identification of a difficulty is the starting point to understanding more fully the circumstances the child was functioning under. Discrepancies between grades and achievement test scores can raise questions regarding under- and overachievement, possible difficulties in the school environment, or emerging test anxiety.

### Medical Records

Pediatric records may have little useful information for the mental health evaluation, but it is wise to obtain confirmation of the child's past general physical examinations and the results of these. Certainly any atypical background with respect to mother's pregnancy, delivery, illnesses, injuries, and development is worth noting. Confirmation of compliance with any prescribed medication regimes is valuable. Although any number of professionals may be aware that a trial of Ritalin was made in the third grade and abandoned after a few months, the mental health evaluator may, unfortunately, be the first person who asks the simple question, "Did you make sure that Jose always took his medication when he was supposed to?"

### Social Service Records

Social work evaluations, family evaluations, social histories, and a variety of other documentation of family, community, and personal functioning and adaptation may be available. If the child has had contact with a social service agency, it is likely that some type of record has been made and is being maintained. Review of these records can greatly enhance the efficiency of your evaluation by eliminating the need to collect again the same background information. Also, cross-checking data that you gained from other evaluations may bring to light other information that had been missed or may clarify apparent contradictions in the record. This information, of course, may not be available for the initial assessment. In this case, one of the outcomes of the initial evaluation may be to identify relevant records that need to be accessed.

## Juvenile Court Records

Juvenile court case histories are a special case of social service records. The reviews, typically prepared for the presiding juvenile court judge, may provide extensive background data on a youth, his family, his home life, school performance and adjustment, medical history, treatment history, and vocational history, as well as the perceptions of the officer, child, parents, teachers, and, if relevant, victim(s). As documents of the court these reports may be governed by somewhat different rules than those covering other mental health reports, but it is often worth making the effort to assess these data if they are available.

## Prior Mental Health Records

Surprisingly, a sometimes overlooked source of information in the evaluation of youths are records from prior encounters with mental health professionals. A major problem here often is obtaining the records in a timely manner, as they will inevitably be covered by confidentiality guidelines restricting access. In any preliminary contacts with caretakers, it is useful to determine whether prior contacts have been made with other mental health professionals. When it is likely that prior records do exist, I try to give the parents the task of obtaining these prior to my initial evaluation meeting with the youth. During my first meeting with the family, I obtain the necessary written consent to communicate with previous therapists or counselors.

# 4 Evaluating Cognitive Problems in Children

## THE DOMAIN OF COGNITIVE FUNCTIONING: DEFINITIONS, DEVELOPMENTAL FEATURES, ISSUES

The child's cognitive functioning—his or her overall mental abilities—is an important general area of evaluation. The development of youths is expressed, in part, in the ever-expanding capacity to intentionally attend and to sustain mental focus; to learn new information and skills and retrieve them as needed; to understand and operate with relationships between objects, people, and ideas; and to solve problems of increasing complexity and challenge. These are the domains of cognitive functioning. Difficulties in these mental abilities were among the first symptoms recognized as differentiating psychopathology, and difficulties in these abilities remain one of the important areas of assessment in mental health evaluation. Disturbances in level of consciousness, memory, and executive function make up the category of cognitive disorders (delirium, amnestic disorders, dementia). Several further categories of mental abnormality (mental retardation, learning disorders, language disorders) are defined in terms of or in relationship to general intellectual functioning. Intelligence has been demonstrated to be both a risk (lower intelligence) and a protective (higher intelligence) factor for a variety of behavior disorders in youths. Few topics in human functioning have commanded as central and as controversial a position as human intelligence.

The formal assessment of intelligence relies on standardized psychological testing, a topic well beyond the purview of this book. On a more preliminary level, however, the topic of evaluating the child or adolescent's general intellectual functioning is always a consideration in mental health assessment. Tested IQ is of consequence only if there has already been some indication of difficulty with adjustment that calls into question the child's mental abilities. Intelligence tests are time-consuming and expensive; these labor-intensive evaluations are not administered without a clear indication of need. A question has already come up about the youth's ability that involves concerns about his or her intelligence. The question often arises in response to difficulties in academic performance or failures to show expected adaptive learning and behavior. This initial assessment of learning and information processing capacity is our current concern and focus.

## FACTORS THAT MAY DISRUPT THE COGNITIVE FUNCTIONING OF CHILDREN

Accurate assessment depends on obtaining good data, good in the sense of being truly representative of the client's responses or abilities. The validity of data refers to the degree to which they reflect the construct we are interested in. In this context the quality of the data we can elicit about children's cognitive abilities in a mental health assessment will covary with our care in considering possible alternative explanations of their performances. A number of factors can influence clients' performances on ability testing. The variable we are interested in is ability, but in order to know that it is actually the child's capability that is primarily contributing to his or her score, we must consider and exclude other possible contributors. It is helpful to consider these deleterious factors in terms of those that are more acute and transient and those that are more chronic and enduring.

### More Acute Disruptive Factors

*Fear and Performance Anxiety*

With clients of all ages, but more especially with the very young client, performance anxiety and fear of the evaluation situation can interfere with the efficient application of the mental abilities the child possesses. This is not a very useful observation, because exactly the same effect could be demonstrated in all of us—anxiety interferes with cognitive efficiency. The more pertinent question is, How much does performance anxiety disrupt this child's mental processing? Part of answering this question requires a demonstration of what the child is capable of when anxiety effects are minimized. The prior discussion about building rapport and setting the proper situation for a valid assessment is relevant here. Taking a few minutes to establish a positive relationship with the child and making him or her as comfortable as possible within the testing environment is an investment that pays off in more meaningful assessment data. Maintaining a positive and supportive interaction with the child during assessment likewise helps to maximize the informative value of the results secured.

## Inadequate Task Motivation

The youthful client may be insufficiently motivated to put forth his or her best effort during ability testing. This can contribute to a false and misleading assessment. Although most children are usually motivated to perform for adults when asked, this is not universally the case. Children with externalizing behavior problems may resist assessment, either in a passive manner or through more active rebellion against testing. It is vital that the examiner make every effort to elicit the child's best performance in order to obtain the most valid interpretation of the results. At times assessments may need to be delayed, interrupted, or prolonged in order to reduce as much as possible the effects of negative attitudes or insufficient task motivation.

## Oppositional Behavior

Active resistance to testing is in some ways a lesser concern than passive underachievement, because it is obvious and can be directly addressed. If necessary, assessment can be terminated until a better situational attitude can be effected. Even if postponement cannot be achieved, it is clear to the examiner that valid results have not been obtained. It may be helpful to attempt to understand as clearly as possible the basis of the youth's objection to the assessment. If the resistance is occasioned by the "stupid" or demeaning level of the questions, you may want to point out that you know these are "baby" questions but that everyone is asked the same questions and that cooperation will get both of you through the exercise as quickly as possible. With some adolescents it may help to actually begin with items or probes that are difficult or clearly beyond the youth's ability level, then to work backward to tasks on which the youth can succeed. Your task as examiner is to remove as much as possible the effects of limited motivation, so that the obtained results yield a good sampling of the young person's capacity for mental processing.

## Illness, Hunger, and Fatigue

Well known to most caretakers and examiners alike are the limiting effects of state variables such as illness, hunger, fatigue, schedule disruption, and similar "real life" issues. You can take the important precaution of inquiring of both the young person and the available caretakers whether a meal or nap was missed in order to get the youth to the appointment, whether there has been a recent illness, or whether any unusual occurrences have transpired in the family or child's life coincident with the evaluation. The quality of the conclusions reached from the evaluation is fixed by the quality of the data obtained. It is far better to reschedule an appointment than to have to try to sort out what limitations result from mental processing deficits and what limitations resulted from a concurrent cold.

## Drugs, Medication, Seizures, and Pain

State effects on intellectual functioning include chemicals and painful conditions. It is vital to know what prescription and over-the-counter medications the child has been given. Many medications are psychoactive, often affecting the child's level of alertness, attention and concentration, and sustained mental effort. It may not be possible to assess the child in a chemical-free state; indeed, his or her natural state may be one reflecting a certain level of chemical effect. The examiner can, however, always take note of the presence of chemical agents and temper diagnostic conclusions drawn from behavioral data. Medical conditions or treatments that have associated pain or other noxious effects may impede the youth's task performance. Again, it may not be possible to wait for the child to be pain free. Unfortunately, some children will never be pain free. It is possible to be highly sensitive to the effects of the pain. Pain is a highly fatiguing experience. Working with clients in physical pain requires sensitivity to their need for frequent rest breaks and an active resistance to the temptation to "get just one more thing done before stopping." In assessment, bad data are far worse than no data at all—bad data are often uninterpretable, whereas the absence of data reminds us that more information is called for. For children who experience seizures, subtle postictal effects may occur over a significant period of time. My policy is not to conduct a general intellectual assessment of individuals within 72 hours of a major motor seizure.

The issue of chemical influences on mental processing is, of course, not limited to legitimate medications. Especially with adolescents, the examiner must consider the possibility that the youth is under the influence of illicit drugs at the time of ability testing. There is obviously no guaranteed procedure to prevent this possibility. Giving preliminary attention to clarifying the reasons for the evaluation and securing the youth's active cooperation and participation should help reduce these problems. My preference is to delay any formal testing if the youth has used any illicit psychoactive chemicals on the day of the appointment. At times I have accepted with little attendant inquiry a young person's request that certain areas of evaluation be postponed until a subsequent appointment. The issue of drug abuse is, obviously, an important topic in itself and needs to be addressed; the matter at hand, however, is eliciting performance data that validly reflects the general cognitive abilities of the young person. Knowing what the youth is capable of when he or she is not "high" is a vital component of understanding the young person. It is also tremendously important to know if the current state of his or her life is such that this type of evaluation cannot be obtained outside a controlled environment.

## More Chronic Disruptive Factors

Topics such as pain, medication, and seizures begin to expand the discussion of disruptive effects from transient influences to more long-standing or even permanent conditions. A wide range of deleterious factors can result in the enduring constriction of a young person's cognitive processing. Traumatic brain injury, toxic exposure to lead poisoning, encephalitic infections, and cranial radiation therapy for tumors are only a few of the many potentially harmful influences that can limit a youth's functioning intelligence. These chronic influences cannot usually be directly affected by the evaluator, but we can work to remain sensitive to the reality that the child has been injured, that this injury probably affects his or her mental capability, and that it also probably increases his or her susceptibility to other limiting influences, such as fatigue, illness, and medication side effects.

## OTHER CONSIDERATIONS IN THE INTERPRETATION OF MENTAL STATUS DATA FROM CHILDREN

### Cultural, Ethnic, and Socioeconomic Status

The possible role of background factors unrelated to the child's general mental functioning that might affect his or her performance on cognitive functioning tasks needs to be considered. Although some data from adults suggest that certain aspects of mental status appraisal are relatively unaffected by ethnic background and socioeconomic level (see the discussion of the Mini-Mental State Examination in Lezak, 1995), comparable data do not exist to support the robustness of mental status measures with youths from diverse backgrounds. Both minority status and low socioeconomic status appear to affect the prevalence of psychosocial dysfunction (Murphy, Reede, Jellinek, & Bishop, 1992; Murphy & Jellinek, 1988). The field of neuropsychology has begun to actively consider the possible influences of culture on cognition (Perez-Arce, 1999) and on cognitive appraisal (Llorente, Ponton, Taussig, & Satz, 1999; Ponton & Ardila, 1999; Rey et al., 1999), but the current literature pertains primarily to adults. Sattler (2001) carefully considers the intellectual assessment of "culturally and linguistically diverse children." His overall conclusion is that the arguments that have been made against the use of intelligence tests with children from ethnically diverse backgrounds have not been supported by empirical examinations. At the same time he presents a compelling case for sensitivity to cultural variables in the service of establishing rapport and reaching the most valid final assessment.

### Possible Dissimulation and "Faking Bad"

The possibility of malingering as a factor influencing the youth's performance should be borne in mind, especially in circumstances that would encourage exaggeration of symptoms. In assessment that stems from Social Security determinations and in forensic evaluations to establish acquired injury as a foundation for damages and compensation, the client may be caught in the difficult position of having to "appear worse to do better." There appears to be evidence that children (Faust, Hart, & Guilmette, 1988) and adolescents (Faust, Hart, Guilmette, & Arkes, 1988) can fake believable deficits during neuropsychological testing and that clinicians are overconfident regarding their ability to detect dissimulation. The youth may have been subtle or overtly encouraged to perform at less than his or her best. On some occasions it may appear that the child has been coached regarding how he or she should perform. A harsh reality to consider, given the largely discouraging results seen in efforts to validly detect malingering, is that evaluators probably become aware of only the most inept and foolish instances of "faking bad" (House & Lewis, 1985). In the cases in which this concern has come up in my practice, my impression has usually been that the individual was in reality compromised but had chosen to exaggerate their limitations. It is a good policy to speak frankly to parents, adolescents, and older children in cases in which financial or placement outcomes appear to rest on testing results, pointing out how they will be best served by the youth's making his or her best effort on all tasks. This policy will allow the examiner to express his or her results with the greatest confidence, and decisions pertaining to the child will be based on the best evidence. Certainly not all instances of "faking bad" will be eliminated, but the number of unfortunate cases in which a truly disabled youth tries to magnify his or her problems out of concern that the examiner will not notice his or her difficulties may be reduced.

## MAJOR AREAS OF MENTAL FUNCTIONING

### General Intellectual Functioning

Part of an initial mental health appraisal should consist of an evaluation of the child's overall mental capability, his or her working intelligence. This appraisal may be impressionistic and subjective, based on your summary appreciation of the young person's resourcefulness and adaptability during the session. A better practice is to systematically consider at least the major areas of mental performance—attention and concentration, language performance, constructional abilities, learning and memory, and executive functions. If caretaker report, informal assessment, or mental status evaluation raises any serious questions about mental abilities, it is prudent to obtain formal psychological assessment. Tested intelligence is one major element in the definition of such diagnostic categories as mental retardation and learning disorders. Before any formal diagnosis of mental retardation or learning disorder could be entertained, the results of testing with an individually administered, comprehensive measure of general intellectual functioning would need to be documented. Brief mental status examination is not a substitute for intellectual testing; rather, it could provide one possible indication that such testing is needed.

## Attention and Concentration

The capacity to focus mental attention, ignore distractions, and concentrate on the problem at hand is one fundamental element of efficient information processing. Attention and concentration are developmentally acquired abilities—in general, an 8-year-old can pay attention longer than a 4-year-old. Attention and concentration fluctuate over time for any given child and vary with novelty, interest in the task, and motivational inducements. Attention and concentration can be influenced by chemical action, either intentionally (the use of central nervous system stimulants to treat attention-deficit disorders) or unintentionally (the sedating side effects of many anticonvulsants). Attention and concentration are prerequisite capabilities for efficient application of other mental abilities; impairments in attention lead to impairments in other areas of performance as well (Rowe & Rowe, 1992). Moreover, attention problems are relatively nonspecific and occur with a variety of behavioral, emotional, and cognitive disorders in children (Halperin, Matier, Bedi, Sharma, & Newcorn, 1992).

### Level of Consciousness

One element of concentration is general cortical arousal—the individual's level of consciousness. If the child is fatigued to the point of falling asleep, sedated by medication or drugs of abuse, or obtunded by neurological disorder, then there is little point in continuing with further mental status assessment. At the other extreme, little is going to be learned from attempting to evaluate the adolescent in a manic episode who is showing flight of ideas, pressured speech, and looseness of associations beyond the obvious; he or she is not thinking straight. In the vast majority of cases the simple notation that the child is "alert" will be sufficient. For the small minority of cases in which the child's level of consciousness is at issue, a variety of rating scales are available. Table 4.1 displays one simple view of the continuum of level of consciousness (cf. discussions in Berg, Franzen, & Wedding, 1994; Strub & Black, 1993; Othmer & Othmer, 1994). The concept of "behavioral states" (Bucy et al., 1999) addresses the same basic continuum of arousal and agitation.

| TABLE 4.1 | Levels of Consciousness |
| --- | --- |
| *Hyperarousal* | Agitated, excessive arousal and tension, oversensitive to stimuli, thinking disrupted and behavior impulsive |
| *Normal* | Alert, attentive to environment, purposeful thinking |
| *Lethargy* | Reduced arousal, thinking not well organized, responds to strong stimulation, tends to drift into sleep when not actively engaged |
| *Obtundation* | Intermediate state between lethargy and stupor, difficult to arouse, confused when aroused |
| *Stupor* | Minimum arousal, no purposeful thinking, minimal response to strong stimulation, sometimes referred to as "semicoma" |
| *Coma* | Completely unarousable, nonresponsive to painful stimulation |

The Glasgow Coma Scale (GCS; Teasdale & Jennett, 1974) is probably the most commonly used measure of impairment in level of consciousness (Yeates, 2000). With very young children (for instance, under 3 years of age) a number of modifications of the GCS have been constructed, including the Pediatric Coma Scale (Simpson & Reilly, 1982) and Yoon Hahn's Children's Coma Scale (Hahn & McLong, 1993; see also the discussions in Nelson, 1992, and Spreen, Risser, & Edgell, 1995). The Glasgow Outcome Scale (Jennett & Bond, 1975) has also been modified for use with infants and children (Ewing-Cobbs et al., 1998). These measures have their primary application in medical settings for the evaluation of traumatic brain injury and other severe lesions of the central nervous system.

## Sustained Attention

Attention and concentration can be conceptualized into several elements. One of the most important features of mental focusing is the capacity to sustain attention on a task or target. Sustained attention, or concentration, is very limited in infants and increases over the developmental years, probably reflecting neurological maturation. Inattentiveness in children is associated with poor academic performance and negative attitudes regarding school achievement (Rowe & Rowe, 1992). Whether considered in terms of informal observations or through the child's performance on mental status items, the reference point needs to be the expected performance of a *child of this age*. The average performance of age peers provides the metric of interest. Digit or letter repetition in chains of increasing length, letter or number or symbol cancellation tasks, and mental arithmetic problems have all been used as tasks to assess attention. Informally, the child's ability to maintain a topic of conversation during the interview and to stay "on task" are important observations to make, as well as noting any indication of unexpected distractibility.

## Orientation

Questions regarding orientation to time, place, person, and situation are used in many mental status protocols. The Temporal Orientation Test format of Arthur Benton (Benton, Sivan, Hamsher, Varney, & Spreen, 1994) provides one standardization of inquiry into temporal orientation. As would probably be expected, young children do not demonstrate consistent orientation to time. By the fifth grade, however, the temporal orientation of most children begins to resemble that of adolescents and adults (Benton et al., 1994). When temporal orientation is adequate, there is usually reasonable appreciation for person and place.

## Interaction with Other Abilities and Disabilities

Although attention deficits seem in many ways to be a relatively nonspecific symptom reflected in a wide variety of childhood disorders, there are reports of specific patterns of difficulty that involve attention deficits. The most well known, of course, is ADHD, discussed elsewhere in this book. Hellgren, Gillberg, Bagenholm, and Gillberg (1994) provide an interesting discussion of ADHD symptomology in the broader context of children who show deficits in attention, motor control, and perception (DAMP). By drawing attention to the extended covariates of ADHD, such as motor control problems and perceptual dysfunction, Hellgren et al. (1994) recall a previous literature in which attention problems and overactivity were seen in concert with a number of other behavioral and cognitive differences as an indication of minimal brain damage (MBD). Although the concept of MBD proved of little value and has been discarded, the empirical cluster of difficulties previously associated with the idea may have clinical usefulness. Hellgren et al.'s (1994) follow-up data suggest continuing psychiatric difficulty and heightened risk for personality disorder diagnoses in children showing DAMP. The usefulness of this view remains an open issue. The association between motor control and perceptual problems, for instance, has been questioned (Henderson, Barnett, & Henderson, 1994). Although DSM-IV includes the relatively new category of developmental coordination disorder, the clinical utility of this category and the nature of its relationship to other diagnoses, such as ADHD, remain to be clearly demonstrated. I have found it useful both to observe children for signs of motor clumsiness and to inquire of caretakers as to histories of poor coordination and sensory or perceptual difficulties. The multiple indications of problems in these areas should raise our level of concern for the child and alert the evaluator to the possibility of atypical developmental features.

## Language Abilities

Symbolic communication is a basic human activity and is most commonly expressed though language. Difficulties or disturbances in language use have serious implications for normal development. Children with language use problems are at greater risk for a multitude of other behavioral disturbances, including anxiety and depression, social withdrawal, and sleep problems (Carson, Klee, Perry, Muskina, & Donaghy, 1998). An assessment of speech and language performance is a fundamental element in evaluating the youth's mental status.

### Speech

Observation of the child's spontaneous speech can provide valuable data with respect to the clarity of articulation, the flow and amplitude of speech, and any unusual qualities of voice that could affect the child's communication or social interaction. Any significantly unusual features of oral language can be explored further with the parents. If there is indication of a functional impact on communication effectiveness or interpersonal relationships, a referral for a speech evaluation can be very useful for a comprehensive evaluation of speech and language performances. Arthur Benton's rating scale for speech articulation from the Multilingual Aphasia Examination (Benton & Hamsher, 1989) is easy to use and provides a basic quantification of speech clarity that can facilitate comparisons over time and communication with other professionals.

## Interview Segment 4.1. Brief Cognitive Evaluation of a Young Child: Jason

The following segment illustrates the screening of mental functions in a young child. Jason is a 5-year-old referred by his mother because of concerns regarding his behavior at home and with other children in the neighborhood. He lives with his mother, an older brother, and his maternal grandmother in the grandmother's home. He attends a morning kindergarten program and is in day care in the afternoons.

EXAMINER: How is that seat for you? Are you OK at the table?

JASON: (*Nods affirmatively.*)

EXAMINER: OK, I want to see all the things you know and can do. Is that ok?

JASON: (*Nods.*)

EXAMINER: Good. Tell me your name. What's your name?

JASON: Jason.

EXAMINER: Very good. What's your last name, Jason?

JASON: Jason.

EXAMINER: Yes, you are Jason. What is your whole name.

JASON: Jason Goodfellow.

EXAMINER: That's right. How do you spell "Jason"?

JASON: J, A, S, O, N.

EXAMINER: Good job. How do you spell "Goodfellow"?

JASON: (*No response.*)

EXAMINER: Jason, would you write your name for me. Write your name right here on the paper. Good job. Jason, would you draw a circle for me? Right here. Now draw a triangle.

JASON: (*No response.*)

EXAMINER: OK, Jason, can you copy this figure for me [triangle]. Great. Copy this one [Greek cross], [overlapping pentagons], [key].

EXAMINER: Jason, how old are you?

JASON: Five.

EXAMINER: Right! Jason, when is your birthday?

JASON: May [correct].

EXAMINER: What day in May is your birthday?

JASON: May.

EXAMINER: Jason, what is your address?

JASON: (*Shakes head no.*)

EXAMINER: Jason, what is your telephone number at home?

JASON: 555-1212 [correct].

EXAMINER: That's right. Good remembering. Can you write your phone number for me here?

JASON: (*Draws several numbers, begins drawing picture.*)

EXAMINER: (*Retrieves pencil and paper.*) OK, Jason, I want you to tell me the names for some things. What is this [comb], [keys]?

JASON: Comb. Keys.

EXAMINER: Jason, if you were at home by yourself and something bad happened, how could you use the telephone to get help?

JASON: Call.

EXAMINER: Yes, who would you call?

JASON: Mom.

EXAMINER: OK, how would you call your mom with the telephone?

JASON: Call Mom.

EXAMINER: OK, Jason, how many eyes do you have?

JASON: Two.

EXAMINER: Good. How many fingers do you have?

JASON: Six.

EXAMINER: How many?

JASON: Five.

EXAMINER: Jason, how many fingers do I have on this hand?

JASON: Five.

EXAMINER: Right. Jason, how many pencils are on the table here [three]?

JASON: Three.

EXAMINER: Good. How many pencils are there now [two groups, three and four]?

JASON: Six.

EXAMINER: OK, Jason, how much is one plus one?

JASON: Two!

EXAMINER: Good. How much is two plus two?

JASON: Four!

EXAMINER: How much is one plus two?

JASON: Two!

EXAMINER: How much is two plus one?

JASON: Four!

EXAMINER: OK, Jason, what color is this [red], [blue], [green], [red], [yellow], [blue], [brown], [green], [yellow]? Great job.

Jason, can you write all the letters for me? Write your alphabet here. Good, now write the numbers from one to ten here.

Jason, you're working really hard. We'll have to tell your mom how hard you worked. She'll be very proud of you.

JASON: (*Smiles.*)

EXAMINER: Jason, what is your teacher's name at school?

JASON: Mrs. Wood [correct].

EXAMINER: What is the name of your school?

JASON: I go to kindergarten.

EXAMINER: That's right. What is the name of the school where you go to kindergarten?

JASON: School.

EXAMINER: Where do you go after school?

JASON: Day care [correct].

EXAMINER: And who is your teacher at day care?

JASON: Teacher.

EXAMINER: Right, what is teacher's name?

JASON: Teacher.

EXAMINER: What do you like to do at kindergarten?

This exchange showed a brief mental screening suitable for a younger child. It could be expanded depending on the child's responses and the referral questions being evaluated. In addition to the verbal content, this sequence allowed observation of Jason's attention and concentration, speech, gross vision and hearing performance, motor coordination, compliance to commands, task behavior, and interpersonal responsiveness. Note that in a one-on-one situation with constant adult attention Jason is highly compliant and that he appears responsive to social reinforcement. At this point it appears that Jason's cognitive abilities are within the normal range for his age and probably are not a major factor in the oppositional behavior that has brought him to attention.

### Receptive Language

The child's ability to listen to and understand oral language is a vital skill for normal social and educational development. Oral comprehension is necessary to the reciprocal interaction of social transactions, as well as to following directions from parents, teachers, and other authorities. Any indication of problems in oral comprehension exceeding those expected at her or his age should be followed up to determine the limits of the child's understanding of what is being said to them. Answering basic questions, following simple commands, and appropriately following a conversation can demonstrate a basic foundation of normal oral comprehension. Given the dynamic quality of language development, children with essentially normal language development can show at least minor lags in receptive language skills. Children from language-rich environments especially may use words whose meanings they do not fully appreciate. Given the ease with which most children learn to appear as if they understand more than they actually do, the examiner would do well to have a very low threshold for suspecting comprehension limitations. It is relatively easy to adjust the level of one's own communication to facilitate understanding. Making appropriate adjustments can pay off in much higher quality of interview data obtained.

### Expressive Language

Naming deficits in children can reflect a wide range of difficulties, including neurological problems in linguistic processing, learning problems, and early environments that do not adequately stimulate speech and language development. Reduced verbal fluency is a highly sensitive but nonspecific indication of a verbal problem. Further evaluation is always necessary to determine the cause and associated conditions present when there are greater naming problems than expected for the child's age.

## Pragmatic Communication

The ultimate goal of speech and language is usually not just to produce verbal language but to communicate, to influence the social world, to relay information, desires, feelings, and inquiries. Poor pragmatic communication can severely limit a child even in the face of intact molecular language skills. The excessive wordiness of some hearing-impaired children or youth with nonverbal learning disabilities and the stilted and empty speech of some autistic children show deficits in the pragmatic aspects of language—the use of oral language to interact with the world. In contrast, the agrammatical and jargon-riddled speech of streetwise children of low socioeconomic status often shows poor formal language characteristics but is dramatically effective in the real job of language—to affect our world. How well does the child get his or her point across or message communicated? This is the question addressed by the pragmatic aspects of language use. In my experience good pragmatic communication is a powerful and positive prognostic variable. Effective symbolic communication, even in the presence of speech or language limitations, reflects the intact operation of vital cognitive processes and predicts relatively good outcome. Li, Walton, and Nuttall (1999) have discussed the challenges of assessing young culturally and linguistically diverse children.

## Reading Skills

The formal evaluation of reading skills goes well beyond the focus of this book, but at least an informal assessment of the child's level of reading ability is important in evaluating cognitive development. A young person's oral reading of letters, numbers, brief phrases, and sentences; his or her demonstration of being able to follow simple, written commands; and his or her explanation of newspaper headlines and advertisements can offer at least an overview of the child's progress toward becoming a literate citizen. The purpose of such screening devices is not to formally diagnose reading problems but to identify cases needing further assessment. As such, all screening measures should be used with a low threshold to maximize sensitivity for possible reading problems. False positive cases—children with normal reading skills who failed the screens—will be easily eliminated by more systematic evaluation. The important aspect is to ensure that the number of false negative cases—children with reading problems who pass the screens—is minimized. For children with whom there is any real question of learning or attention-deficit problems, the use of reading screening tools has no value. The reading skills of all of these children should be comprehensively evaluated with reliable and valid formal measures.

### Writing and Spelling Skills

A sample of the child's writing is valuable to obtain, both as a constructional performance (see the next section) and as a way of assessing the child's capacity to use this medium of communication. Writing to dictation is often used as an assessment of this aspect of language, as in the oral repetition, explanation, and writing item, "He shouted the warning," from the Aphasia Screening Test (Reitan, 1984). An alternative device that allows sampling of the child's generative written language is the use of a "story starter" (Shapiro, 1996). The youth is given a sentence to use as the first sentence of a short story, asked to think about the story for a minute, and then asked to write the story. After three minutes the story is collected and the number of "correct" (recognizable) words counted. Shapiro (1996) offers a number of story starters and norms for elementary grades.

## Visual–Spatial Abilities

### Constructional Performances

Possible perceptual–motor difficulties can be inferred from children's drawing and copying of designs, other constructional activities (building toys), and reports of the child's play activities and coordination. Observation or reports of visual–spatial processing problems severe enough to negatively affect academic learning or social development should be assessed with age-normed measures, such as the Berry Test of Visual–Motor Integration or the Rey Complex Figure.

### Writing

Along with having the child draw and copy at least a few basic shapes and figures, you should obtain a sample of the child's handwriting.

Asking the child to write his or her name and the alphabet or a brief sentence creates a permanent record of his or her graphomotor performance at the time of assessment. Difficulties in printed or cursive letter formations, spelling, and punctuation can contribute to a fuller understanding of academic difficulties. Drawing and writing exercises also provide an opportunity to observe the child's use of a pencil or pen. The young preschool child grasps a crayon or drawing utensil with a fisted grip. Over the next few years, children develop competency with a pincer or tripod grasp, which allows for precise movements. Dunn (1999) reviews fine motor development of grasping patterns. The adequacy of the child's motor control of the writing instrument can be considered in terms of his or her writing experience and the quality of the product.

## Learning and Memory

As with reading, any specific questions or concerns about learning problems should lead directly to formal testing and evaluation. For many children seen in a mental health setting, however, these issues are not primary, and assessment of learning and recall is not necessary. Informal observations of the child's acquisition and retention of information can contribute to our understanding of the child's situation. The ease with which young children master the names of their teachers, their ability to relate information about family members, and their recall of your name and any details of your practice they have been given—such as whether you will see them more than once, where the restroom is, and so forth—provide some insight into their incidental learning and recall. With older children and adolescents a discussion of current events, the status of their favorite team, and who is on top of their preferred music chart can give a similar perspective on the youth's effective learning and memory. Obviously, the reports of older children and teenagers about factual events need to be checked against an independent source, unless you actually do know what the score of last night's ball game was. Emotional and psychiatric factors that might be interfering with learning and memory appear to operate primarily through their impact on attention and concentration (Adams, Stanczak, Leutzinger, Waters, & Brown, 2001). If questions regarding a possible memory deficit became an issue, it would be important to attempt to maximize the child's attention to any learning task presented.

## Executive Functions

One of the most important, complex, and difficult to describe or measure aspects of cognitive functioning is captured by the phrase "executive functions." The capacity for critical thinking, problem solving, planning, utilization of feedback and results for self-correction, abstract reasoning, and judgment are all facets of this domain of mental functioning. The thinking of children and mentally limited individuals tends to be concrete. Their capacity to generalize from specific cases to a general rule is limited and often flawed. Their controlled, successive elaboration and focusing of analysis tends to derail before a final solution is reached. With development these self-governing aspects of mental processing become increasingly efficient and automatic. Young children often equate a good intention with actually having completed a task; the adolescent has begun to appreciate that thoughts and actions are separate and not equal. Effective evaluation of executive functions lags behind our ability to measure general intellectual functioning, arithmetic skills, or even constructional performance; but deficits in one or more aspects of executive abilities are increasingly implicated in a wide range of cognitive, emotional, and behavioral difficulties in young people, such as mental retardation, autism, ADHD, conduct disorders, and some personality problems. Neither formal psychological tests nor client interviews have proved especially helpful thus far in evaluating executive functions in a clinically satisfactory manner. We hope that this situation will change with ongoing efforts and the growing appreciation of how vital this topic is to effective human behavior. For the time being, interviews with informants who have had a great deal of opportunity to observe the youth's day-to-day level of functioning probably gives us our best view of the child's level of executive functioning. Good executive functions are reflected in consistency of performance, in carrying tasks through from beginning to completion, in learning from experiences, in effective planning and execution, and in controlling impulses.

## Reality Testing

A final aspect of mental processing worth discussion is the child's level of reality testing, his or her effective differentiation of the objective world from inner experience. Under the right conditions, even young children will distinguish between their imaginary friends and other people; between stories and actual events; between private thoughts and overheard speech. The differentiation between inner and outer realities, however, is less rigid and distinct in children much of the time. Their capacity for vivid imagery, emotional absorption in play, and role taking tend to be higher than those seen in adolescents and adults. At times it can be challenging for an examiner to determine whether there is actually a difficulty in reality testing that rises to the level of a clinical concern. One illustration of this is in the syndrome called shared psychotic disorder (*folie à deux*). In this syndrome a child may demonstrate apparent delusional thinking that, in actuality, represents the modeling of psychotic thinking evidenced by an adult the child has a close relationship with. Actual hallucinations in children may be more common than often suspected (Schreier, 1999) and may not necessarily carry dire prognostic significance. Hallucinations in children may occur in association with migraine headaches and other relatively frequent neurological phenomena in youth. Such experiences need to be considered within the context of the child's life and adjustment.

## Brief Screening Instruments

A number of screening instruments have been developed for the brief assessment of cognitive functioning in individuals suspected of neurological damage or dysfunction. One commonly employed device is the Mini-Mental State Examination (MMSE; Folstein et al., 1975), which assesses performance on 11 tasks that sample orientation, verbal repetition, attention, verbal recall, object naming, following instructions, reading, writing, and copying a design. The MMSE is frequently used in hospital settings and in outpatient medical practice as a screen for dementia and to assess the possible impact of trauma and other neurological events on the patient's cognition. A Modified Mini-Mental State Examination intended for use with children was developed by Besson and Labbe (1997). The issue with all short screening measures is the level of false positive and false negative errors and the resulting positive and negative prognostic values. Standardized cognitive screening has the great potential advantage of using normative data to establish empirical standards of judgment, but until the variables that affect results are well understood, our confidence in such criteria is guarded. Age and education have been found to be associated with scores on the

**Interview Segment 4.2. Seeing Chickens**

Joan was a preschool child brought by her mother to a public health clinic for her school vaccinations. During the brief interaction between Joan and the pediatric resident, the physician became concerned over possible visual hallucinations. Joan commented about baby chickens that had followed the family from their apartment to the hospital and were "pooping" on the doctor's desk. The resident could see neither the chicks nor the mess they were reportedly making and decided to consult a mental health practitioner. Joan cheerfully told me about the chickens, the mess they made, and other unusual aspects of their family life. When I spoke with Joan's mother about her observations, the mother emphatically agreed that the invisible chickens were making a real mess of the waiting area and that we needed to get busy cleaning the place up. A telephone call to Joan's grandmother revealed that Joan's mother had a history of paranoid schizophrenia, usually well controlled with neuroleptic medication. The following interaction occurred with Joan, as the limits of her "hallucinations" were explored:

EXAMINER: Joan, can you still see the baby chicken up on my desk?

JOAN: I can see it. It's right there.

EXAMINER: Right. And you can see my coffee mug on the table, too?

JOAN: Sure. I see good.

EXAMINER: I'm glad you see good. Tell me, can you see the baby chick just like you can see the coffee mug?

JOAN: Well. . . . You have to look more to see the chick.

    The final impression was that Joan was not experiencing visual hallucinations but was manifesting *folie à deux*, modeling the hallucinatory symptoms of her mother.

---

MMSE (Anderson, 1994; Lezak, 1995), and Besson and Labbe (1997) found that these variables were also correlated with scores on their Modified MMSE. An examiner using the Modified MMSE would need to attend carefully to the age and educational background of the child in interpreting results. If continued studies of the Modified MMSE support its reliability and validity in children, it could become a useful addition to the repertoire of professionals who assess youths.

## ENVIRONMENTAL CONTEXT

Another consideration in evaluating the cognitive functioning of youth is to consider the environmental context in which their learning, problem solving, and applied thinking occurs. With low-birth-weight infants, for instance, maternal intelligence has been found to be a critical variable in predicting cognitive development. Bacharach and Bandmaster (1998) found that the mother's intelligence was correlated with the child's tested intelligence and also interacted with other predictive variables for the child's mental development, such as marital status, income level, and home environment. With all children and adolescents, it is very important to consider the characteristics of the worlds they function within and of the significant actors in these settings if a full appreciation of the youth's situation is to be gained. It is critical to avoid the perception of the child's mental status as a static variable that "resides" within the youth. The individual's mental functioning is the overt manifestation of a dynamic interaction between that person's central nervous system, learning history, and current environments. Only by attending to all elements of this equation can we fully appreciate their strengths and limitations.

## SELECTED CATEGORIES OF DISTURBANCE IN WHICH COGNITIVE CAPABILITY IS A MAJOR FOCUS

Problems of intellectual functioning can be an associated and complicating feature of almost all problems of youth. In some cases, however, the cognitive difficulties are one of the primary foci of concern. Several of these are discussed here, and two others (mental retardation and autism) are reviewed in Chapter 8.

### Learning Disabilities

Learning disorders are one of the most common manifestations of cognitive problems in children. Despite ongoing contention regarding basic definitional issues (Beitchman & Young, 1997; Hooper & Willis, 1989), this is a classification of high prevalence. Half of all children receiving special education services are qualified by the status of learning disability (U.S. Department of Education, 1997). Although many fundamental questions regarding learning problems remain unanswered, a great deal of progress has been made in this area (Beitchman & Young, 1997), and it is hoped that continued effort will increase our clarity of understanding of these frequent difficulties.

Learning disorders are not usually diagnosed without the benefit of psychological assessment of intelligence, academic skills, and related cognitive abilities and emotional adjustment and functioning. The initial evaluation serves primarily to identify learning disorder as an area of concern, to gather associated information, and to screen for frequently comorbid emotional and behavioral problems. Many children come to an evaluation with the presenting concern of academic underachievement, and the family's express purpose is to have an assessment of possible learning problems done. In extreme cases, the parents may have concluded that the child must have a learning disability and are looking to the evaluation with an expectation that this impression will be supported by the evaluator. It is important to recognize that not all cases of academic underachievement can be explained. This is a source of great frustration for concerned parents, teachers, and the informed public, as well as the evaluator. Nevertheless, it is the current state of affairs, and on some occasions the best we can offer a family is a clear and frank description of a situation for which no explanation can be made.

Even if academic problems are not introduced as part of the presenting clinical picture, you should inquire into this possibility. Learning difficulties are common in children and are often premorbid to other problems that clients may focus on in initial presentation. A straightforward screening question usually draws forth any concerns: "Can you tell me about any problems Johnny/Mary has in school?" As a follow-up to discussion of academic difficulties, it is usually helpful to request that the parent have a copy of the child's or adolescent's school records sent in for review. These are valuable data to consider whenever there is a question of the youth's cognitive functioning. In addition to classroom grades, there is typically information from standardized achievement tests, which are usually administered every few years in most school systems.

Learning disabilities are a special case of academic failure not accounted for by general intellectual ability. Intelligence is one among several variables associated with academic success and failure. For instance, among inner-city adolescents, past school performance but not tested intelligence tends to predict which high school youth are at greatest risk for academic failure and dropping out of school, along with other risk factors such as distress and drug involvement (Ripple & Luthar, 2000). The potency of other risk factors associated with behavior problems, such as poverty, may be influenced by ethnic or racial differences (McLeod & Nonnemaker, 2000). The appreciation of how various risk and protective influences (personal, familial, and cultural) interact in individual lives remains one of the fundamental challenges of mental health assessment.

## Traumatic Brain Injury and Other Neurological Conditions

Traumatic brain injury (TBI) in children can cause both short-term and chronic changes in cognitive processing, emotional and behavioral adjustment, and associated medical conditions (motor problems, seizures, physical deformities). Adequate assessment of cognitive problems in youth following TBI requires comprehensive evaluation of the domains of mental ability: attention and concentration, visual–spatial processing, language processing, learning and memory, and executive functions. Associated competencies in sensory or motor performances or both often need to be assessed. Other neurobehavioral syndromes (cerebral vascular disorders in youth, fetal alcohol syndrome, central nervous system infections and tumors, etc.) require similar, extensive psychological testing. The reader is referred to the constantly expanding literature on neuropsychological assessment of children and adolescents (Aylward, 1997; Franzen & Berg, 1989; Spreen, Risser, & Edgell, 1995; Teeter & Semrud-Clikeman, 1997).

Assessment of the behavioral and emotional adjustment of children with TBI and other neurological abnormalities is an equally important and challenging task. Brain injury in youths in general is a risk factor for behavioral and emotional problems; this risk is especially evident for moderate and severe TBI (Bloom et al., 2001). There is significantly less certainty regarding the relationship between mild injury and subsequent adjustment problems (cf. House, 1999, and Kinsella, Ong, Murtagh, Prior, & Sawyer, 1999, for discussions). Although it would be neither accurate nor helpful to assume that all children exposed to TBI will develop subsequent adjustment problems, it certainly is prudent to consider the possibility of adaptive problems following major neurological events and to screen for these. The reports of Brown (Brown, Chadwick, Shafffer, Rutter, & Traub, 1981), Max (Max & Dunisch, 1997; Max et al., 1997a, 1997b, 1997c, 1998b), and Bloom (Bloom et al., 2001) all show elevated rates of novel psychiatric disorders in children following a history of brain injury. Symptoms of ADHD and depression were especially frequent (Bloom et al., 2001; Max et al., 1998a). The attention disorders were more persistent than the depressive disorders in Bloom's sample. Max also reported a relative high occurrence of an organic personality syndrome (27%); Bloom commented that this finding probably reflected the use in that study of an interview instrument designed to evaluate changes in personality (cf. Max et al., 1998b). This finding highlights the problem of being able to find only what we are prepared to look for. The evaluator of a child or adolescent who has sustained a significant head injury should be alert to the possibility of personality changes following the trauma.

Problems of social adjustment can be as difficult for the youth and his or her family following a TBI as the cognitive difficulties that may present. Limitations in social skills may be especially disabling. Russman's (1997 doctoral dissertation, cited in Clark, Russman, & Orme, 1999) found that parents of children with a history of TBI reported their sons and daughters as having difficulty with handling teasing, being excluded by others, accepting "no" for an answer, solving arguments and problems, and exercising self-control. These problems may reflect, in part, the disruption of executive functioning in the brain-injured youth. Severely injured children and children who experience brain damage at a young age appear to be at the greatest risk for problems of social adjustment (Bohnert, Parker, & Warschausky, 1997).

Kinsella and colleagues (1999) highlight the importance of family resources and response as one determinant of behavioral sequelae in children following TBI. The postinjury family environment was one of three factors that predicted outcome for children with severe and moderate brain injury in a study by Taylor and colleagues (1999), along with preinjury factors and TBI severity. Consistent with these findings, my own experience has been that the family to which the brain-injured child returns is a very powerful influence in that child's eventual adaptation to any residual mental or physical changes.

One key aspect of evaluation that the mental health professional can contribute is an assessment of the family's readiness to accept and process information that the health care professional provides about a child's situation and prognosis. In the aftermath of a major injury to one of their children, the typical family is in a state of shock, anxiety, and confusion. At the same time they are desperately seeking information from doctors, nurses, social workers, and ward secretaries; they are often scarcely capable of processing a fraction of what they are being told. The parents may seize on bits of a conversation with the child's doctor and forget most of the remaining, often including the context of and provisos on what they do recall. Handouts and informational brochures that are thrust into their hands by well-intended hospital staff are often mislaid, forgotten, or lost. Psychologists and other mental health professionals are often in a position of being able to spend enough time with parents and other family members to have a reasonable assessment of how much of the information being presented to them is being processed, understood, and remembered. This assessment can be very valuable in adjusting the scheduling of discharge planning and family education efforts.

As HIV infection and AIDS continue to grow as major public health challenges, the likelihood of mental health practitioners having contact with affected children grows. Recent reports show children, adolescents, and young adults accounting for 21% of individuals infected with HIV and 13% of those with active AIDS in the United States (Brown, Lescano, & Lourie, 2001). From 20% to 40% of HIV-positive children show evidence of central nervous system disease (Brown et al., 2001). Tested intelligence, academic performance, language functioning, and visual–motor abilities are reported to be the typical areas of difficulty manifested (Brown et al., 2001). These cognitive difficulties have a direct negative impact on the child's progress in school. School success may be further undermined by absences secondary to their illness.

In addition to their risk for cognitive dysfunction, other psychiatric disorders often occur in concert with HIV infection in children. Interpretation of prevalence data is complicated because information on premorbid occurrence of behavior problems is often lacking, but emotional and behavioral problems appear to be overrepresented in youth struggling with HIV infection. Rates of major depression were found in 25% and 34%, respectively, of two groups of children and adolescents with HIV, and a history of suicide attempts was reported in 28% and 33%, respectively, of two other samples (Brown et al., 2001). Anxiety symptoms and anxiety disorders, as well as attention problems and attention-deficit disorders, are reported to be common in HIV-positive children (Brown et al., 2001). Rates of conduct disorders and substance abuse disorders are very high among HIV-positive youths; the directions of these associations are not clear—the risky behavior often seen associated with conduct disorders and substance abuse may have contributed to increased likelihood of infection (Brown et al., 2001). Regardless of the causal relationships, youths who are HIV-positive need a careful review for possible mental health problems.

Sickle cell disease refers to a group of genetic hematological disorders seen most often in individuals of African descent, although sickle cell disease occurs at lesser frequencies in children from a wide range of genetic pools. Children with sickle cell disease are at risk for neurological disease, including stroke. However, even in the absence of stroke or other overt neurological disease, there may be evidence of neurocognitive deficits that can contribute to academic problems (Bonner, Schumacher, Gustafson, & Thompson, 1999). Although many children with sickle cell disease do well in school, others show learning problems, difficulties with social adjustment, and behavior problems (Bonner et al., 1999; Thompson & Gustafson, 1996). Given the various educational and adjustment risks faced by youth with sickle cell disease, professionals need to be aware of the potential for difficulty and evaluate as necessary (Bonner et al., 1999).

Traumatic brain injury, HIV infection, and sickle cell disease are merely three of a wide range of medical disorders and adverse events that significantly affect the cognitive functioning and emotional and behavioral adjustment of a youth. As our understanding of brain–behavior relationships and of the differing phenotypical expressions of biological influences advances, there will undoubtedly be increased recognition of the physiological foundation of problems with learning and cognition. Exciting new linkages between medicine, child development, and psychological adjustment are being explored, such as the concept of pediatric autoimmune neuropsychiatric disorders associated with streptococcal infections (PANDAS; Swedo et al., 1997). The potential for deleterious impact on central nervous system development and functioning associated with biologically based disorders creates possible difficulties in mental functioning. The initial assessment with many of these youngsters is used to plan the more systematic evaluation of mental ability and personal functioning needed for optimum treatment and rehabilitation.

## Evaluation of Exceptionally Talented and Gifted Children

At the other extreme of the continuum of cognitive ability lie the youths whose mental abilities are above average. Conceptual and applied definitions of talent, creativity, and giftedness are not as consensually agreed on as they are for mental disorders (which has no shortage of definitional problems in itself), and our appreciation of both the associated characteristics and prevalence of exceptional ability are somewhat limited by this lack of agreement. With some frequency, however, children with positive exceptionalities cross our paths. In one such circumstance, the parents or school system already have a question of possible giftedness and are seeking an evaluation to aid in their determination. The qualifications for enrichment or acceleration decisions vary in different states and school districts and influence the nature of the assessment tools used. Although there has been some effort toward developing broader and more inclusive views of positive exceptionality, much of the emphasis has remained on high intelligence as measured by intelligence tests (Kamphaus, 1993). Kamphaus (1993) discusses some of the issues involved in the assessment of intellectual giftedness.

In a second possible case, the evaluator comes to suspect that above average talent or ability may be contributing to other adjustment issues that have brought the child in for evaluation. Although most gifted children also enjoy good social and personal adjustment (Clark, 1997; Howe, 1999; Gottfried, Gottfried, Bathurst, & Guerin, 1994), some experience difficulties. They may have difficulty adjusting to us or we may have difficulty adjusting to them, especially if their exceptional talents have not been generally recognized by the caretakers and school personnel they interact with. James T. Webb, a psychologist who has worked with gifted children for two decades, believes that gifted children are often misdiagnosed as showing any number of psychiatric problems due to the intensity of their emotional reactions (Webb, 2000). Webb (2000) also suggests that when gifted children do have emotional and behavioral disorders, it is important to appreciate how their talents and abilities interact with their problems to shape unique expressions. Like cognitive limitations, exceptional mental abilities are by definition rare. Nonetheless, it is certainly prudent to keep in mind the possibility that perhaps, as a mother once suggested, "She acts up because she's just bored with the work the class is doing."

# 5 Evaluating Emotional Problems in Children

*E*liciting valid information from a youth regarding emotional concerns requires the examiner to create interpersonal circumstances that promote honest self-disclosure of personal and distressing material. This is one of the most challenging aspects of assessing young people. In reviewing these concerns, the paramount need is to demonstrate attitudes of respect, concern, and ultimately confidence in the client's ability to participate in the assessment process. This process begins with the establishment of a working relationship between the mental health professional and the youth.

## ESTABLISHING RAPPORT AND TRUST

### Attitudes of the Examiner

The accurate assessment of problems that revolve around primary emotional states of the child or adolescent is one of the most difficult demands placed on the clinical evaluator. Difficulties arise from the need to establish the conditions in which veridical reports can be obtained from the young person and informants, as well as from the limited communication ability many people within our culture possess with respect to feelings and moods. We lack a precise vocabulary and conceptualization of emotions; this condition limits both our potential understanding of how these relate to more obvious problems in our lives and our ability to communicate any understanding we have. Much of our communication about feelings is by analogy, metaphor, simile—the (literally) picturesque language of abstract verbal expression. Children may have only begun to effectively discriminate internal states, adolescents may just have begun finding the language to express these inner currents, and neither may feel motivated to share this most private experience with an adult. The examiner and caretaker may empathize together on how difficult it is to know the heart of a young person, but this moves the assessment ahead very little.

I believe this is one of the areas of evaluation in which the attitudes of the mental health specialist are especially critical in either facilitating or inhibiting accurate assessment. My experience has been that certain basic values, if reflected in behavior, actively promote the self-disclosure of the youth to the degree that he or she is able. Careful and open self-inquiry prior to undertaking the mental health evaluation of others can be very valuable in enhancing our ability to effectively relate to another person. I believe that key among the several important attitudes are honesty, directness, respect, and humility.

Typically, the young person has just met the examiner, usually under circumstances that have created at least some level of tension within the youth's natural environments. Such conditions as these are not inherently associated with trust and self-disclosure. The young person, to the limit of his or her capacity, is probably very sensitive to any inconsistency or vagueness in communication that could signal mendacity. I believe the only effective response to these almost universally limiting initial conditions is a high level of honesty on the part of the examiner. Age-appropriate clarity regarding the purpose of the interview and assessment will help put the youth at ease. To achieve this, however, you as a professional must consider how much value honesty has for you: Do you really believe children and adolescents deserve to know the truth? There are any number of circumstances in which of us would choose to withhold the complete truth from the other person in a relationship—to protect him or her from distress; sometimes to protect ourselves. How much "protection" should be undertaken in a psychological or psychiatric evaluation? The precise limits of our judgments here depend on many factors: our own moral values, professional training, discipline, and theoretical positions. Yet even while acknowledging these critically important particulars, the general question can and should be considered. To what degree should the examiner be as honest as possible with the person being evaluated? My impression is that the more deliberately and consciously honest we are, the more open and valid are the responses we obtain from youths regarding their emotional experience and problems.

A related issue is the directness in our communication. If we are deliberately vague about certain topics or attempt to "talk around them," it usually has a direct effect on the quality of information we elicit from others. At a simple level, one can see that it is difficult enough to obtain responses regarding very personal experiences when the client understands precisely what is being asked. If the inquires are vague, it both leaves the client uncertain of what is being requested and provides great opportunity to avoid disclosing information that is uncomfortable. A basic reality is that most of our clients can deliberately deceive us successfully if they wish to do so. My experience has been that usually clients, including children and adolescents, prefer not to lie to us; but they can be very selective in the information they offer. If our questions allow for multiple interpretations, they will choose to answer the question easiest to deal with. Because we have heard an answer to our question, we often believe that it was an answer to the question we wished to know about. There is a clear use for very general, non-directive inquiries, but these often need to be followed up with very specific questions if we want to know what is really going on.

In my clinical practice I have recurrently realized the value of a basic respect for the client and his or her experience and attempts to cope. Respect for the child or adolescent being evaluated is more than an abstract philosophical consideration—it underlies effective communication with other human beings. It seems to me to be very difficult for most of us to successfully obscure our fundamental attitudes toward others. One of the most basic elements of the social skill training we have all experienced at the hands of our culture is learning that trust cannot always be automatic. We have all gone through extensive shaping through our everyday life in learning the cues and situations that suggest that confidence is or is not justified. I believe that even the most limited of us have often been taught to be sensitive to any indication of a lack of respect as a signpost that the person should not be trusted. Consider your own experience with teachers as a child—most students had teachers who were gruff and strict, who were compassionate and caring, who were demanding, or who were easily pleased. Whom among these did you feel trustful of? Possibly all and possibly none; for the answer to trust does not come from nurturance, reserve, expectations, or many other human characteristics, but from a respect for who you are. As psychological examiners of young people, we can each do well to periodically examine our own attitudes toward the population we purport to serve.

A final important value in a mental health examiner is humility. There is no phenomenon in the known universe more complex than human behavior. The truth is always more complicated than it appears to be, than can be understood or communicated. There are limits to what the very best psychological evaluation yields. Appreciating this truth helps balance our very human tendencies to want to be more certain, more confident, more resolved regarding a case than is justified by the data we have in hand. We seek a certainty, a resolution of a question that will allow meaningful planning and action; but the nature of human experience is often ambiguous and uncertain. Our appraisals are but approximations, the most useful interpretations given what is currently known. A tolerance for such ambiguity helps us to remain open to new data that may become available in the future.

## Interpersonal Behavior of the Examiner

The positive and beneficent attitudes of the examiner can be helpful only if they are overtly manifested in her or his behavior. The interpersonal actions and responses of the evaluator must be consistent with the values that promote trust and the self-disclosure of emotional experiences. Basic interpersonal skills that promote communication and understanding include: attention and observation, accurate empathy, feedback, directed introspection, acceptance, and unconditional positive regard. The clinical and empirical literature of psychology, psychiatry, and allied disciplines support the efficacy of these interpersonal responses in eliciting active participation from the client in a helping-interview situation (Benjamin, 1987; Cormier & Cormier, 1985; Morrison, 1993; Othmer & Othmer, 1994).

Careful attention to the other person usually facilitates communication. A common difficulty among novices in assessments is that they are so concerned about what they are going to ask next that they fail to listen to the answer offered to the question just asked. Years ago I had the opportunity to observe a live, clinical interview by Joseph Wolpe, one of the founders of behavior therapy. What was most remarkable to me was how carefully he listened to the answers the client offered to his inquiries. If the client did not answer the question, he found another way to phrase the inquiry. *He did not move on until he had an answer.* This deliberate and careful inquiry contrasted with what was then my own often frantic series of question after question in hopes of eliciting some useful data. A true secret to successful assessment is to attend fully and carefully to your clients—their words, tone, gestures, posture, and other behaviors.

Accurate empathy for the emotional experience of the client is another very helpful response of the examiner. To demonstrate your recognition of the feelings of the child or teenager communicates your interest, your respect, your understanding. Seeking confirmation or correction of your perceptions makes a bid for cooperation and collaboration. The youth is the authority on his or her feelings—only he or she is in a position to validate our perceptions. Acknowledging this authority empowers the young person within the session, showing her part of what she has to offer to the encounter. Establishing a legitimate role for the youth helps decrease the motivation for oppositional or defensive behavior.

Giving and receiving feedback from the client begins to define a pattern of cooperative and reciprocal interaction between the evaluator and the youth. As we seek confirmation of the accuracy and validity of our perceptions of the young person's feelings, we simultaneously direct his attention to internal states and reactions he may have had little awareness of or experience in articulating verbally. This directed introspection and discussion has the side benefit of increasing his sense of self-understanding and of self-management of emotional states. Emotions, especially negative feelings, can be frightening to any of us, and more especially to the young person with limited experience in dealing with his or her motivational and affective responses. To learn to identify, label, and relate experiences is to learn how to control these phenomena to a degree. As the child feels less helpless in the face of strong emotions, his or her willingness to share these experiences increases.

Our own willingness to accept and acknowledge the feelings of the youth without prejudgment also greatly affects what is shared with us. Acceptance here does not mean approval or disapproval or imply the inevitability or permanence of the child's responses. Acceptance refers solely to acknowledging what the youth is experiencing now and accepting the validity of this experience. An important lesson in life is that we do not choose our feelings in the same manner in which we choose our actions or thoughts. We can decide to deliberately entertain certain ideas or to deliberately take certain actions; we cannot decide to feel or not feel something. Although there are techniques that can modify our emotional responses, feelings are still to a large extent something that "happens to us" rather than "something we do." Acknowledging the nonvolitional character of feelings frees the youth from feeling the need to justify his or her emotions.

It is also vital that we demonstrate to the youth our capacity to tolerate his or her feelings. If we cannot maintain our own emotional balance when confronted with the intense feelings of a troubled youth, the youth will respond to our anxiety by suppressing or exacerbating his or her emotional communications, thus distorting the data we have to consider. Only by accepting the youth's experience and tolerating the feelings expressed can we facilitate continued emotional exploration and disclosure. A high and unconditional positive regard for the value and integrity of the client facilitates his or her participation in the assessment process.

Hundreds of books, chapters, and articles have been written on elements of effective interviewing. There is an exceedingly rich literature from which the student of human adjustment can draw suggestions and examples. In addition to the previous references, I recommend the following as useful starting points to build knowledge and skills in this area: Cepeda (2000), Cox, Hopkinson, and Rutter (1981), Greenspan and Greenspan (1991), Hopkinson, Cox, and Rutter (1981), Hughes and Baker (1990), Rutter and Cox (1981), and Sandifer, Hordern, and Green (1970).

## GATHERING INFORMATION ABOUT AFFECT STATES

Everyday social training has produced in most of us a sensitivity to several potential sources of data regarding the emotional experiences of others. Within our culture this sensitivity and possible understanding is often not verbally articulated. Bringing this often (verbally) unconscious processing into the domain of language increases the value of our perceptions and the deliberateness of the process of evaluation.

### Observation of Emotions

Although we often acknowledge the inherent privacy of other people's feelings and emotional responses, feelings often can be directly observed, at least to a degree.

The observation of facial behavior provides one set of clues regarding feelings. The empirical literature on judgments of human emotions based on facial features suggests an underlying potential validity to such perceptions, especially if we seek to validate the accuracy of our perceptions through feedback. We can err in ignoring the possible information that may be seen on the face of the youth, and we can err by accepting uncritically our own perceptions. Continence, gaze direction, and overt potential emotional response, such as tears, can provide important clues, but these need to be verbally checked against the report of our client. A number of years ago a colleague related this experience: Her undergraduate class had become especially attentive, respectful, and dutiful in carrying out assignments. Seeking to learn how she had so successfully touched the lives of these students with her pedagogy, she asked them directly one day in class. Their somewhat abashed replies revolved around her frequent tearfulness in class. Assuming she was going through some trying personal crisis, the thoughtful students had tried to be especially good learners so as to lessen the burdens on her at that difficult time. My friend was understandably somewhat reluctant to disclose that her tearful state was the result of a shift to a different type of contact lens.

Inference of emotional states from behavior takes advantage of high base-rate associations: Blank and rigid faces often "cover" a belligerent attitude, sudden shifts of gaze may signal evasiveness, and tears usually connote sadness. But sometimes tears are a sign of tension, or happiness, or dust, or new contact lenses. It is in the process of validating both our perceptions and our inferences that valuable information is generated. This is similarly the case for body posture, gesture, and movement within the session. It is foolish to ignore such potential sources of hypotheses about emotional reactions, but it is equally foolish to jump to the conclusion that our hypotheses are facts.

### Self-Report of Feelings

Establishing setting conditions conducive to open discussion of emotional responses is only the first step toward effective assessment of problems of affect and mood. In an effort to extend beyond our limited ability to make accurate inferences regarding the young person's emotional reactions, we frequently employ other techniques of data collection. The crucial step is eliciting useful information about the client's emotional states and their relationships to thought and actions. This can potentially be accomplished through several avenues.

The most commonly employed technique for learning about almost all clinical topics is the interview. A major challenge in interviewing for affective data is that the personal referents for commonly used "feeling words" ("depressed," "sad," "angry," "hurt," "excited," etc.) may differ profoundly among individuals and within an individual at different points in his or her development. It becomes essential to determine what this child means when she tells us she feels "sad." The limited vocabulary of children, the possibility that their experiences have not prompted them to attend to emotional events, and their developmentally limited cognitive skills (attention, discrimination, memory) all impose significant limitations on the self-report of emotional states that can be expected from youths. Useful probes for drawing out information on feeling states from youths include: "Can you tell me what that was like?" "Tell me about the last time you were. . . . " "How would I know you were feeling . . . ?" "What do you do when you are feeling . . . ?"

Questionnaires and self-report instruments offer another mechanism for evaluating emotional states in youth. Their limitations are the same as those of the interview but have the added complication of reading comprehension requirements. The important advantages of the printed instrument are its fixed nature and the associated possibility of objective norms, its economy of use in terms of both time and expense, and its availability for empirical investigation of reliability and validity. Examples of the variety of instruments used in the emotional assessment of children are the Child Depression Inventory (Kovacs, 1992), the Revised Children's Manifest Anxiety Scale (Reynolds & Richmond, 1995), and the Social Anxiety Scales for children and adolescents (La Greca, 1999), as well as various fear surveys (Gullone, 1999). In addition to printed questionnaire instruments, analog devices such as fear thermometers and 100-millimeter line scales for graphic rating of pain or fear are useful in the assessment of youths.

It is important to recognize that interview and questionnaire assessments of anxiety symptoms are not equivalent. With respect to panic attacks, for example, interview evaluations tend to identify smaller populations of adolescents as having anxiety episodes than does questionnaire use, but these results are complicated by the finding that some teenagers who report panic phenomena in an interview are not detected by questionnaire (Hayward et al., 1997). Open-ended questions, such as "What do you fear most?," were reported by Muris, Merckelbach, Mayer, and Prins (2000) to have a stronger association with symptoms of anxiety disorders than did fear survey schedule ratings. The best evaluation of an individual child, including the particular methods employed, depends on a variety of particular circumstances. In clinical determinations the use of multiple methods is often best because it can provide collaboration in findings.

## Informants

Another approach to evaluating emotional behavior in youths is to assess the perceptions of significant adults who have contact with the child. Unfortunately, adults may be relatively insensitive to negative mood states in children. Low correlations between adult and child reports of anxiety and depression symptoms in youths have been commonly found. Aronen and Soininen (2000) suggested that "children are the best reporters of their emotional well-being" (p. 469). Caretaker (parent–teacher) reports may be more useful in assessing traits—chronic, persistent emotional experiences (e.g., dysthymia) rather than acute feelings that may or may not be openly expressed. Possibly, better correspondence between the reports of adults and children regarding more enduring emotional responses in the child may also be reflected in parental perceptions of their child's mood and affect. Caretakers may be in a better position to report on stable mood states than on the fluctuations of immediate affect.

## MAJOR DIAGNOSTIC CONSIDERATIONS

### Relationship to Environmental Events and Stress

Our understanding of children's responses to environmental stress and trauma has grown significantly over the past few decades. Although the concept of children showing "adjustment reactions" was readily accepted by both the professional and lay communities, there was some resistance to the idea that children might show more severe stress responses, such as posttraumatic stress disorder (American Academy of Child and Adolescent Psychiatry, 1998). Where the exact boundaries are among the more severe stress disorders continues to be problematic, especially in young clients. This uncertainty reflects a more general problem with the diagnostic boundaries between acute stress reactions in adult populations (Harvey & Bryant, 1998). A great deal of continuing work will be necessary for further clarity to emerge in this important area. The development of evaluation instruments, such as the Pediatric Emotional Distress Scale (Saylor, Swenson, Reynolds, &

Taylor, 1999), may help support further empirical clarification of these questions. Stress reactions in youth can be marked by a very wide range of clinical features (American Academy of Child and Adolescent Psychiatry, 1998), and careful individual analysis is necessary to develop a comprehensive assessment for the child who has been exposed to highly arousing circumstances.

Age is a major variable affecting the clinical presentation of stress reactions in children and adolescents (American Academy of Child and Adolescent Psychiatry, 1998). The youth's repertoire of coping and adaptive responses, social network of support, and level of cognitive development all seem to function as moderating factors in reactions of adversity. The nature of the stressful event itself is clearly an influential variable. Our understanding of relatively common stressors such as parental conflict and divorce has continued to evolve with ongoing empirical research (Kelly, 2000). Fletcher (1996) provides a highly useful meta-analysis of data on posttraumatic stress responses in children and adolescents and shows how responses differ with both acute and chronic stressors. Premorbid adjustment problems have been increasingly highlighted as potential moderators in reaction to stress. Deykin and Buka (1997) called attention to the high prevalence of traumatic exposures among youths who are chemically dependent and to an associated high rate of posttraumatic stress disorder.

Most stress reactions in youths are transient and would probably be characterized as adjustment disorders. Adjustment disorder remains one of the most commonly made psychiatric diagnoses in youth (Newcorn & Strain, 1992), despite some efforts to constrain its use in the current DSM diagnostic system (American Psychiatric Association, 2000). Mixed symptom patterns tend to predominate in the clinical presentations of children and adolescents with adjustment disorder, and depressive symptoms are very common (Newcorn & Strain, 1992). Although by definition the long-term prognosis of adjustment disorder is positive, the evaluator should be aware of a reported association with suicidal behavior and a high comorbidity with other psychiatric diagnoses (Newcorn & Strain, 1992). Suicide attempts in children have been reported to be often occasioned not by depression but by adjustment disorder pattern events (Rapoport & Ismond, 1996). Consistent with the broad literature on comorbidity, association of adjustment disorders with other emotional and behavioral problems appears to predict a worse long-term outcome (Kovacs, Gatsonis, Pollock, & Parrone, 1994).

Trauma, including severe traumas that could create the potential for associated stress disorders, are unfortunately not rare in the lives of youths (Giaconia et al., 1995). A potential problem, however, with the diagnosis of posttraumatic stress disorder (PTSD) in youths is that the criteria tend to rely heavily on the verbal reports of clients regarding their experiences and internal states. This is a difficulty in the evaluation of younger children, especially because parents do not accurately estimate the stress responses of their children (Pfefferbaum, 1997). A complex interaction of factors influences adult perceptions of children's distress (Walton, Johnson, & Algina, 1999). Scheeringa, Zeahah, Drell, and Larrieu (1995) have proposed alternative diagnostic criteria that are less dependent on verbal report and that can be used in diagnosing PTSD in children younger than 48 months. In evaluating all children and adolescents with possible PTSD, you should remember that partial symptomatology is common and may be debilitating even if full diagnostic criteria for PTSD are not met (Pfefferbaum, 1997). As is usually the case, comorbidity with other disorders is common (Pfefferbaum, 1997). It appears that a history of other psychiatric disorders is a significant risk factor for PTSD and that PTSD, in turn, is a risk factor for subsequent depression, anxiety problems, and substance abuses.

## Traumatized Children

Traumatizing events are not rare in children's lives, but their relationship to behavior problems can often be missed (Burger & Lang, 1998). Whereas some cases present with clear-cut traumatic stimuli identified and with a full symptomatic picture of PTSD or some other stress syndrome pattern, in many other cases there may not be an initially clear picture of the precipitating trauma nor the classical diagnostic picture of PTSD. The trauma may have occurred long before the youth came to attention, the symptom picture may have attenuated over time, or the presenting concerns may focus on disruptive behaviors or substance abuse or depression. PTSD diagnoses can be easily missed in children and youths unless deliberately considered in the differential diagnosis (Burger & Lang, 1998).

When we evaluate children who have been exposed to potentially traumatizing events and are thus at risk for acute stress disorder and PTSD, as well as adjustment disorders, it is very useful to evaluate as well for the situational and child characteristics associated with resiliency in the face of trauma. Higher IQ is one protective factor that has emerged in empirical investigations (Silva et al., 2000). Tested intelligence has appeared as both a protective (higher IQ) and a risk (lower IQ) factor for a variety of behavior problems. Family integrity and support for the individual appear to have potential as a protective factor. The child's own previous adjustment may also be an important variable in mediating reaction of trauma (Bowman, 1999). The topic of biological susceptibility to PTSD and what may contribute to it continues to be the focus of active debate and research (Yehuda, 1999), and it seems very prudent for clinicians and investigators to resist urges toward premature closure regarding what is known about this area of adjustment and maladjustment. In terms of risk factors, witnessing family violence appears to be particularly associated with increased morbidity (Silva et al., 2000). Abused and neglected children seem to be at increased risk for PTSD, but this history of adversity does not inevitably lead to PTSD (Widom, 1999). Depression is reported to be very frequent in preschool children who have been abused or neglected (Kashani & Carlson, 1987) and is often premorbid with PTSD. The precise interactions between abuse, mood disorder, and susceptibility to PTSD have not been sufficiently clarified for conclusions to be drawn. Of significant clinical importance is a reported relationship between PTSD symptomatology and adolescent suicide ideation and suicidal attempts (Mazza, 2000). It is a wise precaution to carefully review suicide risk in youths who show PTSD or cases in which PTSD is a serious diagnostic consideration.

Sexual abuse is a special case of trauma in the lives of some unfortunate children. This topic is deal with more thoroughly in Chapter 10. It is interesting to note that in this case, as with other traumatic experiences, the child's attributions and perceptions of the encounters and the reactions of people in the child's social environment to the events are powerful determinants of outcome (Cohen & Mannarino, 2000). Nevertheless, sexual experiences with adults are usually traumatic for children from Western cultures (Goodwin, 1985; Miller-Perrin & Wurtele, 1990).

The role and relationship between a childhood history of trauma, the occurrence of dissociative symptoms, and diagnoses of several mental disorders remains unclear (for an interesting comparison, see Carrion & Steiner, 2000, and Marshall et al., 2000). It has been my experience that is nearly impossible to know a priori the impact of a wide range of noxious and abusive events that children may have had to endure. It is a disservice to our clients to fail to inquire into possible histories of abuse, neglect, and trauma; these are powerful forces affecting the lives of many youths. By the same token, it is a disservice to automatically assume that such forces affect all children in identical ways and lead to uniform outcomes. I have consistently been impressed by the range of human adaptation and the almost infinite variety shown in the lives of children exposed to highly similar circumstances. It is my considered opinion that allegiance to this empirical variability, even at the expense of our treasured theoretical beliefs, is essential to properly serve our clients.

## Depressive Symptoms

Depression in children is often overlooked or not fully appreciated by caretakers (Puura et al., 1998). Severe depressive symptoms appear to be relatively stable (Edelsoh, 1992) and carry increased risk for later emotional and behavior disorders (Aronen & Soininen, 2000; Lewinsohn, Rohde, & Seeley, 1998). Both chronic dysthymic syndromes (Kashani, Allan, Beck, Bledsoe, & Reid, 1997) and major depressive syndromes (Kashani, Holcomb, & Orvaschel, 1986; Kashani & Carlson, 1987) can be identified in preschool children. Given the difficulties in assessing internalizing symptoms in children, the use of multiple informants is invaluable (Kashani et al., 1997). In children, especially in very young children, depression may present largely in terms of complaints of physical symptoms and somatic concerns (Callahan, Panichelli-Mindel, & Kendall, 1996; Kashani & Carlson, 1987). Hopelessness is a particularly sensitive indicator of depression in children (Callahan et al., 1996), and it is a symptom that should be inquired into in school-age children and adolescents. The development of unexplained problems in academic performance or social participation can be a behavioral manifestation of depression (Callahan et al., 1996). Certainly many children begin experiencing school difficulty without being depressed, and children may become socially withdrawn without having a mood disturbance; but depression is one of the possible explanations and should be deliberately ruled either in or out.

Diagnostic boundaries often appear less distinct in children than in adolescents and adults, noticeably with regard to internalizing problems. The DSM-IV syndromes of major depressive episode and dysthymia may not be well differentiated in children (Goodman, Schwab-Stone, Lahey, Shaffer, & Jensen, 2000). Despite this possible problem, there may still be value in struggling with such differentiation. Dysthymia appears to function as a pathway (risk factor) for later major depression in children and adolescents (Lewinsohn et al., 1998). The comorbidity of a severe depressive episode and a history of chronic depression appears to identify a more seriously disturbed and impaired population of children (Goodman et al., 2000). As is often noted, the appearance of multiple problems in a child's life usually has serious implications for current functioning and future adjustment. This is notably the case with depressive disorders in youth. The comorbid occurrence of other problems along with depression in children is a common occurrence, and the manifestation of depression plus other disorders is associated with greater functional impairment in the youth than the handicap seen from a mood disorder alone (Lewinsohn et al., 1998). In evaluating children and teenagers with evidence of depressive symptoms, it is crucial to review carefully for other areas of possible emotional and behavioral disturbance.

Life stresses play an important, but not omnipotent, role in the etiology of depressive states in youths. As the young person passes through puberty, other events come into increasingly strong play, especially in females. The increase in depressive disorders in females following puberty appears to reflect, to some degree, a greater genetic role in the onset of depression, whereas males continue to display depression largely in response to negative life events (Silberg et al., 1999). Recognizing a genetic role in the pathways leading to depression does require uncritical acceptance of an organic model of mood disorders; environmental factors continue to have a demonstrably important influence. It would be foolish, however, to totally ignore the probable role of heredity influence in many cases. Obtaining a brief history of the extended family's mental health can be very useful in evaluating affective disorders in a youth. Helping the family understand the child's difficulties in the context of their family history can act to reduce secondary negative reactions to recognition that the young person has a "mental disorder."

## Bipolar Spectrum Symptoms

Assessment of possible periods of mania or hypomania in teenagers often proves to be an especially difficult task for evaluators. It is quite likely that manic spectrum phenomena are underdiagnosed in adolescents, as well as in adults. A retrospective survey of adults diagnosed with bipolar disorder found 59% reporting their perception of an onset of symptoms during youth (Lish, Dime-Meenan, Whybrow, Price, & Hirschfeld, 1994). One major difficulty is that bipolar disorders can present with a variety of initial symptoms, including depression, anxiety, mood swings, insomnia, irritability, fatigue, concentration difficulties, abuse of alcohol or drugs, legal involvement, relationship problems, or impulse control difficulty. Clients with apparently atypical conduct and disruptive behavior disorders should be carefully evaluated for a possible affective component to their behavior control problems. The relationship between conduct problems and bipolar spectrum symptoms continues to be explored (Biederman et al., 1999a) and to prove challenging to clear conceptualization. High rates of mood disorder, including mania, have been found in adolescents in juvenile detention facilities (Pliszka, Sherman, Barrow, & Irick, 2000); a history of involvement with juvenile court should lead to increased scrutiny for a possible affective disorder. Any family history of bipolar disorder should markedly raise our level of suspicion for a possible comorbid mood disorder alongside behavior problems. Efforts are currently underway to develop a Mood Disorder Questionnaire (MDQ), which would screen for behavior characteristic of a manic episode ("Screening Test," 2000). Geller and her colleagues have used a diagnostic protocol for youths that requires current mania or hypomania with elation, grandiosity, or both as a criterion to eliminate the use of criteria that overlap with ADHD (Geller et al., 1998, 2000a). Such tools should help in the evaluation of adolescents with possible bipolar disorder.

The diagnosis of manic behavior in children is even more problematic. The prevailing opinion in the mental health field appears to have shifted from a position that bipolar disorders do not occur in children to an acceptance of the possibility of this manifestation. Isaac (1991) argued a decade ago that bipolar disorders in children were underrecognized. Papolos and Papolos (1999) have made the same case more recently. Isaac's suggestion that children with a history of diagnosed ADHD who begin to show depressive episodes or episodic exacerbation of behavior problems should be carefully reviewed for possible bipolar disorder certainly seems prudent. Bipolar disorder in prepubertal children continues to be underrecognized by mental health professionals (Geller et al., 2000b, 2001). This is of especial concern given evidence of low recovery and high relapse rates in children with bipolar disorder (Geller et al., 2000b, 2001). A high index of suspicion for these problem patterns is advisable in the practitioner.

## Suicide Risk

A particularly critical area of evaluation is suicidal and self-injurious behavior. Suicidal behavior covers a broad range of actions and can be conceptualized on a continuum (see Figure 5.1; see also Moscicki, 1995).

Suicidal ideation—the initial stage of this phenomenon—can vary in terms of frequency, duration, intrusiveness, detail, planning, and authorship. During times of stress, transient, brief, infrequent, and passive thoughts of no longer existing ("Maybe it would be better if I just wasn't around") that are quickly replaced by the ongoing stream of behavior and thought are probably relatively common in adolescents and may occur in older children with little clear psychological significance. Of much greater potential concern are thoughts that are frequent, that intrude on other thoughts or ongoing behavior, and that are of sustained duration, detailed, and active ("I could take the rope

Suicidal Ideation
Infrequent, passive thoughts
to
Frequent, intrusive, active planning

Precursor Behavior
Saying good-bye, giving away possessions,
writing note, communicating intent,
assembling elements of method to be used

Attempts
Low lethality (delayed, little risk, easy to trigger)
Overdoses of "pills"
"Superficial" wounds
Medium lethality (more rapid, destructive)
Specific drug combinations
Slashing wounds
High lethality (rapid, very dangerous)
Hanging
Firearms

Completions
Death

**FIGURE 5.1** A continuum of suicidal behavior.

from the garage and tie it to the beam in the basement . . . "). A key psychological variable appears to be *intent*—has the youth made a decision to kill him- or herself or made an attempt? Intent reflects to what degree there is an unconflicted motivation to die versus the desperate desire to escape from intolerable circumstances. The more clearly articulated the intention to end one's life, the more dangerous the situation.

Another key variable is the degree of planning involved, which often appears to be roughly correlated with the duration and frequency of suicidal thoughts. The more detailed the suicide plan, the more dangerous the situation usually is. I have found it very helpful to carefully review the suicide plans of youths who express any degree of suicidal thinking.

The degree of hopelessness the young person is experiencing is yet another important predictor of risk. Hopelessness has consistently been reported to be a powerful predictor of suicide attempts and deaths. In evaluating suicidal ideation, it is important to elicit sufficient information to allow a full determination of how serious the situation being presented is. The counselor does not want to overreact to suicidal thoughts as a reflection of distress, alienation, and dissatisfaction with major areas of one's life; neither does the counselor want to fail to appreciate the plea for assistance and relief from an untenable position. Only full information and the interaction that generates this allows both the clinician and the youth to make an informed determination of what needs to be done. Linehan's modification of her Reasons for Living Inventory for Adolescents shows promise as a useful measure (Osman et al., 1998).

A client's difficulties in freely discussing the topic of suicidal thoughts should alert the examiner to the possibility of problems in this area. The majority of adolescents (whether they have experienced suicidal thoughts or not) do not have problems talking to you about this. They will freely report that suicide has never been an issue with them or will acknowledge that they have had thoughts such as these in the past or even currently. In this particular subject area, youths appear to take their cues directly from the interviewer. If we bring up suicide in a matter-of-fact manner as another area that needs to be covered, most of our young clients respond in the same manner. Children tend to show more hesitation in discussing suicidal thoughts but usually have no difficulty in telling us if they have not had such ideas. Marked emotional reactions to the topic, withdrawals from active communication or participation in the session, or blank refusals to discuss such a

## Interview Segment 5.1. Asking about the Unthinkable: Carolyn and Karen

Standard practice for mental health professionals today includes a formal evaluation of suicide risk. This is a necessary component of almost any assessment that might be conducted. The examiner may decide not to overtly address the subject based on his or her assessment that the client is not suicidal, that suicide risk is low to nonexistent, and that asking about the subject is not justified in terms of the client's mental age and/or circumstances. With older children and adolescents, as with adults and senior citizens, the prudent advice is to always formally assess and record factors pertinent to suicide risk. This does not need to take up more than a few minutes of the session, as is illustrated by the first example.

Carolyn was a 14-year-old middle school student referred for obsessive–compulsive behavior. There was a family history of depression. She lived with her parents and reported compulsive behavior developing over the past several months.

EXAMINER: Carolyn, have you ever thought about killing yourself?

CAROLYN: Oh, no. I would never do something like that.

EXAMINER: Good. I'm really glad you would never hurt yourself. But have you ever had thoughts about doing this, even though you knew you never would?

CAROLYN: No, I never have thought about suicide.

EXAMINER: Good. I need to ask you just a couple of questions about this. Have you ever done anything that could have hurt or killed you?

CAROLYN: No, never.

EXAMINER: Excellent. Why wouldn't you ever do that? What would stop you?

CAROLYN: Well, I know people sometimes do, even if they don't want to. Mom and I talked about how she gets down sometimes and how that might happen with me. She feels bad about my rituals because she thinks I got them from her. I wouldn't hurt myself because my family really loves me and it would be awful for them if I did anything like that. And I know that bad depressions do get better; and you can get help, like mom did. And I like doing things, I want to grow up and go to school and have a family someday. It would be stupid to kill myself and miss out on everything I want. It's a bad sin in the church, too.

EXAMINER: Those are some very good reasons not to harm yourself. One more question before we talk about other things—what would you do if you began feeling so bad you had thoughts about suicide?

CAROLYN: I'd tell mom and dad, like I did about the rituals once I realized how bad they had become. And I could talk to Coach, too; she talks to us about stuff like eating disorders and drinking and says we can talk to her about anything. I guess I could talk to you, too.

EXAMINER: Absolutely, you could always talk to me about that or anything else that was bothering you.

This exchange took only a few minutes and established a low level of suicide risk for Carolyn, despite some elements in her case that would raise concern (an anxiety disorder on her part, a family history of mood disorder). Carolyn consistently denied any history of suicidal thoughts or actions on direct inquiry. There was no equivocation or evasiveness about her replies. She gave a good response to inquiry into her reasons for living and articulated a good plan to deal with problems if they should develop. The fact that she had a history of going to her parents to deal with mental health problems and that her parents had directly discussed such issues with her further increased the confidence of the examiner that her risk was low.

Depending on the information revealed from initial inquiry, a more extensive evaluation may be necessary, as it was with Karen. Karen was a 15-year-old high school freshman who lived with her parents and siblings in an affluent neighborhood. She attended a parochial school and had been active in sports and civic groups until 2 months previous to examination. She was referred for evaluation of a depression, which had developed over the past 3 months. There was no prior history of mood or behavior problems, there was a family history of heavy alcohol use, and she denied any precipitating events for her depression or abuse in any relationship.

EXAMINER: Now I need to ask you about some other areas. Have you ever thought about killing yourself?

KAREN: I would never do that.

EXAMINER: I'm glad to know that you would never hurt yourself, but have you ever had thoughts about it?

KAREN: Sometimes. I try not to. It's a sin. Sometimes, I just feel like it might be the only way to stop feeling so bad. I don't want to die. (*Looks down and begins to cry.*)

EXAMINER: You must feel really frightened by these thoughts that you don't want to have. I guess that's pretty terrible for you.

KAREN: Yes. It's like I don't have any control over my mind. I think sometimes I must be going crazy. (*Stops crying and resumes eye contact.*)

EXAMINER: I know you probably don't like to talk about this, but it may actually help you feel a little better to get things out in the open. What kinds of thoughts about suicide do you have?

KAREN: That I'm never going to feel good again, that I should just give up and die. Sometimes I think about how to do it.

EXAMINER: How would you do it?

KAREN: My father has a gun. I think about holding it against my chest and pulling the trigger.

EXAMINER: Where does your father keep the gun?

KAREN: He keeps it in a locker in their closet. He thinks we don't know where the key is, but my brothers found it a few years ago and showed the rest of us. They were showing off. My father never found out. The key is still there.

EXAMINER: Have you ever gotten the gun out?

KAREN: I didn't do anything. (*Looks away.*)

EXAMINER: Karen, have you ever unlocked the trunk and gotten the gun out?

KAREN: Only once. I just held it a minute and put it back. I didn't do anything with it.

EXAMINER: Is the gun loaded?

KAREN: No. The box of shells is beside it.

EXAMINER: Are there shells in the box?

KAREN: Yes, it was heavy when I picked it up.

EXAMINER: Did you load the gun?

KAREN: No, I just held it a minute. I picked up the box of shells. Then I put them both back and closed the trunk.

EXAMINER: What were you thinking about?

KAREN: I don't want to talk about this.

EXAMINER: I know, and I feel bad for you, but I really need you to tell me what you were thinking about.

KAREN: That I should just do it.

EXAMINER: Do what?

KAREN: Shoot myself. (*Sobs.*)

EXAMINER: That must have been really awful, to feel that bad.

KAREN: I want it to stop!

EXAMINER: You are going to feel better, and the feelings about hurting your-self are going to stop. Right now, though, the most important thing is to make sure that you are safe. First, we need a plan for what you are going to do if you start feeling that way again; we'll work that out in a few min-utes. Second, you told me a little while ago that a few times lately you have tried drinking alcohol. That is certainly something that a lot of peo-ple your age experiment with, but for right now we need to talk about your not doing any drinking or using any other drugs until all these thoughts and the depression that causes them are gone. Third, there's something else we need to do; do you have any ideas about what that is?

KAREN: Get rid of the gun?

EXAMINER: Yeah, the gun has to go.

KAREN: Are you going to tell my parents?

EXAMINER: We need to talk with your parents about this. The important things are that you need to be safe and that the gun has to go some-where else, just as soon as the three of you get home tonight.

Karen's suicide risk is high: She is depressed and has experienced ac-tive suicidal thoughts; a high lethality method is available that she has actu-ally accessed on at least one occasion; and there is a recent history of alco-hol use. The assessment was terminated at this point without addressing possible inhibitions against suicidal behavior, and an intervention was initi-ated. Karen had shown some evasiveness in responding to inquiry and without direct questioning might possibly have avoided this discussion and remained at risk for a tragedy.

---

"bad" subject should cause the interviewer concern. Children who are not having suicidal thoughts are usually not disturbed by being asked about the topic and usually have no difficulty in directly assuring us that it is not a concern for them.

It is always useful to consider multiple sources of information. The child's response to interview questions about suicidal thoughts can be contrasted with his or her response to self-report questionnaires, such as the Children's Depression Inventory (Kovacs, 1992). If there is an apparent disagreement, it can be clarified through inquiry. In a similar manner, I often directly address the possibility of suicidal statements with parents or other adult caretakers: "Has José ever said anything about wishing he were dead?" If there is significant incongruity between various sources of information, the evaluator needs to further review and resolve the confusion. The examiner may also wish to consider other potential indicators of suicidal risk, such as diagnostic signs in human figure drawings (Zalsman et al., 2000).

An escalation to a more dangerous situation than that reflected in suicidal ideation is seen in what may be called "precursor behavior." These are overt actions that are not dangerous in themselves but that prepare for future suicidal behavior. Examples of precursor behavior are the youth saying good-bye to his or her friends, giving away possessions, or assembling the means for a planned attempt. The adolescent might purchase a length of rope. This action could be taken for a hundred different perfectly good reasons, but it is taken on this occasion because the teenager is planning eventually to use the rope to hang him- or herself. The importance of precursor behavior is that at this stage the action is no longer inside the youth's mind; he or she has moved into the arena of overt behavior. The actions are not dangerous in themselves, but they do represent a graduation from purely mental consideration to behavioral steps taken toward a possible tragic conclusion. Effective probes about precursor behavior can be as simple as asking, "What have you done about these thoughts?" "Have you taken any steps regarding these ideas?" As in many other areas, the evaluator needs to be alert to both the youth's answer and the delivery of this answer. Delays in responding to straightforward inquiry, a loss of eye contact, or equivocal phrasing of replies (e.g., "Not really") all suggest possible conflict in full and open reporting and call for further inquiry.

A suicide attempt is a more dramatic and dangerous escalation. The youth has actually carried out behavior with the intention of self-harm. Suicide attempts can be considered in terms of the dangerousness of the behavior: how likely this action was to end the youth's life; the latency of the effect (how rapidly this action could have killed the person and the personal or cultural acceptability of the actions); how much inhibition must have been overcome to actually trigger this method of attempt. Some methods of attempted suicide are extremely destructive and highly likely to kill anyone who performs these actions. Suicide attempts by firearms and hanging are usually judged to have very high associated lethality. Overdoses of medication, slashing wounds, and jumping from a high place are often judged of lower lethality. A gunshot wound is extremely damaging to the human body, and strangulation can effectively end life—these are very dangerous methods. These are also methods whose effects are almost instantaneous or very rapid—there is limited opportunity for a change of mind or for discovery and outside intervention. These are also methods that are unfortunately "acceptable" within our culture for the purpose of self-destruction. There seems, unfortunately, to be far too little inhibition about pulling the trigger of a weapon aimed at oneself or stepping off a box with a rope about one's neck. In contrast, many adults are insufficiently educated to calculate an effective lethal dose of medication for themselves, and even a "lucky" guess will be followed by a number of minutes during which reconsideration or discovery is possible. Although obviously some individuals do die by cutting their wrists and bleeding to death, it is again a slow process and painful and unpleasant. These are factors that work ultimately for survival. Jumping from a high place carries similar considerations: Will the individual actually trigger the method? Some fear of heights seems sufficiently generalized in most people to create an inhibition that must be overcome. Even for the desperately suicidal, there is something about that first step into nothingness that is, fortunately, often difficult to take.

So on one level, a consideration of the youth's history of suicide attempts is justified. Past behavior tends to predict at some level future behavior, and a history of prior attempts by high lethality methods is clearly of grave concern. Furthermore, any history of suicide attempts is of great concern. Clear documentation of all prior suicide attempts appears to be a clear "standard of care" issue. Establishing a definite chronological history of all attempts, the methods used in the attempts, and the consequences (discovery or not, medical treatment, hospitalization, and resolution of the crisis) is necessary in evaluating youths. Working to document such a history also makes clearer the actual situations. Sometimes a client reports as an attempt behavior that falls short of common understandings of such an event. One teenager I interviewed reported as an attempt an episode in which he was sitting at his desk for a long period, looking at his prescription medications, and thinking about taking an overdose. He never actually took any extra pills. This was definitely a dangerous episode and of marked emotional and therapeutic significance, but it was not an "attempt" as I conceptualize such actions.

The end of the continuum of suicidal behavior is the actual death of an individual through his or her own behavior. Phrases such as "completed suicide," "successful suicide," and "suicidal death" are seen in the literature. Our ability to further evaluate and intervene with the youth is at an end, although the needs of the survivors of such tragedies may be many.

Assessing risk factors for suicidal behavior in children and adolescents has been the focus of considerable clinical work (Berman & Jobes, 1992; Moscicki, 1995; Pfeffer, 1986). A distinction between immediate or "proximal" risk factors and background or "distal" risk factors is often made (cf. Moscicki, 1995, 1999) and has some clinical utility. Distal risk factors involve demographic, familial, personal, or adjustment characteristics that carry heightened risk for suicidal actions. Examples include such variables as age of the child (increasing risk with increasing age), a family history of suicide (higher risk), trait impulsively (higher risk), and substance abuse (higher risk). A clinical mood disorder, often depression, is one of the most widely recognized and documented distal risk factors for suicidal behavior (ideation, attempts, and completed suicide) in children and adolescents (Flisher, 1999). The increased suicide risk associated with disruptive behavior disorders is beginning to be more appreciated (Groholt, Ekeberg, Wickstrom, & Haldorsen, 2000; Renaud, Brent, Birmaher, Chiappetta, & Bridge, 1999). A prior history of suicidal behavior may act to increase the intensity of a current crisis (Joiner, Rudd, Rouleau, & Wagner, 2000). It is helpful to be aware of the range of family, demographic, personality, and psychopathology factors that have been associated with heightened suicide risk.

Proximal risk factors are immediate, situational influences that are associated with the short-term risk of suicidal actions. Examples if high-risk variables include a breakdown in an important relationship, availability of means of suicide, stressful circumstances, and any measurable blood alcohol level. Proximal risk factors often signal a crisis period of acute risk, although McKeown and colleagues (1998) illustrate that the false-positive rate of predictions from undesirable life circumstances is high. Like life itself, suicidal behavior is a terribly complex phenomenon. Despite our need for simple diagnostic heuristics, a single classification risk profile is probably inadequate (Gould et al., 1998). It is critical that the examiner carefully review a wide range of information in

## Practice Note 5.1. Variables Associated with Higher Risk of Suicide

**Family characteristics**

Domestic violence
Parental maladjustment
   Mood disorder
   Substance abuse
   Psychosis
   Antisocial or borderline personality disorder
Family member with medical disorder

**Demographic characteristics**

Male
Caucasian or Native American
Older child or adolescent

**Personal history**

Exposure to a suicide model
Recent suicides in community
Social isolation
Stress
   Breakdown in communication
   Interpersonal loss or conflict
   Academic failure

**Adjustment history**

History of mental illness
   Depression
   Substance abuse
   Conduct problems/delinquency
   Eating disorder
   Psychosis
   Panic attacks
History of impulsive behavior
History of other "risky" behavior
   Substance use
   Unprotected intercourse
   Fighting
History of previous suicidal behavior
   High frequency of previous attempts
   Greater lethality of previous attempts

**Psychological state**

Intoxicated
Depressed
Hopeless
Alone
Absence of reasons for living

**Access to means**

Presence of firearms in home

evaluating suicide risk. The reader is referred to the extensive literature on evaluating suicide risk (cf. Goldman & Beardslee, 1999: Jacobs,
Brewer, & Klein-Benheim, 1999; Risk Management Foundation of the
Harvard Medical Institutions, 1999; Wise & Spengler, 1997; and the
previously cited references).

Yet another perspective on this important matter is offered in the
recent work of Flisher and colleagues (2000), who present data that
show that suicidal ideation and attempts in youth are related to a group
of "risk behaviors"; these include marijuana smoking, alcohol use, sexual intercourse, fighting, and cigarette smoking. Each of these behaviors was positively associated with each of the others. These authors argue that clinicians should be aware that the presence of one risk
behavior signals the possibility that others may also be present and that
we need to recognize the need to systematically evaluate these other
potential problems.

## Anxiety and Panic Disorders

Anxiety symptoms are common in children and adolescents and in
both males and females (Bernstein & Borchardt, 1991; Costello, 1989).
Anxiety disorders are among the most common psychiatric problems
afflicting children and adolescents (Albano, Chorpita, & Barlow,
1996). Childhood anxiety causes not only individual distress but also a
wide range of functional impairment (Albano et al., 1996). Finally, anxiety problems in youth are often chronic into adulthood (Albano et al.,
1997). Despite clear evidence of need, our understanding of anxiety
disorders in children is limited, in part due to the difficulty of differentiating normal and adaptive from excessive and maladaptive anxiety
and arousal. Comorbidity is common both within anxiety disorder
diagnoses and with other emotional and behavioral disturbances
(Albano et al., 1996), especially mood disorders (Lewinsohn, Zinberg,
Seeley, Lewinsohn, & Sack, 1997), as well as substance abuse (Deas-
Nesmith, Brady, & Campbell, 1998). The simultaneous occurrence of
anxious ruminative thinking and suicidal thoughts may identify a
subpopulation of highly disturbed children (Allan, Kashani, Dahlmeier, Beck, & Reid, 1998). Comorbidity is common in both male and
female children (Beidel, Turner, & Morris, 1999) and adolescents
(Lewinsohn et al., 1997). The boundaries between specific anxiety
disorders in children and adolescents continue to be investigated
(Compton, Nelson, & March, 2000).

Panic attacks and panic disorder occur in adolescents and in children in a symptom pattern essentially identical to that seen in adults (Biederman et al., 1997; Kearney, Albano, Eisen, Allan, & Barlow, 1997; Moreau & Weissman, 1992). Until recently there was little appreciation of childhood onsets of acute anxiety episodes, and most children, in my experience, do not spontaneously report these to unknown adults. A brief but systemic inquiry into possible anxiety experiences, gauged to the child's developmental level, is necessary to elicit information about possible experiences such as these. Questions such as the following can be helpful: "Have you ever felt really scared, but for no reason?" "Do you ever have trouble getting your breath?" "Tell me about those times." A possible interesting developmental difference between children and adults in the pattern of comorbidity of panic disorders is the reported association with disruptive behavior disorders (Biederman et al., 1997). A strong association with depression has been reported for children who experience panic episodes (Kearney et al., 1997).

Agoraphobia, the conditioned avoidance reactions that develop as an attempt to control anxiety attacks in some clients subject to panic, is not usually seen in children or young adolescents. Panic attacks are a well-established risk factor for the development of agoraphobia, often conceptualized as a "fear of fear." Craske, Poulton, Tsao, and Plotkin (2001) have provided support for a possible etiological pathway. Their study of a cohort from Dunedin, New Zealand, supported a model that emotional reactivity in early life provided a vulnerability and that early respiratory disturbance was a common sensitizing event in individuals who developed panic disorder and agoraphobia by 18 or 21 years of age. This association between early asthma and later anxiety attacks was strongly evident for their male subjects. Craske and her coauthors (2001) make several important points: First, different symptoms were more or less prominent at different points of the children's life spans— they commented on the greater fluidity of diagnostic status in children than in adults. Second, even mild asthma may have a significant mental health impact on youths at risk for panic disorder and agoraphobia. Third, there may be important differences in the risk profiles of males and females for anxiety disorders, differences that potentially could have implications for treatment approaches.

Whether anxiety is conceptualized as "neuroticism," "anxiety proneness," "avoidant attachment," or "behavioral inhibition," there is increasing evidence that some children are more vulnerable than others to anxiety and mood disorders (Hayward, Killen, Kraemer, & Taylor, 1998). As the Craske et al. (2001) findings illustrate, experiences that may have little or no long-term significance for most children may dramatically affect the development of youths with this anxiety diathesis. Sensitivity to early individual differences and inquiry into developmental responses during the first few years of life can yield clues to the foundation from which later problems emerged.

A similar situation exists with respect to obsessive-compulsive disorders (OCD) in children. Both full clinical syndromes and subclinical presentations of obsessive-compulsive disorder are seen in children (American Academy of Child and Adolescent Psychiatry, 1998; March & Leonard, 1996), as well as in adolescents. A review of some of the more common obsessions and compulsions in youth (March & Leonard, 1996) can form at least a rapid screening for these problems. Anxiety problems in parents should alert the evaluator to the possibility of anxiety problems in children. It is important to assess not only the presence of anxiety symptoms but also the functional impairment associated with them—the amount of time taken up by compulsions or the interference with other desirable activities. As with panic attacks, I have found questions such as, "Do you ever . . . ?" followed up by inquiry to be helpful in evaluating these phenomena.

Specific fears are common in children and adolescents (L. Miller, Barrett, & Hampe, 1974), as are phobias (Milne et al., 1995). Some care needs to be taken in evaluating possible phobic disorders due to the high frequency of transitory fears in youth that may have limited functional significance (Milne et al., 1995). It is also prudent to be cautious in the diagnosis of phobias during the period in which the stimulus may be a developmentally typical concern (Albano et al., 1996; L. Miller et al., 1974). Talking with children about fears requires some tact and special sensitivity to the needs of the child to maintain both a sense of control and a sense of dignity. Normalizing the experience of having fears is often quite helpful and promotes a more realistic perspective on fear behavior. Briefly discussing fears experienced by other children you have known or sharing some of your childhood anxieties can have a pronounced effect on the willingness of children to disclose their own fears. A study by Muris and others (2000) found that open-ended questions regarding fears (e.g., "What do you fear most?") led to more data more closely associated with anxiety disorder symptoms than did having children respond to fear surveys.

Social anxiety in children affects not only their emotional states but also their functional adjustment (Beidel et al., 1999). These chil-

**Practice Note 5.2. Inquiry into Early Temperament: Anxiety and Behavioral Inhibition**

When caretakers from the child's earliest years are available, it is often valuable to attempt some evaluation of the youth's early temperament. Whereas in research activities it is reasonable to devote a great deal of time to this enterprise and to make use of extensive structured interviews, in applied settings these inquiries need to be relatively brief. The supplemental information elicited can be of use in conceptualizing the development of the child's current problems. A relatively simple set of inquiries such as the following may suffice.

**Interview probes for emotional lability and behavioral inhibition**

*Preliminary*: Establish to your confidence that the respondent was regularly involved in the youth's life during the child's first 2 to 4 years.

> "Whom did Jonathan live with after he was first born? Who was around?"

*Preliminary*: Set all questions in the context of the first 2 to 4 years of life.

> "I would like to ask you some questions about what Jonathan was like as a baby and toddler."

*General temperament probes:*

> "What was Jonathan like as an infant? As a very young child, when he was just walking? What do you remember about his mood? About his curiosity? About how sociable and loving he was?"

*General behavioral inhibition probe:*

> "As an infant and toddler, how did Jonathan react to change, to a new person coming around ,for instance?"

*Specific behavioral inhibition probes:*

> "Compared with other infants and toddlers, did Jonathan seem fearful?"

> "Compared with other infants and toddlers, did Jonathan 'hang on you more,' have trouble separating?"

> "Compared with other infants and toddlers, did Jonathan seem more withdrawn and guarded?"

*Critical event probes:* If previous interviewing has not already established the presence or absence of critical events during the first 5 years of life, these issues should be addressed:

> "Did Jonathan have any major illness or injury early in his life? Could you tell me about these?"

> "Was Jonathan separated from you early in his life? Could you tell me about that?"

---

dren are often socially isolated and lonely and make excessive use of avoidance coping techniques. Other anxiety problems and psychiatric symptoms are frequent, as are limitations in the children's social skills (Beidel et al., 1999). This last finding is potentially very significant in understanding the maintenance and long-term morbidity associated with social phobias in youth. When you are evaluating anxious children, it is worthwhile to make a careful review of their friendship patterns, frequency of association with other children, and social skills.

Finally, generalized patterns of anxiety occur in children and have long been recognized in clinical populations. Previous conceptualizations of "overanxious disorder of childhood" are currently viewed as juvenile-onset cases of generalized anxiety disorder (GAD). Current (DSM-IV) diagnostic criteria appear to be reasonably satisfactory for use with children (Tracey, Chorpita, Douban, & Barlow, 1997). A major phenomenological aspect of GAD in children is worry. These children tend to be threat sensitive and concerned—they ruminate about negative possibilities and outcomes. Rapoport and Ismond (1996) suggest that these children usually show anticipatory anxiety, especially in situations in which the child's performance or appearance will be appraised, and they comment that perfectionistic tendencies are often present. Comorbidities with other anxiety disorders, mood disorders, and substance use problems, as well as with stress-related physical complaints, are reported (Rapoport & Ismond, 1996). I have found these youths to often manifest a great degree of personal distress—they frequently appear as abjectly miserable. I have also seen fairly debilitating constriction of age-appropriate activities and social functioning in these children. A careful review of adaptive behavior and social adjustment is warranted in children with GAD.

## Interview Segment 5.2. Tell Me about the Darkness: Ted

Fully appreciating the prevalence of anxiety disorders in youths has taken a great deal of time within the mental health community. Most adults would like to believe that childhood is a time of sunshine and carefree indulgence, even if their own memories are not fully compatible with the wishful daydream. Understanding the dynamic of tension and fear in children's lives requires us to be open to its existence and also to help a child find the words to convey the darkness that lurks around the corner. Ted was a 10-year-old child living with his divorced mother; he was shy and had few playmates; and his academic progress was above average. He was referred for evaluation after extensive medical assessment failed to explain his frequent somatic complaints and an emergency room internist suspected panic attacks.

EXAMINER: Can you tell me why your mother brought you here to talk with me?

TED: I get sick a lot (*soft voice, clear articulation*).

EXAMINER: Yes, that's what your mother said. Tell me about being sick.

TED: I feel bad.

EXAMINER: Yes, that's how people feel when they are sick. And there are different ways people feel bad. Sometimes it helps to know exactly how a person feels bad, in order to help them feel better. Tell me about how it is with you when you're feeling bad; maybe we can figure out how to help you feel better.

TED: Do you have to take blood?

EXAMINER: No. No, I am not that kind of doctor. You and I are going to going to talk and figure out what is making you feel bad, and then do something about it so you feel better.

TED: All right.

EXAMINER: Your mother told me you had to have some blood samples taken. Bet that wasn't much fun.

TED: I threw up (*very soft voice*).

EXAMINER: I guess it hurt a lot.

TED: I was scared (*teary eyes*).

EXAMINER: The way you felt at the lab, where they took the blood sample. Did you feel bad there?

TED: Yes. I feel bad a lot.

EXAMINER: All the time?

TED: No, not all the time.

EXAMINER: At the lab, before you threw up, can you tell me how you were feeling.

TED: Bad.

EXAMINER: Yes, what else?

TED: I wanted to go home.

EXAMINER: You really wanted out of there.

TED: Yes! I wanted to go home. Then I threw up. The nurse was nice, though.

EXAMINER: That's good. I know a lot of nurses; most of them are nice.

TED: Not the one at school.

EXAMINER: What's she like?

TED: She's not very nice when I go to her office.

EXAMINER: What does she do that's not nice?

TED: She doesn't like me coming to her office. Because I go there a lot. My teacher sends me there when I tell her I'm sick.

EXAMINER: You were telling me about how you felt when you were sick. When did you go to the nurse's office last?

TED: Friday.

EXAMINER: What was the first thing you noticed on Friday when you didn't feel well?

TED: I was hot. The nurse said I didn't have a temperature but I was hot. It was hot in the room. She acted like I was making it up and I wasn't. It was hot.

EXAMINER: Sometimes it seems like people don't listen when we try to tell them things.

TED: Yeah. The nurse made a joke about it. I think she was making fun of me.

EXAMINER: I don't like people making fun of me.

TED: Yeah.

EXAMINER: You said you were feeling really hot on Friday. What was that like?

TED: It was hard to breathe.

EXAMINER: Hard to breathe.

TED: Yeah, like when I got wrapped up in my sleeping bag at Joey's. I couldn't get anyone awake to help.

EXAMINER: You felt like that Friday?

TED: Yeah.

EXAMINER: How are you feeling now?

TED: OK (*tentative*).

EXAMINER: Not feeling bad now?

TED: No (*firmer*).

EXAMINER: How about when you first came in, you seemed like you might be feeling a little bad then?

TED: A little. You have carpet.

EXAMINER: Carpet?

TED: Once I threw up at a doctor's office. They had carpet and the nurse got really upset. I didn't mean to. They were mad.

EXAMINER: Right. I don't think that'll be a problem for us. No blood tests today, remember?

TED: Yeah. (*Smiles.*)

EXAMINER: So, sometimes when you feel bad, you are feeling really hot and it feels hard to get your breath, like you're wrapped up too tight in a blanket?

TED: Yeah! Like that. I feel bad.

EXAMINER: Yes, and if it goes on and gets even worse, you get sick to your stomach.

TED: Yeah.

EXAMINER: And if you can get out of the place where you feel bad, then what happens?

TED: I feel better.

EXAMINER: Like you feel better now than when you first came in today?

TED: Yeah.

EXAMINER: OK, we've made some good progress. Now let's talk a little more about the kind of places you get to feeling bad in.

A good deal more discussion was necessary, but the case data increasingly supported a view of panic episodes superimposed on a chronic state of high arousal and tension. The final diagnosis was of panic disorder, generalized anxiety disorder, and traits of social phobia. As is often the case with anxiety disorders, the client showed evidence of several comorbid anxiety problems. As is often the case in children, Ted showed both fully manifested anxiety syndromes (panic disorder, generalized anxiety disorder) and partially manifested subthreshold syndromes (agoraphobic and social phobic traits). Typical of both anxiety and mood disorders in children was the presentation primarily in terms of somatic complaints, as well as the frustration at adults who often seem to judge but seldom seem to listen.

## Somatization

As noted previously, depressed children may present with more somatic complaints than phenomenological symptoms of negative mood (Kashani & Carlson, 1987), and adults may respond more readily to complaints of pains and physical symptoms in children (Puura et al., 1998). Pediatric somatization refers to children or adolescents who present with physical symptoms that cannot be medically explained or adequately accounted for on the basis of physical findings (Campo & Fritsch, 1994; Garralda, 1996; Shapiro & Rosenfeld, 1987). Campo, Jansen-Williams, Comer, and Kelleher (1999) found that children who were classified as "somatizers" were at risk for psychiatric disorder, family dysfunction, functional impairment, and frequent use of medical services. They conclude that medically unexplained physical symptoms may be important indications of emotional disorder and should be followed up with careful evaluation. Medically unexplained symptoms are common in youths (Garralda, 1996), but diagnosis of somatization disorder is unusual and may reflect developmentally inappropriate diagnostic criteria in the current classification manual (Fritz, Fritsch, & Hagino, 1997). Campo found that classification of a youth as a somatizer was more common with adolescents, with female clients, with minority subjects, in urban practices, with children from nonintact families, and with children whose parents had achieved lower levels of formal education. The possibility of bias operating here is a real concern, and examiner caution is advised.

## Undifferentiated Somatoform Disorder

Children may often experience and communicate emotional distress in terms of physical symptoms and complaints. When an appropriate medical workup fails to adequately explain the basis for physical symptoms, it is reasonable to look for alternative formulations. Depressive and anxiety syndromes should be carefully considered. If mood or anxiety disorder conceptualizations fail to capture the essential features of a child's situation, you might review the category of undifferentiated somatoform disorder. The eventual usefulness, reliability, and validity of this classification remains to be demonstrated, but it does offer an opportunity to identify patterns of behavioral disturbance in some children that are not adequately characterized by other diagnoses. This diagnosis would not usually be based on a single evaluation contact or be convincingly demonstrated in an initial assessment.

## Conversion Disorders

Conversion disorders in children and adolescents are seen from time to time in a clinical practice, especially if physician referrals or consultation to medical services contribute significantly to the client population. The most important diagnostic consideration is to ensure that the conceptualization is based on positive psychological findings, as well as on the absence of any medical findings that would account for the results. A careful evaluation is always prudent and, of necessity, extends beyond an initial assessment contact. Forming a strong working relationship and therapeutic rapport with the child is vital to being able to conduct a valid assessment. Careful evaluation of situational stresses, family dynamics, and associated psychopathology in the youth are all necessary to develop a complete conceptualization to guide treatment efforts.

Although some interesting work has been done, most of the literature on conversion disorder and related somatoform disorders in youth, such as body dysmorphic disorder, remains at the case study level (Fritz et al., 1997; Phillips, Atala, & Albertini, 1995; Siegel & Barthel, 1986). One active area of investigation is that of body image in children, especially as it is related to eating disorders (Sands, Tricker, Sherman, Armatas, & Maschette, 1997).

Recurrent abdominal pain and headaches are the most frequently reported somatic symptoms in children and in adolescents (Fritz et al., 1997). Open-ended inquiry to the youth, after some rapport has been developed, will often elicit these concerns if they are on the mind of the youth: "How are you feeling today?" "What have you been to the doctor for recently?" In my own practice, concerns about possible somatization usually lead to my actively pressing for another careful review of the child by his or her pediatrician. I am cautious in accepting a referral from a physician as *prima facie* evidence for a "psychological disturbance." Consistent with the adult literature on identified conversion disorders, studies of children diagnosed with conversion disorder have found that unacceptably high percentages, 27% to 46%, are eventually diagnosed with a physical disease (Lehmkuhl, Blanz, Lehmkuhl, & Braum-Scharm, 1989). I advise caution in accepting too readily psychological explanations of physical symptoms, especially given concerns of possible biases in population identification.

The assessment of pain is a difficult clinical enterprise, especially in children. It is difficult for most examiners to maintain objectivity in the face of a child's suffering. Providing sufficient time and emotional support for the child to relate her experience at her own pace and in her own manner helps reduce the stress of the interview. One type of commonly encountered chronic pain problem in children is headaches. Viswanathan, Bridges, Whitehouse, and Newton (1998) provide a very useful set of data on childhood headaches, as well as a headache questionnaire that is helpful with a juvenile population.

# 6 Evaluating Behavior Problems in Children and Adolescents

## THE EVALUATION OF AGGRESSION, DISOBEDIENCE, AND RULE BREAKING

Problems with oppositional and defiant behavior, poor impulse control, and aggressiveness are among the most frequent referral concerns of parents in mental health settings and of teachers in educational settings. The assessment of this domain of problem behavior is a vital skill for the mental health counselor. These problems have been labeled with a variety of names: acting out, disruptive behavior disorders, externalizing symptoms, antisocial or psychopathic or undercontrolled behavior. The essential elements in evaluation are to assess the nature, frequency, severity, and pervasiveness of the problem behavior, the pattern of development, the social influences at play, comorbid problems, and associated prognostic factors.

A wide range of specific behavioral symptoms involving oppositional defiance of adult instructions, rule breaking, and aggression have been found to frequently covary. It is important to establish, usually from an adult informant, exactly what problems the child in question is exhibiting. Given the diversity of our cultural, ethnic, social, and personal backgrounds, even the use of seemingly objective terms such as "aggressive" and "disobedient" can show appreciable variation from individual to individual. Asking for specific examples is usually the most helpful response of the examiner: "Can you tell me about the last time Suzy was 'hateful'? What was happening and what did she do? Tell me about the time it happened before that one. Tell me about some other times she was disrespectful. What exactly did she do?" Similar patterns of questions can be directed to the child: "When you 'lost your temper' yesterday, what exactly did you do?" The general interview strategy of beginning with open-ended, less directive questions and moving to more focused inquiry is usually the most productive, moving from "Tell me what happens when you 'get into a fight' " to "How many times did you hit people with your fist yesterday?" "What kinds of weapons have you actually used in fights with somebody?"

The emphasis in mental health assessment is on identifying recurrent patterns of behavior. Most children strike another child sometime during childhood; a few children repeatedly hit their schoolmates and other children. Observational studies of normal children in homes show what appears a rather high frequency of disobedience of parental commands, but normal children tend to be very selective in the parental instructions they choose not to comply with. Children with acting-out problems tend to be as likely to disobey the third repetition of a command (which is likely to be followed by punishment in their homes) as they are to disobey the first or second statement of that instruction. It is the pattern of problem behavior, the recognition of repetitive instances of poor behavior control, that is the focus of our interest. Determining the pattern of consequences of the child's disobedience is as informative as establishing the frequency of ignoring adult commands.

Determining the frequency of disruptive and aggressive behavior is very important because families and teachers very widely in their tolerance for these actions. In some families a child may be seen as having a problem with aggression if he or she has been in two fights during the past year; in another family the child is not seen as having any difficulty despite almost daily complaints from the neighbors regarding the child's assaults on other children in the area. "How often has this been a problem in the past week, month, 6 months, year?" is a valuable series of questions in establishing behavior parameters for meaningful comparison with age peers.

The severity or seriousness of the conduct problem behavior is also an important aspect to assess. Using a weapon to inflict harm on another person is a much more problematic action than being a few minutes late for curfew. The consequences or potential consequences for the victim is a fundamental consideration in judging severity. Also meaningful is the overall density of aggression within the context of antisocial behavior. Frequent reliance on aggression as a coping response appears to be a powerful and negative prognostic variable in terms of children's future adjustment and functioning.

Establishing the pervasiveness of the conduct problems in the child's world is another significant determination in evaluating behavior difficulties. Acting-out problems limited to a single environmental setting may reflect marked conflict within that area of the child's life, but not necessarily generalized maladjustment. The more widespread problems have become in the child's world the greater the concern for long-term maladjustment. Reviewing the child's adjustment at home (with various combinations of caretakers if several adults are involved in the child's life), in the neighborhood, at friends' homes, in school classrooms, on the playground, while shopping, and in other important settings is useful in obtaining an appraisal of how widespread the behavior problems are.

Much more difficult to reliably evaluate are emotional and qualitative aspects of acting out: guilt, remorse, anger, revenge, satisfaction. My experience is that children have a far greater reluctance to honestly discuss the motivations and emotions accompanying aggression than to discuss the actions themselves. They may freely admit that they cut a classmate with a lab knife during a scuffle in biology but have great difficulty sharing the feelings that preceded, accompanied, and followed this event. Helping the youngster voice these emotions may help the examiner understand the context in which aggressive acting out is more likely to occur. Self-reports of trait anger, for instance, were found to be more strongly associated with incidents of aggression in an incarcerated sample of male adolescents than either the youngsters' histories of violence or staff ratings of the adolescents' apparent anger (Cornell, Peterson, & Richards, 1999). Although the drive to increase the reliability of psychiatric diagnosis has led to a decreased emphasis on internal states in the classification of behavior problems, a fuller understanding of the child's situation and the difficulties to be overcome often requires an effort to know the inner world of the aggressive child. Achieving this knowledge depends on balancing a matter-of-fact objectivity about misbehavior with an empathy for the experience of children who both victimize and are victimized more often than normal children.

As final important consideration, we must recognize how differences in prevalence and age of onset of ADHD and conduct disorders between males and females has shaped our empirical database regarding these problems and exercise due caution in the assessment of young girls. Both ADHD and early-onset conduct disorders are significantly more common in males than in females; adolescent-onset conduct disorders show a closer to even balance in prevalence between the sexes (Hinshaw & Anderson, 1996). These differences in age of onset may ultimately play a profound role in our development and evaluation of etiological models of disruptive behavior disorders (Zahn-Waxler, 1993; Zoccolillo, 1993). For the present, these differences have implications for both detection and evaluation of behavior problems in females (Hartung & Widiger, 1998). Girls may show not only differences in the age of onset of acting out but also differences in patterns. Females with conduct problems are reported to show less overt aggression (Crick & Grotpeter, 1995; Webster-Stratton, 1996) and more covert antisocial behavior, such as truancy (Zahn-Waxler, 1993). Early sexual maturation has been reported to be a predictor variable for antisocial behavior in females (Clarizio, 1997; Simmons & Blyth, 1987), possibly by promoting differential association with males who may model aggressive behavior (Caspi, Lynam, Moffitt, & Silva, 1993). The association with comorbid problems, especially internalizing ones, appears stronger in females; the adult outcome is poor, but not as dire as it is for males; and potential negative sequelae include poor parenting skills in adulthood (Lewis et al., 1991; Robins, 1986). A good deal more work needs to done on understanding the development of disruptive behavior problems and related social problems, such as gang delinquency (J. Miller, 2001), in young women.

## ESTABLISHING RAPPORT AND TRUST

Discussing behavior problems with children is often best done following a more general review of the child's life and establishment of a nonjudgmental and supportive pattern of interaction between examiner and child. I may make some passing reference to the referral issues, with little attempt to gain any comment from the child, and then pass quickly into inquiry about less threatening topics: "I understand you have been having problems getting along with the other children on your street. We will talk about that in a few minutes, but first I would like to get to know more about you. What do you like to do?" Children often experience the undivided attention of an adult who does not tend to criticize or advise as a novel and interesting experience, and conversation can usually be initiated. These first few minutes may or may not be "productive" in the sense of eliciting data of diagnostic value or thematic importance, but the time is well spent nevertheless. A few moments of calm and nonthreatening attention tend to reduce the child's anxiety and defensiveness and help establish a pattern of free communication that can be maintained as the interview moves into more problematic areas.

Interviewing the adolescent about conduct problems can be much more challenging and frustrating for all involved than discussing these matters with the preadolescent or child. The teenager is often acutely aware of possible negative consequences to sharing information with even well-intentioned adults and may have little inclination or reason to trust the good motives of the examiner. Patience, forthrightness, and a slow pace of inquiry have been vital to any success I have enjoyed in evaluating adolescents with histories of conduct problems. Adolescents may, of course, lie to you outright; but they are even more likely to equivocate, dodge, state a half truth, or answer part of the question you posed to see if that will satisfy you. The examiner who is hurried in his or her attempt to complete an agenda or fill out an intake sheet will often find him- or herself having been led down a path to very limited understanding of the young person. It has been productive for me to begin with an interview style of inquiry, then move on to other areas, then return to a subject for clarification, then shift again to other topics, then return to the subject for review and further clarification, repeating the pattern as often as needed. Inconsistencies can be presented objectively and calmly to the youth for explanation.

A difficulty that may occur as frequently as dissimulation in teenagers is the exaggeration of deeds and misadventures. Especially with some patterns of conduct problems, they may intentionally or "spontaneously" elaborate on stories of defiance, rule breaking, or aggression. Sometimes this behavior represents deliberate lying in order to boost one's reputation or imagined status. Even more often, the self-aggrandizement occurs without forethought or even conscious intent. The youth's role in the story grows with the telling and may sound very sincere. In my own professional practice I proceed as if all my clients are attempting to cooperate and to be as honest with me as they can until I have clear data suggesting that this is not the case. This does not necessarily mean, however, that I accept everything my client tells me as having actually happened in the way he or she recalls it having occurred.

## GATHERING INFORMATION ABOUT ACTING OUT

The literature suggests that there is often a higher correspondence between the verbal reports of children, parents, and teachers regarding

### Interview Segment 6.1. Tell Me about Mic's Fighting

Mic was 15 years old when he was evaluated in a juvenile detention center in preparation for placement at a residential facility. He had a history of oppositional behavior going back to his preschool days. He had been a constant discipline problem in school since kindergarten and had been in behavior disorder classes throughout his school years. He has a juvenile court record of shoplifting, curfew violation, vandalism, cruelty to animals, two cases of arson, and assault going back to the early elementary school years. In junior high school he had escalated to armed violence, assault with a deadly weapon, assault to inflict bodily harm, and sexual assault.

EXAMINER: Mic, would you tell me something about the fights you get in?

MIC: I don't get into fights much anymore.

EXAMINER: But you're back in detention for fighting.

MIC: Yeah, but that shouldn't have gone that way, it was bogus.

EXAMINER: How do you mean, "It was bogus"?

MIC: I got arrested because Ms. Salaski came around the corner just as I decked Raul. She didn't even ask what had been going on, just ordered me to the counselor's office, and the next thing the cops are there.

EXAMINER: Would you tell me what happened?

MIC: Well, Raul and Johnny had been getting into it all week over Johnny's girl, because she used to be with Raul. I was staying away from it all, because I was on probation and knew I'd be in it if I got caught up in anything. It's stupid to fight over a skirt.

EXAMINER: What happened?

MIC: OK, well, Johnny's being pretty cool, because he didn't need any trouble either. And Raul just keeps picking at him. Anyway by then Johnny had had it. Raul said something and Johnny jumped him. Johnny's kind of a wuss and Raul got him in a corner. So that was it.

EXAMINER: And how did you get involved?

MIC: Well, Johnny was going to get cleaned.

EXAMINER: And?

MIC: Johnny's with us. I'm not going to let some [ethnic slur] shitkick him!

EXAMINER: What did you mean, "Johnny's with us"?

MIC: Well, a bunch of us kind of hang together.

EXAMINER: Like a gang?

MIC: No! No, nothing like that. We just pal around, you know. It's not like the LK or Bloods, we just do things together.

EXAMINER: So, you were standing up for Johnny?

MIC: Right. That's how it was.

EXAMINER: What did you do?

MIC: I just hit him.

EXAMINER: Where did you hit him?

MIC: In the kidney. He dropped like a rock, just as Ms. S came up.

EXAMINER: Your record says you've been in fights in the neighborhood, too.

MIC: Sometimes. Not as much this year as last year.

EXAMINER: Have you ever used a weapon in a fight?

MIC: Yeah.

EXAMINER: What did you use?

MIC: Just a piece of board.

EXAMINER: When was that?

. . .

EXAMINER: What other weapons have you used?

MIC: Only a box opener.

EXAMINER: How many times?

MIC: Only one time, twice, two or three times.

. . .

EXAMINER: Have you ever used any other kind of weapon in a fight?

MIC: I hit a kid with a bottle once. Busted it over his head. He bled like a pig.

EXAMINER: Ever use a bottle as a weapon any other time?

MIC: Don't think so.

EXAMINER: When was the first time you used a weapon in a fight?

MIC: Last year, well, the bottle was in the sixth grade. Then nothing until last year.

EXAMINER: Altogether, how many times have you used any kind of weapon in a fight during the last year?

MIC: I don't know, maybe . . . maybe a dozen, a few more maybe.

EXAMINER: Now at home, ever hit anyone in your family?

MIC: My brother and I get into it once in a while.

EXAMINER: How serious do the fights get?

MIC: Well, sometimes one of us gets mad. We busted up the family room once. Mom was burning.

. . .

EXAMINER: You ever threaten to really hurt your brother?

MIC: I never did anything to him.

EXAMINER: You never cut him, even once?

MIC: That thing last spring wasn't what they said.

. . .

EXAMINER: Mic, did you ever hit your mom?

MIC: No, she just says I do.

EXAMINER: Did you ever push her?

MIC: I pushed her, because she was going to hit me and I wouldn't let her, and then I was going to leave, to cool down, and she got in my way and I just moved her aside.

EXAMINER: You pushed her.

MIC: Because I wanted to go outside before things got out of hand.

EXAMINER: Was that when her arm got broken?

MIC: Yeah.

. . .

EXAMINER: Ms. M, can you tell me about Mic's fighting?

MS. M: He's always fighting. That boy has always been a handful. No one would play with him for years, it always wound up in a fight. People embarrassed me in the neighborhood because he was a bully. I've had to call the police three times. He threatens his brother, and he means it. He's hurt Fred in the past. You know, all boys fight. But Mic can't control himself. He hits everybody in the family, and hard. I'm afraid of him some times. He's bigger than I am now. After last spring, I'm not going to stand up to him.

EXAMINER: What happened last spring?

Ms. M: He had threatened his brother with a knife. It was over some stupid game. He had a paring knife and said he was going to cut Fred.

EXAMINER: What happened?

Ms. M: I came in the kitchen and told him to put the knife down.

EXAMINER: And?

Ms. M: He put the knife in the sink, and then said he was going out.

EXAMINER: What happened?

Ms. M: He was on probation and had an 8 o'clock curfew. It was past 10. I told him he had to stay home.

EXAMINER: Mmmm?

Ms. M: He went and got his jacket and was heading out. I stood in front of the door and told him he wasn't going out. That was the first time he hit me.

EXAMINER: What exactly happened?

Ms. M: What I said, he hit me.

EXAMINER: How did he hit you?

Ms. M: With his fist. He hit me right in the face. I thought my jaw was broken. It knocked me down. When they X-rayed my arm, it was broken. My jaw just hurt like fire, but my arm was broken.

EXAMINER: What happened with Mic?

Ms. M: He had left. We didn't see him again until the weekend. My neighbor took me to the hospital. I made Fred come with us. I was afraid Mic would come home while I was gone and hurt him.

---

externalizing symptoms than has been reported to be the case for internalizing symptoms, such as anxiety or depression. Nevertheless, there are clearly many instances in which it would not be safe to rely on the word of the youth alone. Usually multiple sources of information are necessary to establish a clear picture of what has been occurring. The self-report of the youth is only one of these sources of data.

Observation of children during the assessment may make a limited additional contribution. Even though there is support for noting test behavior in addition to test performance (DeWolfe, Byrne, & Bawden, 1999), I have found such observations to be specific but not sensitive. Occurrence of impulsive or inattentive behavior during your session is usually clinically meaningful, but many youths with clinical behavior problems do not manifest these symptoms in an initial session. A commonly heard lament from parents of oppositional or hyperactive children is that the child has behaved better in your office than anywhere ever before. Although this is probably an overstatement, the underlying message is usually correct: You have not seen a representative sample of this young person's typical behavior. The combination of a novel setting, usually one-on-one attention from the examiner, a typically relatively short duration of session, and probably better than average skills on the adult's part in eliciting and reinforcing compliance and cooperation combine to help the child present his or her best face. Occurrence of significant inattention, noncompliance, or out-of-seat and physically destructive behavior in the clinical situation has important diagnostic implications—the child is probably even worse everywhere else—but is unusual even in clinical cases.

Potentially much more informative are opportunities to observe interactions between parent and child in the waiting area, during transitions in the evaluation process, and during departure from your office. Few mental health counselors have available the resources to carry out extensive home visits for assessment; possibly no observations will be conducted in natural settings. It is important to make the most of opportunities that occur during the office visit to watch the interactions between children and caretakers. It is very informative to make note of the frequency and quality of instructions from adults to children, as well as adults' responses to the child's compliance and noncompliance with directives. As has been frequently commented on in the behavior therapy literature, child noncompliance tends to be associated with patterns of adult behavior. The parents of oppositional children often given more frequent commands than parents of normal children, their instructions are often vague and may not actually meet any operational criterion for a command, and they often do not respond differentially to compliance or noncompliance. Bursts of commands may be evident: "Sit down. Quit bothering the doctor's things. Behave. Michael, look at me while Mommy's talking. Put that down. Please be good. Don't sniff. Sit up in the chair." "Commands" may be so unclear that compliance would be impossible to produce or evaluate: "Do you want to be good now?" The adult may fail to notice that the child actually did the first three things he or she was asked to do, ignored the fourth command, and hit his or her younger sibling during the repetition of the first command, which had been followed already.

In addition to making these behavioral observations, you should be sensitive to the emotional tone of the interaction between parent and child. Parents who must contend with hyperactive, oppositional, and aggressive children are frequently frustrated and unhappy. There may be indications of anger, fatigue, resignation, or depression in their voices, tones, or manners. Parents may have difficulty acknowledging the emotional reactions their children pull from them, but this is an vital area of evaluation. Sending parents home to carry out a positive reinforcement program when they can barely look at their children without becoming angry is self-defeating for all involved unless these emotional reactions are addressed. It is possible to teach angry and frustrated parents how to reinforce their children effectively, but only if they recognize the need to learn to do so.

Productive interviewing of parents, teachers, and other informants about acting-out behavior in children and adolescents follows the same general guidelines as does interviewing the youth. We assist parents in providing good information for us by asking them specific questions and giving them the opportunity to illustrate their answers with examples. It is often helpful to ask the caretaker to describe the last time the youth had problems with fighting, destruction of property, and so forth. The emotional impact on the family of acting-out behavior is also important to establish. Parents of severely disruptive children may be exhausted by the constant struggles with the youth. They may be frustrated and angry over having to respond to calls from teachers, retail merchants, and the parents of the child's playmates. The siblings may reject the disruptive child as a source of irritation and the one who "spoils" family events, and sometimes brothers and sisters may be afraid of the potential for violence and aggression. Practice Note 6.1 illustrates sample questions that may be productive in interviewing parents of children with behavior disorders.

## DOMAINS OF CONDUCT AND ADJUSTMENT

When evaluating acting-out behavior problems, it is especially important to systematically review the child's adjustment in all the major settings in which he or she participates and to review the range of problematic behavior that can be seen in children. Very dramatic symptoms, such as aggression or overactivity, can capture our attention as evaluators and lead to the heightened risk of several potential errors

## Practice Note 6.2. Asking Caretakers about Acting-Out Behavior

General behavioral interviewing attempts to establish the nature of problematic actions that occur, as well as to gain data on the frequency, pattern, and environmental circumstances of symptoms. Requests for examples, illustrations, and clarification are used as needed to gain a clear picture of the actions that have caused difficulty for the youth. The following are examples of interviewing probes that be productive.

"What kind of problems have you had getting Suzy to mind at home?"

"How does Suzy's minding you compare with her brothers and sisters?"

"How does Suzy get along with her brothers and sisters?"

"What kind of trouble does Suzy get into at home?"

"What happens when Suzy plays with other children in the neighborhood?"

"How well can Suzy occupy herself for awhile?"

"How does Suzy do during meals in your home?"

"How does Suzy do with her chores at home?"

"Have you had any problems with Suzy talking back to you, calling you names, threatening to hurt you?"

"Have there been any problems with Suzy being accused of stealing, playing with fire or setting fires, being mean to animals, using a weapon or object in a fight?"

"Have you ever felt afraid of Suzy? Have your other children?"

---

in assessment. We may assume a degree of generalizability regarding the child's problems that is not actually supported by the child's real-life behavior. The first time a child turns your office upside down, despite all your best efforts at effective management, it is almost impossible to imagine that such an out-of-control little hellion could be much better behaved elsewhere. The research literature on child behavior problems, however, tends to indicate that high situational specificity is the rule and not the exception in child behavior. For an accurate assessment it is vital not to assume too much regarding the child's misbehavior in different settings. A deliberate inquiry into behavior at home, in the classroom or playground, before and after school, in the neighborhood, in other people's home, in stores and recreation areas, and in the car while traveling can help delimit the boundaries of the child's self-control and adaptation.

Also recall the high degree of comorbidity reported between externalizing behavior problems and other patterns of maladjustment. Both ADHD and conduct disorders have high associations with each other and with learning problems in childhood and substance use problems and mood disorders in adolescence. Oppositional problems that fall short of conduct disorders are frequently comorbid with ADHD and other adjustment difficulties. Identifying one pattern of behavior problem should not halt a careful review of other potential areas of difficulty. Multiple problems are much more common than isolated maladjustment.

We should also realize that children who show acting-out behavior are at higher than base-rate risk for a variety of other difficulties with potential implications for development and outcome. Children with behavior problems are at greater hazard for head injuries, especially as adolescents when they begin to drive. It has also been demonstrated that youths with ADHD have more driving accidents than the average teenager, which can contribute to a wide range of injuries (Woodward, Fergusson, & Horwood, 2000). Exceptional children in general, including youths with behavior problems, are at greater risk than unremarkable youths for child abuse by caretakers. The family situations of many youths with antisocial behavior patterns are more disorganized, fragmented, and conflicted than those of typical children of the same ethnic and sociocultural background. The parents of children who act out frequently have their own histories of adjustment problems. All these potential risk factors should be considered when evaluating the youth with behavior problems. The need to survey a wide range of the child's life to generate the most comprehensive and meaningful assessment possible is a recurrent theme in this book.

## IMPORTANT AREAS FOR ASSESSMENT

Several behavioral domains are of interest in evaluating youths with behavior problems; these are briefly outlined in this section. At the same time, it is important to realize that most of the clinically relevant behavior will never be seen in your office. Although some children "let it all hang out" and provide the examiner with many instances of inattention, overactivity, distractibility, impulsivity, destructiveness, non-compliance, and aggression to report on, the majority of children, even those with severe behavior problems, are well behaved and compliant in your office. The most common lament of the bewildered, frustrated, and desperate parents seeking guidance in dealing with a challenging child is, "But, Doctor, he's never this good at home." Small wonder, given that most evaluations take place in a novel setting with unfamiliar people, with highly structured but brief activities, and with almost constant one-on-one attention. Disruptive behavior disorder symptoms tend to be situationally specific, often confined to only a few general settings of the child's environment. Furthermore, these behaviors are frequently low base-rate occurrences, even though it may not seem so to the adults charged with caring for the child. Low-rate, high-amplitude behaviors, such as fire setting, assaults on others, and suicidal behavior, are especially difficult to evaluate. For both of these general reasons, the office evaluation, although invaluable and necessary, is seldom sufficient for assessment of children with behavior problems. At a minimum, behavior rating scales completed by informants familiar with the child's typical behavior in major settings should be obtained and augmented whenever possible with additional sources of data.

## Inattention

Problems with sustained mental focus can interfere with a wide variety of academic, vocational, and recreational activities, as well as render such everyday acts as driving a car or mowing the lawn dangerous. The cognitive capacity for sustained attention grows over the developmental years, and the relevant comparison group when questioning a child's ability to pay attention is always his or her age peers. Informal observations that contribute to an impression about ability to concentrate are the child's ability to follow a conversation, to focus on requested activities, and to deal with mental status items such as counting or mental arithmetic. More formal assessments may involve dedicated instrumentation such as the Gordon Diagnostic System (Gordon, 1983) or software, such as continuous performance tasks (Riccio, Reynolds, & Lowe, 2001). Attention difficulties, however, are nonspecific symptoms found in many behavioral and emotional presentations (Halperin et al., 1992). Children with ADHD usually have problems with attention, but so do children with conduct disorders, depression, anxiety, autism, schizophrenia, mental retardation, and so forth. Distractibility can occur as part of many behavior disorders and can contribute in turn to a range of cognitive and academic disturbances in a nonspecific pattern. Attention-deficit problems seldom occur in isolation or without having affected multiple areas of the child's life.

## Impulsivity

As with attention limitations, impulsivity in responding is developmentally normal in the very young. With increasing maturity the child's responding becomes more organized, planned, reflective—characteristics of executive functions. Conceptually, impulsivity may be closely associated with another attribute of interest, rule-governed behavior. As impulsivity decreases, rule-governed behavior tends to increase, and visa versa. Impulsivity during the evaluation can be noted in how children respond to tasks, as well as how they conduct themselves in your office as they learn (or fail to learn) the rules and conventions of your practice. Impulsivity may be functionally associated with hyperactivity, consistent with the current DSM-IV conceptualization (Pillow, Pelham, Hoza, Molina, & Stultz, 1998). In children with ADHD, the symptoms of hyperactivity and impulsivity appear to carry increased risk for adult criminal behavior (Babinski, Hartsough, & Lambert, 1999).

## Overactivity

Like inattention and impulsivity, overactivity can sometimes be directly observed in your office. The child may be unable to remain seated, may move about your office in a restless pattern, or may fiddle with every object within reach. There may be a "nervous hum" about the child, but often there is not. Motor overactivity is one of the symptoms of ADHD that most clearly reduce with advancing age. The child who could never stay seated in elementary school sits through his or her high school class; he or she just can't attend sufficiently to learn anything. Through careful observation you will note the drumming of fingers, pulling of ear lobes, twisting of hair, removal and return of pens, comb, slips of paper, and various objects from shirt pockets and jeans and so forth, as the child twists and stretches and repositions. But these more subtle signs of motor restlessness, although probably more frequent than those displayed by other youths of the same age, are no longer clearly outside the normal range. Many high school children are restless and wait impatiently for the bell. Continued severe motor restlessness is an important symptom that has rather direct implications for adjustment and functioning, but its absence is not remarkable and does not necessary mark overall clinical improvement. The high school student who can now sit through class is not necessarily learning while there or learning at the same rate as his or her age peers.

In evaluating caretaker reports of hyperactivity, we need to consider how generalized the problem is across different activities and settings. The more pervasive the difficulties with self-regulation of activity level are, the more likely it is that the child has a clinical problem, especially at younger ages (Stormont & Zentall, 1999). Assessment of activity and impulse control across different settings is also of diagnostic importance since DSM-IV brought the United States in line with the majority of nations in requiring a pervasive manifestation to classify a child as showing ADHD. Due to the rapid developmental changes in activity and impulse control, behavior rating scales that allow for comparisons of parental rating of hyperactivity against appropriate age and gender comparison groups is invaluable in assessing overactivity in children.

## Aggression

Evaluation of a youth's aggressiveness, especially instrumental or "proactive" aggression, is of critical importance in considering the child's current adjustment and risk for future behavior problems. Proactive aggression is goal-oriented behavior that is used to achieve an aim. It does not require provocation or anger (Vitaro, Gendreau, Tremblay, & Oligny, 1998); it is a tool that the child is using to influence his or her world. The difficulty with this particular tool is that it tends to be seductive—few or no other interpersonal tactics work as well over the short term as violence for achieving reinforcement in childhood—but ultimately very limiting. The "costs" of aggressiveness tend to be delayed, which further increases the temptation to rely on this means of influencing others. An extensive literature documents the developmental risks associated with hyperaggression (Patterson, 1982; Patterson, Reid, & Dishion, 1992). The more aggressive children in an age cohort are at risk, compared with their peers, on virtually every outcome that has ever been measured.

## Interview Segment 6.2. Winnie at 15: "Eat Shit and Die"

Winnie was 15 years old when she was admitted to the psychiatric unit of a community hospital for unmanageable behavior, suicide threats, and delinquency. Her history was of relatively severe oppositional behavior from preschool through the present. Her behavior problems had escalated over time to serious aggression and destruction of property. Although there was no indication of attention or learning problems, she had done poorly in school due to misbehavior. At the time she had been expelled for beating another girl up in the rest room. She reported having smoked since she was 9, and she drank alcohol when it was available. She preferred to associate with a group of older high school youths and young men out of school. There was a great deal of conflict within her home but no indication of any history of abuse. Her presentation in the initial interview was provocative in dress and behavior, flippant, and superficially cocky. There was a great deal of posturing, deliberately offensive language, and verbal sparring to control the interaction. Youths with conduct problems are often reluctant to engage a counselor in emotionally open interactions. Their self-reports, further, may be deliberately distorted to minimize problems or exaggerate exploits. A combination of direct behavior inquiry and initial uncritical acceptance of their stories will often yield some level of productive exchange. As information accumulates, the examiner can begin to confront in a nonthreatening manner the inconsistencies in their accounts.

EXAMINER: Can you tell me about the problems that brought you into the hospital?

WINNIE: It's a lot of bull.

EXAMINER: What do you mean?

WINNIE: My mom just wanted me out of the house for awhile.

EXAMINER: What kinds of problems have you and your mom been having?

WINNIE: Nothing really.

EXAMINER: I don't understand why your mom would want you out of the house if you're not having any problems.

WINNIE: It doesn't matter.

     The interview continued in this manner for several minutes. An area of productive inquiry was developed around Winnie's conflict with several peers in school.

EXAMINER: You said there had been trouble before between you and the girl the fight was with in the rest room.

WINNIE: Yeah, Zelda's been a bitch since kindergarten. I told her to stay out of my face.

EXAMINER: What started it that morning?

WINNIE: She did. She made this whole thing about the jacket. Like it was any of her fucking business anyway.

EXAMINER: I'm lost, what jacket?

WINNIE: This leather jacket she wore to school. Her daddy gave it to her (*sarcastic*).

EXAMINER: What happened about the jacket?

WINNIE: Nothing!

EXAMINER: Wait, I thought there was some trouble between you two involving the jacket.

WINNIE: Not her jacket. My jacket. I didn't have one. I had one but it was lost. I was going to get a new one. I heard one of Zelda's little mouses (*sic*) saying something about it. And then Zelda asks me where my jacket was. Like she cared anyway.

EXAMINER: Then what happened?

WINNIE: I told her to "eat shit and die."

EXAMINER: And?

WINNIE: She told the teacher. I got another detention. But I really clubbed the snot out of her in the can. She'll still have a fat nose after I'm out of this place.

Patience and persistence can usually lead to productive information from youths with even severe conduct problems. One key is establishing an atmosphere of uncritical discussion in which the expectation is of honest disclosure. Approaching the child to help you clear up your confusion about apparent inconsistencies tends to be more productive than directly confronting them with accusations of lying, evading, and minimizing. I have found this same style continually useful in more directly "therapeutic" interactions with youth. Few of us respond well to being labeled dishonest, even when we have been distorting; the situations in which this is the most productive tactic are limited.

## Rule Adherence and Compliance

Problems with noncompliance and oppositional behavior are among the most frequent concerns about children presented by parents and teachers to mental health professionals (Wenar & Kerig, 2000; Wicks-Nelson & Isreal, 2000). Oppositional behavior is a risk factor for later disturbance in at least some children (Speltz et al., 1999). One difficulty in evaluating these concerns is that noncompliance and oppositional behavior occurs at a certain frequency and intensity in normal children; indeed, this behavior is usually considered a part of normal development (Wenar & Kerig, 2000). As Rey (1993) pointed out in his discussion of the diagnostic category of oppositional defiant disorder (ODD), the reliability of clinicians' assignment of this classification could be improved by establishing a threshold for assignment of symptom presence. Angold and Costello (1996) made a start toward this kind of classification. They published data on the frequency of ODD symptoms in a large community sample of children aged 9, 11, and 13. Their data suggest that some of the ODD symptoms (deliberately annoying others or being angry or resentful, for instance) show relatively high frequencies of occurrence, whereas others (blaming others or spiteful and vindictive behavior) have relatively low base rates in children. Based on these, Angold and Costello (1996) recommend that frequency threshold criteria be considered for the evaluation of DSM-IV symptoms of ODD. They suggest counting reported occurrences of "spiteful or vindictive" or "blames others for his or her mistakes" as positive if these problems have occurred at all in the past 3 months. The symptoms "touchy or easily annoyed," "loses temper," "argues with adults," and "defies or refuses adults' requests" are accepted as symptomatic only with reports of occurrences twice or more a week. The symptoms "angry or resentful" and "deliberately annoys others" are counted as present only with reports of occurrences four or more times per week (Angold & Costello, 1996).

Additional specificity of classification can probably be obtained by emphasizing the extent to which possible symptoms of noncompliance and oppositional behavior are associated with impairment in the child's adjustment and functioning (Rey, 1993). The fourth edition of the DSM took a similar position in emphasizing the need for potential disorders to be associated with significant personal distress or functional impairment (American Psychiatric Association, 1994, 2000). Although many children may become angry with others or annoy their parents at times, some children respond in these ways so often and intensely that the quality of their relationships is adversely affected. Indications that such a pattern has developed should raise alarm regarding the child's adjustment.

Qualitatively, there are observable differences in the oppositional behavior shown by normal and by disturbed children. Although noncompliance with adult instructions is a common occurrence in both control-group children and youths with disruptive behavior disorders, normal children tend to be selective in the commands they ignore. In the common parent–child interaction pattern of commands being repeated several times before becoming "critical," control-group children show a remarkable ability to accurately estimate how much they can get away with (see Figure 6.1). One repeated observed difference in clinically diagnosed children is their poor performance in knowing how far they can push the caretaker without consequences. Children with behavior problems may also be poor in knowledge of which commands are more important to their parents and which instructions can be ig-

| Parent | Normal child | Problem child |
|---|---|---|
| *Command* | *Noncompliance* | *Noncompliance* |
| "Joey, come pick up your game." | No response. | No response. |
| *Repeated command* | *Noncompliance* | *Noncompliance* |
| "Joey, I want you to pick up your game." | No response. | No response. |
| *Repeated command* | *Noncompliance* | *Noncompliance* |
| "Joey, I'm waiting. Come get your game." | No response. | No response. |
| *Repeated command that will be followed by a consequence* | *Compliance* | *Noncompliance* |
| "Joey, get your game or else!" | Goes to retrieve toys. | Continues ignoring and is punished. |

**FIGURE 6.1** Instruction–reaction loops between caretaker and child. In many families the history of interaction has taught children "how much they can get away with." The point at which parental commands are actually followed by consequences may vary with the number of times the command has been repeated, the nature of the request, or the mood of the parent (possibly suggested by voice tone and manner). Children without behavior problems can usually estimate very accurately at what point compliance becomes imperative if punishment is to be avoided. Children with behavior problems often are much less accurate at this discrimination. This skill difference may reflect inconsistencies in parental behavior, poor attention and learning in the child, limited reactivity by the child to usually employed consequences, or unknown influences.

nored with relative impunity. Some data suggest that youths with disruptive behavior problems may have become relatively insensitive to the consequences dispensed by their parents. An observational comparison of control-group and oppositional children by House (1975) found that the normal children were more likely to disobey commands when their mothers did not have them in view, whereas the oppositional children showed no difference in probability of compliance when their mothers could see what they were doing. Sensitivity to these types of difference can be useful when interviewing caretakers about oppositional behavior.

The use of behavior rating scales by caretakers to evaluate noncompliance and oppositional behavior is helpful because these instruments allow comparisons against the average ratings of age- and gender-matched samples. Such comparisons are absolutely essential with problems such as ADHD, in which the contributing symptoms are strongly influenced by developmental age of the child. A large number of these instruments have been developed and are available; useful examples can be found in Barkley (1998b, 1997a), as well as in the work of Conners, Siltarenios, Parker, and Epstein (1998a, 1998b). Kazdin (1995) reviews a number of measures using the reports of significant others in the evaluation of conduct disorders. I often have parents complete one or more of these types of instruments while I am initially meeting with the child. Behavior rating scales are typically brief and easily completed by parents, and they can provide a good starting point for discussion with the parents, as well as a quantified measurement of their perception of the child's actions.

Although more difficult to objectively assess than behavior patterns, the child's attitudes and perceptions are also important in understanding his or her patterns of response and rebellion. Aggressive children tend to be more sensitive to threat and to attribute more hostile intent to the actions of others. Children who engage in risky behavior tend to perceive less risk in their actions than more cautious children (Hillier & Morrongiello, 1998; Morrongiello & Rennie, 1998). My experience is that children who are more likely to disobey and violate standing rules see fewer consequences as likely to follow from these transgressions. In some homes this perception may be factually accurate—the parents are not effective at reliably providing differential consequences to the children based on behavior. In other homes there may actually be a history of reasonable monitoring and reacting differentially to actions of the children, but the child with behavior problems seems relatively oblivious to this. Asking the youth a few questions such as "What happens when you don't do as you are told? What happened the last time you did [a prohibited behavior]?" can be illuminating with respect to the child's view of his or her world.

## Behavior Control

The relationship between deficiencies in executive functioning and problems with hyperactive and oppositional behavior is becoming a major theme in conceptualizations of disruptive behavior disorders. Barkley (1997b, 2000) has articulated a model for ADHD in which executive dysfunction plays a central role. Problems in executive functioning are more closely related to difficulties in interpersonal relationships in young, "hard-to-manage" children than is empathy with peers or emotional understanding (Hughes, White, Sharpen, & Dunn, 2000). Executive function difficulties have also been implicated in conduct disorders (Moffit, 1993). Despite the apparent relevance, findings in the search for a link between executive functions and disruptive behavior disorders have been negative (Leung & Connolly, 1998; Wiers, Gunning, & Sergeant, 1998). One difficulty in this literature is that there is no agreed-on definition of executive functions nor a well-accepted set of standardized measures to capture the variable (Wiers et al., 1998). Part of the challenge is the very nature of "executive functions"—metacognitive activity directed toward planning for the achievement of selected purposes, carrying out these plans, utilizing feedback for persistence and/or self-correction, and verification of final results. Above-average executive functions may be a potent protective factor in youth; below-average executive functions appear to be a major risk factor. Some understanding of the child's cognitive maturity may be gained from observations of purposeful planning, goal-directed persistence, active utilization of feedback, and abstract thinking; from caretaker reports of such activities; and from more formal measures, such as the Tower of London (Shallice, 1982) or the Wisconsin Card Sorting Test (Heaton, 1981).

On a more general level, lower general intelligence appears to be a risk factor for children with disruptive behavior disorders (Aman, Pejeau, Osborne, & Rojahn, 1996). Higher intelligence may be a positive prognostic indication.

## Interview Segment 6.3. Macon W

Macon was a 10-year-old boy with a history of serious antisocial behavior (House & Stambaugh, 1979). He illustrated many aspects of youths with early onset conduct disorders, including a set of cognitive beliefs and attitudes that tended to inhibit his receptivity to change. Macon also showed good verbal skills, had above-average tested intelligence, and was usually cooperative in discussing his view of the world—features not usually characteristic of the unsocialized–unaggressive pattern of conduct disorders that he otherwise exemplified. Although his behavior control improved relatively rapidly under a token economy, his worldview remained chilling for some time.

EXAMINER: So, how has your program been going?

MACON: It's OK. I like being able to get out of surveillance. [Purchasing periods of time off "constant observation" was an option Macon could purchase in the reinforcement economy he was under.]

EXAMINER: The nurses have been a lot happier with your behavior this week.

MACON: Yeah, I guess. They're all right.

EXAMINER: Several seem to have taken quite a liking to you. They are really interested in how you are doing.

MACON: Yeah, well, you know, they get paid.

EXAMINER: Do you think that's all they care for?

MACON: Well, sure. What else would they care about?

EXAMINER: Helping people? There were probably lots of jobs they could have had other than nursing.

MACON: Sure! I mean, get real. They're losers. If they could do better, they would.

EXAMINER: You really don't think they would be doing this if they were able to get better jobs?

MACON: Well, no. I mean, I know I'm supposed to say so, but you said we could be real. All that helping people stuff is crap. Everyone is just looking out for themselves. You wouldn't be here if you weren't getting paid.

EXAMINER: Well, I am getting paid, but some internships are unfunded. I don't know if I could have taken this position without some funding, but I would probably be somewhere.

MACON: Yeah, you might have, but it's just so you can rake in the big bucks later. At least you're not a fool, trying to "do good and help others."

EXAMINER: Sorry, I am one of those fools.

MACON: Oh, no. Not that crap. I thought you were different. This hasn't been like all those other counselors I saw. You don't put up with any shit. Are you going to start ragging me about the golden rule?

EXAMINER: Not right now. But I am interested in what you think. Don't you believe that anyone ever does things just to help someone else out?

MACON: I guess. No. I don't. You look out for yourself. That's what's real. There's always an angle.

EXAMINER: What about when you stood up to the bully, the one who picked on your sister? What was your angle?

MACON: That's different. She's blood. OK, maybe you would for your family, but for other people, no way. That's not real. No one really cares about what's good for someone else. You care about what's good for you. So do I. There's no difference.

## Life Circumstances

A final area of great importance in evaluation of the youth with a disruptive behavior disorder is his or her psychosocial environment and the available emotional support for prosocial and antisocial behavior. Patterson (Patterson, 1982; Patterson et al., 1992) has carried out extensive investigations on the family circumstances associated with conduct problems in youths. His findings have been consistent with a broad empirical literature showing an association between conduct problems in youths and a pattern of impaired parental behavior—poor monitoring of children's behavior, inconsistent discipline, and an overreliance on coercive methods of control. Antisocial behavior in family members is a negative prognostic variable for children with ADHD (Faraone, Biederman, Mennin, Russell, & Tsuang, 1998), as is parental substance abuse. In addition to evaluating the difficulties of the youth with a behavior disorder, we should also assess the environment in which the child is functioning and the behaviors these settings act to encourage. It is also important to be cognizant of research that suggests that raters may systematically underestimate the psychosocial adversity of children with ADHD relative to their evaluations of family conflict in children with conduct disorders (Overmeyer, Taylor, Blanz, & Schmidt, 1999). Although it is a relatively new instrument, there may be great potential clinical utility in the Risk and Protective Factors Scale developed by Looper and Grizenko (1999) for evaluation of youths with disruptive behavior disorders.

In evaluating adolescents with conduct problems, we need to bear in mind the relationships between conduct difficulties and other risky behavior. Conduct disorder in females is a risk factor for adolescent pregnancy (Zoccolillo, Meyers, & Assiter, 1997). Being prematurely thrust into the role of parent layers additional psychosocial demands on young people who are already struggling to maintain adjustment. For both females and males, impulsive and unprotected sexual activity exposes youths to the risk of disease and other complications from their behavior that can add to the difficulties they face in their daily lives.

## DIFFERENTIATION OF DIAGNOSTIC CATEGORIES

Differential diagnosis among disruptive behavior disorders can present an evaluation challenge for the examiner. ADHD is frequently comorbid with ODD and with conduct disorder. In my experience, very few children who meet DSM-IV criteria for ADHD do not also meet criteria for ODD. This differential is important because the absence of comorbid diagnoses is a good prognostic feature. Conversely, the presence of problem aggression, as is the case in most children who show both ADHD and conduct disorder, is an important negative prognostic feature for children with ADHD. Most children who meet the criteria for conduct disorder concurrently meet criteria for ODD, and for this reason the DSM-IV criteria preclude the diagnosis of concurrent ODD once a diagnosis of conduct disorder is satisfied. Alternatives to the DSM-IV diagnostic criteria for disruptive behavior problems have been proposed and may have utility under some circumstances. Barkley (1990) proposed diagnostic criteria to be used in addition to the DSM-III-R criteria to identify children showing ADHD symptoms, which are "developmentally deviant, pervasive across situations, and developmentally stable" (p. 174). Some of Barkley's recommended additions are reflected in the changes that took place in DSM-IV, but his suggestion that scores at least 1.5 standard deviations above the mean on standardized behavior rating scales be required still represents a more con-

## Interview Segment 6.4. Winnie at 16: "It Just Hurts"

Winnie was readmitted to the hospital a year later. A moderately serious suicide attempt precipitated the admission. Her behavior problems had continued largely unabated since her previous admission. Careful inquiry revealed that she had been sexually assaulted while drunk at a house party a couple of weeks prior to her suicide attempt.

The denial, avoidance, and bravado of youth with conduct disorders can hide the degree of anxiety, fear, and distress they often experience. Although some acting-out children completely lack emotional reactions to the events of their lives, most show a mixture of both externalizing and internalizing symptoms. Their defiance of rules and conventions, deviant peer associations, and other behavior problems also often place them at risk for victimization, exploitation, assaults, and other traumatizing experiences. As Patterson (1982) has noted, the child who most frequently hurts others tends, in turn, to be the most hurt by others also. It sometimes requires discipline to remind ourselves that the adolescent who has terrorized others without apparent remorse can experience perfectly normal emotions in response to his or her own mistreatment.

EXAMINER: What happened afterward?

WINNIE: They all left. I laid there awhile. It was quiet, so I got up and found my clothes and went out the back. I just walked around a long time and then went home.

EXAMINER: You must have been feeling really hurt.

WINNIE: I was just numb. I didn't want to think about it ever again. I got in the shower at home until all the hot water was gone. I was standing in the shower freezing but I just wanted to stay there and never get out. My mom came in, she knew something was wrong. She saw the bruises and started asking me questions. I just wanted to disappear (*crying*). . . .

EXAMINER: What was it like on Monday, back at school?

WINNIE: It was like being in a dream. I don't remember anything, until I passed Chad in the hall. He acted like nothing had happened. I just stared at him, and then my teeth started to chatter, and then I started shaking. I dropped my books. Everybody was looking at me. The next thing I knew I was in the nurse's office. I heard her call the hospital. That was when I broke the glass and cut my arm.

EXAMINER: What were you feeling then?

WINNIE: I wanted to die. I never wanted to come here again or talk about any of this ever again.

EXAMINER: How about now?

WINNIE: I don't know. Maybe.

The evaluator continued to assess both Winnie's symptoms of depression and her suicide risk, as well as symptoms of acute stress disorder secondary to her assault. Although the causal pathways between conduct problems and emotional disturbances of anxiety and depression continue to be explored, the mental health evaluator needs to remain vigilant to the frequent comorbidity in young people.

---

servative criterion than that of DSM-IV. As inevitably occurs when a diagnostic criterion is changed in a more conservative/restrictive direction, the results of adopting such additional standards would be that (1) a smaller population of children would be identified as showing ADHD, (2) this smaller population would show a higher average level of impairment than was the case in the original population of identified children, and (3) the new population will be more homogeneous in characteristics.

A more recent alternative diagnostic conceptualization of ADHD, based on a signal detection analysis of diagnosis, has been suggested by Mota and Schachar (2000). They suggest a diagnostic algorithm for ADHD (without considering subtypes) based on the optimal sensitivity and specificity of the DSM-IV diagnostic symptoms. They point out that not all symptoms are equally informative and that using a receiver operating characteristics (ROC) analysis allows selection of the most effective combinations of symptoms for diagnosis. Their analysis suggests that the indication in a teacher's report of any of the following symptoms may be indicative of ADHD: avoiding tasks requiring sustained mental effort, often losing things necessary for activities, or having difficulty waiting for one's turn. In their analysis of parents' reports they found that the combination of one symptom from each of two four-item clusters optimally classifies children. Cluster 1 comprises the following symptoms: having difficulty sustaining attention in tasks, avoiding tasks that require sustained mental effort, being forgetful, and blurting out responses. Cluster 2 comprises the following symptoms: not listening when spoken to directly, not following through on directions, having difficulty organizing tasks and activities, and talking excessively. Mota and Schachar (2000) note the predominance of symptoms of inattention in both parent and teacher ROC algorithms. This dominance of distractibility symptoms would seem to be a potential difficulty, given other findings that suggest the relative nonspecificity of inattention problems in disturbed children (Halperin et al., 1992). Nonetheless, the examiner of children might find it productive to be especially sensitive to the symptoms highlighted by Mota and Schachar (2000) in detecting potential cases of attention deficits and hyperactivity in children.

## THE ISSUE OF COMORBIDITY

Comorbidity of behavior problems of behavior problems with other emotional and cognitive difficulties is the rule rather than the exception for youths (Lewinsohn, Rohde, & Seeley, 1995). It is unusual to encounter children and adolescents who meet the criteria for only a single mental disorder. Most youths who meet criteria for one mental disorder will concurrently meet the criteria for other disorders. The theoretical and applied questions and implications of the high level of comorbidity between diagnostic categories in youths are many, and go well beyond the purposes of the present discussion. A few practical consequences, however, require attention. The first has already been stated: Comorbidity of problems is common. Some diagnostic systems encourage comorbid diagnoses (DSM), some tend to discourage comorbid diagnoses (ICD), some may preclude comorbid classifications (IDEA); but the children usually do present with multiple difficulties. As evaluators we need to remain aware that our job is not necessary concluded because we have identified "a problem"; there may be multiple problems. A second practical consequence is that comorbidity is associated with increased morbidity of impairment (Babinski et al., 1999; Gresham, MacMillan, Bocian, Ward, & Forness, 1998; Spencer et al., 1998), as well as increased utilization of mental health services and increased difficulty with intervention (Stahl & Clarizio, 1999). Multiple problems are common "out there" in the everyday world of youth, and they are even more common among that limited sample of troubled children who find themselves in our offices. Combinations of problems often reflect more serious clinical presentations and adjustment impairment (Hinshaw & Anderson, 1996). In addition, multiple problems can greatly complicate our efforts to provide services; the number and duration of services necessary may vary with comorbidity (Stahl & Clarizio, 1999).

As noted elsewhere in this book, comorbidity is especially likely among children who show one of the disruptive behavior disorders. Among the disruptive behavior disorders ADHD and conduct disorder as well as ADHD and ODD are frequently comorbid. Approximately 25% of children with ODD will develop conduct disorder (which then supersedes the ODD diagnosis). ADHD, conduct disorder, and ODD are often comorbid with learning disorders, speech and language disorders, and other cognitive and developmental problems. In adolescence, ADHD and conduct disorder are often cormorbid with substance abuse and sometimes substance dependence. Further, conduct disorder and ADHD also show comorbidity with affective disorders during adolescence, including bipolar disorder (Biederman et al., 1999a; Pliszka et al., 2000). A history of bipolar disorder in one or both parents of a child identified as showing ADHD may be a potent risk factor for development of bipolar disorder in the child (Faraone et al., 1997; Sachs, Baldassano, Truman, & Guille, 2000). Finally, gender may be an important modulating variable for comorbidity. Keenan and Loeber (Loeber & Keenan, 1994; Keenan, Loeber, & Green, 1999) have called attention to the heightened risk for comorbid adjustment difficulties in girls with conduct disorder, especially for internalizing pattern problems.

Disentangling positive correlations between behavior problems can be challenging, especially with multiple comorbidities. Both early conduct problems and early ADHD, for instance, are positively correlated with later substance use problems (as well as with each other). It increasingly appears that the relationship between early ADHD and adolescent substance use problems is entirely mediated by the association between conduct problems and ADHD. Based on their New Zealand sample, Lynskey and Fergusson (1995) suggest that attention-deficit problems, absent conduct disorder, show little association with later substance abuse; early conduct problems, however, do function as a risk factor for later substance use difficulty. Conversely, although both conduct disorder and ADHD are associated with academic underachievement, the relationship between conduct disorder and academic failure seems largely mediated by the comorbidity between conduct disorder and ADHD—ADHD is a primary risk factor for scholastic underachievement; conduct disorder (in the absence of ADHD) is not (Frick et al., 1991; Hinshaw, 1992). The use of multivariate statistics and large samples is slowly changing the face of what we "know" about disruptive behavior problems. With the emerging empirical database, the individual practitioner can be increasingly confident over the coming decade in the profession's understanding of the basic pathways to behavior problems in youths.

Disruptive behavior disorders show frequent comorbidity not only with other externalizing behavior problems but also with internalizing problems such as anxiety and depression. Children with ADHD or conduct problems may also show excessive fears, worry, dysphoria, or social withdrawal. These emotional manifestations may appear to be reactions to the behavioral conflicts with parents and teachers or seemingly independent problems that wax and wane according to their own schedules. The functional pathways between disruptive behavior patterns and comorbid disturbances of anxiety, depression, and somatization are only beginning to be understood. What is clear at this point is that many of the children who have difficulty conforming their behavior to external expectations are also at risk for emotional distress and suffering. These emotional problems may or may not cross the threshold, justifying additional mental health diagnoses. If the criterion for other DSM-IV diagnoses are met, these additional classifications should be made. But falling short of a diagnostic criterion does not eliminate these issues from the child's life. The comprehensive formulation of the youth's situation is enriched by attention to mood and affective responses, and these may prove especially useful in treatment planning and implementation.

A particularly difficult comorbidity to unravel is the association discussed in the last chapter between ADHD and bipolar phenomena. The prevalence of diagnoses of bipolar mood disorder in adolescents and young adults who were classified as children with ADHD is greater than would be expected and suggests an association between these problems. How best to understand this association is the subject of ongoing study and debate. Are some childhood cases of apparent ADHD really unrecognized juvenile manifestations of bipolar I or II disorder? Is childhood ADHD a risk factor for later bipolar disorder? Are some cases of apparent bipolar disorder in adolescents or adults misdiagnosed residual cases of disruptive behavior disorders? Do both ADHD and bipolar disorder share common genetic or environmental risk factors? We do not yet have confident answers to these and related questions. It does appear that bipolar disorders occur in adolescents and children and frequently go unrecognized and undiagnosed. Some of these cases may be misidentified as ADHD or disruptive behavior disorder not otherwise specified, in part because of the symptom overlap in the diagnostic criteria for ADHD and hypomanic syndromes. As reviewed previously, Geller and her coworkers have used a classification protocol that minimizes the overlap between these phenomena by requiring elation or grandiosity as one criterion (Geller et al., 1998, 2000a, 2000b, 2001). The evaluator can also be suspicious of apparent ADHD that appears to worsen and remit unrelated to interventions or environmental circumstances. A family history of mood disorder, especially bipolar disorder, should raise the possibility of a previously unrecognized mood disorder in the youth. A poor response to typically efficacious treatments for ADHD, to pharmacotherapy with central-nervous-system-stimulant medications, or to a well-executed behavior modification program should prompt a review of the diagnostic formulation. Finally, there remains the possibility of a true comorbidity—some children with ADHD appear to also develop a bipolar disorder. Their ADHD symptoms tend to be stable and pervasive, and their mood cycles are superimposed on this background. It is difficult to accurately assess and to effectively treat such behavior problems.

As a general position, the evaluator should remain suspicious of "simple" presentations of a single behavior problem until it is clear that there are no associated difficulties. I have repeatedly found that a continuing, careful evaluation and review of problems until all major areas of functioning and difficulty have been covered is a highly useful assessment strategy.

## EVALUATION OF EXTERNALIZING BEHAVIOR IN SPECIAL POPULATIONS

### Diagnostic Assessment in the Very Young

An ever-increasing consideration in the evaluation of behavior problems in youths concerns the assessment of these problems in very young children. Both the empirical literature (Patterson, 1982) and clinical experiences suggest that disruptive behavior problems may begin very early in life. Age of onset is an important prognostic variable in conduct problems. These considerations focus attention on indications of emerging behavior problems in the preschool child. Thomas and Clark (1998) provide a thought-provoking discussion of the application of the Zero to Three (Zero to Three/National Center for Clinical Infant Programs, 1994) modification of the DSM-IV classification system to assessment of disruptive behavior problems in very young children. There seems to be clear potential for clinically useful conceptualizations in this approach to early childhood evaluation. At the same time, the evaluator needs to be sensitive to the potential for stigmatization of youths who do not have a diagnosable condition. Although it appears undeniable that very young children who are at a statistical extreme for disobedience, rule breaking, and "aggression" are at risk for later classification with a conduct disorder, it is also true that this prediction would have less than perfect accuracy and that most of the "diagnostic" observations would, considered in isolation, be clearly "within the normal range." As is frequently the case, caution and humility are highly recommended in evaluations of very young children.

Distinct from the evaluation of identified behavior problems in the very young child is the assessment of early temperamental differences in youths that may contribute to their risk for later behavior problems. Consistent with the report of many parents, the findings of investigators suggest that some of these young people have been different from their age peers from the very earliest years. The continuing interest in possible early temperamental differences between children who come to be classified as showing a behavior problem and their relatively problem-free age peers contributes to one effort at understanding possible etiological factors to these cases. As in the case of anxiety disorders, disruptive behavior problems do not spring into existence without precursor phenomena. Establishment of early behavior patterns is also important for the disruptive behavior disorders because of the need to document early onset of at least some symptoms for certain diagnoses (at least some symptoms of ADHD must be evident prior to age 7) or subclassifications (the childhood-onset type of conduct disorder requires at least one symptom evident prior to age 10). When informants are available who had direct experience with the youth during his or her first few years of life, the evaluator should spend a few minutes exploring with them early personality features that may have contributed to the child's current difficulties (see Practice Note 6.2).

## Evaluation of Adolescents with ADHD

With increasing recognition that ADHD can be a lifelong disorder, there has been a corresponding increase in the presentation of adolescents for evaluation with respect to ADHD. The motor overactivity that may have made it impossible for the youth to stay in his or her seat in

**Practice Note 6.2. Inquiry into Early Temperament: Accommodation and Compliance**

Disruptive behavior disorders often emerge from an early history of disorganized and noncompliant behavior. When caretakers from the child's earliest years are available, you should attempt some evaluation of the youth's early temperament. A few questions will help provide a context in which later and/or current problems can be considered.

**Interview probes for sustained attention and organization**

*Preliminary*: Establish to your confidence that the respondent was regularly involved in the youth's life during his or her first 2 to 4 years (unless already done).

"Whom did Marie live with after she was first born? Who was around?"

*Preliminary*: Set all questions in the context of the first 2 to 4 years of life.

"I would like to ask you some questions about what Marie was like as a baby and toddler."

*General temperament probes* (unless already done):

"What was Marie like as an infant? As a very young child, when she was just walking? What do you remember about her mood? About her curiosity? About how sociable and loving she was?"

*General behavioral organization probe:*

"As an infant and toddler, what was Marie's play like? How did she occupy herself?"

*Specific behavioral organization probes:*

"Compared with other infants and toddlers, could Marie keep herself entertained?"

"Compared with other infants and toddlers, could Marie sit through a meal?"

*Specific compliance probes:*

"Compared with other infants and toddlers, did you have a lot of trouble getting Marie to mind you?"

"Compared with other infants and toddlers, did Marie get into a lot of trouble?"

*Specific aggression probes:*

> "Compared with other infants and toddlers, did Marie get into fights with other children often?"
>
> "How did Marie react when you punished her?"

*Critical event probes:* If previous interviewing had not already established the presence or absence of critical events during the first 5 years of life, these questions should be addressed:

> "Was Marie ever abused or mistreated as an infant or child? What can you tell me about this?"
>
> "Was Marie ever treated with medication for her behavior as a child? Tell me about that."

---

elementary school has probably modulated to some degree. He or she can probably sit through high school classes, although it needs to be determined how much learning is occurring. The youth may show subtler signs of motor restlessness—fidgeting, shifting postures, handling objects on the desk, or touching himself and objects. His or her capacity for sustained attention continues to be below normal relative to age peers, although it is probably better than it was at younger ages. Impulsivity and difficulty with organization and planning usually continues to create significant problems in his or her life. Because many adolescents may complain (or be complained about) regarding distractibility, restlessness, and especially impulsivity, it is important to establish the functional impairment caused by these characteristics in the young person's life. Given the high comorbidities reported between ADHD and mood and anxiety disorders, the examiner needs to carefully review possible affective problems. Similarly, possible substance use and other "risky behavior" (unprotected sex, reckless driving) need to be evaluated carefully. Adolescents with ADHD are at higher risk than normal-age peers for automotive moving violations and accidents (Barkley, Guevrement, Anastopoulus, DuPaul, & Shelton, 1993). Interview probes such as those in Practice Note 6.3 may be productive.

## Evaluation of Youths in the Juvenile Justice System

Delinquency is a legal term referring to youths who have come into conflict with the laws of their community. Delinquency can be "identi-

**Practice Note 6.3. Sample Questions for Interviewing Teenagers about Symptoms Associated with ADHD**

"Let me ask you some questions about how you are doing at things, compared with other people your age at school. How do you do at keeping your mind on jobs? Has that caused you problems? How about keeping your mind on your schoolwork? How has that affected your grades?"

"How are you at sticking with things you are doing, compared with the other people you know? How has that made a difference in your life? Do you ever avoid doing things that require you to really 'keep at it?' Tell me about that."

"How are you at planning things out, so that you know what you're going to do before you start something? How has that worked out?"

"How organized do you keep your belongings, compared with your friends? How much trouble have you had finding things you need or losing things? Has this been more of a problem for you than for other people you know?"

"Compared with the other kids, do you take a lot of chances? Tell me about that. Has anything bad ever happened or almost happened because you took chances? Tell me about that."

"Have you started to smoke? How about your friends?"
"Have you started to drink alcohol? How about your friends?"
"Have you started to drive? What's your driving record like?"
"Have you started to have sex? Do you use protection every time?"
"Have you ever taken a drug even when you didn't know exactly what it was?"
"Have you ever done things on a dare that you knew were stupid or risky? Tell me about that."

fied" or "hidden" (undetected), "alleged" or "adjudicated," and can be based on felonies, misdemeanors, or "status offenses" (acts that are illegal solely on the basis of the individual's age—e.g., buying cigarettes). Delinquency could be based on a single act, a series of related acts, or a habitual criminal lifestyle. The topic of delinquency is vast and of great importance to our society, but it is largely outside the scope of this book, except for the fact that many delinquents have mental health problems. Grisso, Barnum, Fletcher, Cauffman, and Peuschold (2001) cite unpublished data from Teplin, Abram, and McClelland suggesting that up to 70–80% of youths in the juvenile justice system have mental disorders if conduct disorder and substance abuse disorders are included and that 40–50% still have mental health diagnoses when these two categories are excluded. High rates of mood disorders, such as major depression and bipolar disorder, have been reported in incarcerated samples of adolescents (McManus, Akessi, Grapentine, & Brickman, 1984; Pliszka et al., 2000). Posttraumatic stress disorders may be especially likely in female juvenile incarcerated offenders (Cauffman, Feldman, Waterman, & Steiner, 1998). Finally, substance abuse disorders may have a strong association with recidivism in adolescent offender populations (Kataoka et al., 2001).

Because of the high base rate of psychiatric disorders in juvenile offenders and the prognostic significance of emotional and behavior disorders, especially substance abuse for juvenile offenders, these populations frequently merit a mental health evaluation. A younger age at first arrest, repeat offenses, and arrest for more serious offenses increase the likelihood of a referral for mental health evaluation and treatment (Kataoka et al., 2001). The increase in violent crimes among female offenders has led to more attention being paid to mental health issues in this group (Kataoka et al., 2001). Grisso and colleagues (2001) have developed a screening questionnaire to assist in the evaluation of youth in the criminal justice system, the Massachusetts Youth Screening Instrument—Second Version (MAYSI-2).

Psychological evaluation of youths within the criminal justice system is complicated by the immediate situational contingencies. Their cooperation, or at least superficial compliance, is usually high, due directly to the powerful and aversive consequences that will probably follow overt rebelliousness. Their openness and forthrightness, unfortunately, is often low—there is the real possibility (from their perspective) that honesty on their part may complicate their lives. The mental health evaluator in this setting needs to be especially careful to communicate clearly the limits of any perceived confidentiality in the relationship. My experience has been that cooperation usually appears to increase when an effort is made to be direct and open with the youth about who will have access to the information being requested. This cooperation may occur for several reasons. First, it is likely to be congruent with the youth's own assessment of the situation. Second, a good case can usually be made that cooperation with the evaluation has greater potential to help than hurt the youth's ambitions. Finally, there may be a certain "novel appeal" to dealing with an adult who is objectively honest and straightforward with the young person. Although assessing populations of offending adolescents can confront the examiner with unique challenges and frustrations, it is possible and often greatly needed.

# 7 Evaluating Relationship Problems in Youths

$S$ocial relationships are among the most important and defining features of human behavior. Responding to social cues, interacting with another person, and learning how to make and keep friendships are some of the critical developmental tasks that challenge almost all of us during our formative years. Difficulties in social relationships can have a pervasive effect on the quality and character of our lives. Problematic peer relationships during childhood, for instance, place youths at risk for a wide range of negative outcomes in adolescence and adulthood (Woodward & Fergusson, 2000). Understanding the social world of a child or adolescent provides one of the most useful foundations for understanding his or her strengths and challenges of adjustment.

The developmental literature suggests that infants show individual differences in temperament early in life and that these characteristics interact with characteristics of their families to contribute to the growing child's unique personality and functioning. Very basic aspects of our nature, such as the regularity of our biological rhythms, the average intensity of our reactions to events, our adaptability, and our prevalent mood all act to color our behavioral responses to events and learning experiences. The attachment between caretaker and child that is necessary for normal development grows out of the interaction between the needs, feelings, and actions of each member of the dyad. Extroversion, our need for stimulation, especially social contact and engagement, appears probably to be at least partially determined by our genetic inheritance. We can learn to be social; it is less clear to what extent we can learn to *want* to be social. Our fundamental capacity to appreciate another person's perspective, our empathy for their needs and feelings, is shaped by our learning history but may also have its roots in a biological predisposition that has served our species over its development. Child and adolescents, just as much as the rest of us, are in many ways unique and distinctive; the basis of this individuality may stem from characteristics that are only partially mutable, if at all.

Yet if some aspects of our social presentation develop out of biological processes that alter little over our lives, it is nevertheless clear that most social action is learned. Human beings are the most behaviorally adaptive organisms on our world, and much of the adaptation reflects our responsiveness to social contingencies, models, expectations, and beliefs. We all may, to some degree, be "hardwired" to socially interact just as we may be neurologically prepared to use a symbolic communication system; but the content of that interaction, like our native language, is filled in by the experience of social teaching and learning within our society and culture. We learn how to interact with others to fulfill our various needs and desires; we learn problem solving and social skills to sustain our relationships; we form our very identity in the context of our social relationships (Vygotsky, 1962, 1978). Leadership, assertiveness, persuasiveness, altruism, kindness, responsibility, entrepreneurship, and other aspects of personality exist only in a social dimension, as do violence, rebelliousness, exploitation, prejudice, and jealousy. But some children may show problems in forming, managing, and sustaining relationships.

It is worth considering that in all aspects of development it is typically the interaction between multiple variables which yields the final manifestation in behavior. Attachment and self-esteem in children, for instance, appear to be sensitive to the child's emerging developmental level—early neuromotor impairments can apparently contribute to emotional conflict with the potential for disrupting interpersonal relations (Wintgens et al., 1998). As much as we all at times desperately desire the universe to be a simple place of straightforward and unidirectional influences, the reality is that the universe is complex, and human social behavior is on the first tier of multidetermined phenomena.

## PROBLEMS IN FORMING RELATIONSHIPS

### Shyness

Children and adolescents may have difficulty in establishing satisfactory and reciprocal social relationships due to social anxiety. Fear of rejection, humiliation, and embarrassment is not an unusual problem in our society, and the evidence is that often such difficulties begin early in life. The extreme manifestations of such problems are social phobia and avoidant personality disorder. These are internalizing syndromes, and evaluation for them should follow the general outlines covered in Chapter 5. The differentiation of acute clinical syndromes that reflect excessive anxiety (social phobia or subclinical problems with peer or family relationships) and enduring and pervasive patterns of worry and threat sensitivity (avoidant personality disorder and high trait anxiety) is often difficult, and this diagnostic distinction may ultimately prove to have little validity. Specific anxiety syndromes in children are often embedded in a context of chronic high arousal and reactivity of negative affect. Understanding specific symptoms may be much easier if the child's overall pattern of response is appreciated, as with the case of Brannan in Interview Segment 7.1.

## Aloofness

A very different clinical picture from that of the shy, socially anxious child is presented in the youth with true schizoid characteristics. A small fraction of the human species does not appear to experience a primary drive toward social affiliation and gregariousness. As with shyness, these characteristics seem to arise early in life, but the intrapersonal dynamic is entirely different. The young people are not worried about rejection or fearful of embarrassment in interpersonal encounters, they are simply not strongly motivated to participate in social activities. During childhood they will often tolerate a certain amount of interpersonal activity because it is encouraged by their parents, teachers, and other agents of society. Schizoid youths often seem to accept the path of least resistance until they are in a position to make their own choices—then their own preferences become quite evident. They choose to spend large amounts of time alone or in only superficial interactions with others; they choose solitary activities and vocations; and they usually do not choose to seek counseling to change their preferences.

Clinically, the socially anxious and socially schizoid youth may present with a similar history—both having few friends, largely isolated, and probably showing social skill deficits related to their limited social interaction. The critical distinction is their experience of this state of affairs and their motivation to change their relationships. The shy child would like to have friends but is frightened of the activities involved in

**Interview Segment 7.1. Help Me Understand**

One difficult aspect of evaluating relationship difficulties with children and adolescents is that the topic is much more complex than most other areas of inquiry. Simply eliciting the factual history of actions, characters, and roles is important but does not answer the most basic questions of human adjustment; these depend more on perception, interpretation, and meaning. The reciprocal interactions of human social behavior are difficult to reduce to a handful of data points, and youths may lack the vocabulary to express their feelings, motivations, and attitudes. The phenomenological approach of George Kelly has much to recommend it in making sense of this complicated and subtle dance of emotion and act. Kelly (1955) stressed the value of assessment that works to help us understand the world as it is perceived by the client instead of insisting that the client be understood through the lens of our cognitive constructs. In more formal assessments, his repertory grid technique can be very useful in mapping out the social–psychological worldview of the client. But even in brief initial evaluations, there is great value in remembering that it may be helpful to try to understand things from the perspective of the child.

Brannan was an 8-year-old whose parents had been divorced since very early in his life. Despite rather intense personal animosity between them, both parents had struggled to keep their son removed from their problems and to cooperate in matters of his rearing. Brannan had always known two homes, two bedrooms, two sets of toys, and two loving parents—one in each home. Both parents attended his games, school parents' nights, teacher conferences, and birthday parties. The announcement by his father that he was planning to remarry took both Brannan and his mother by surprise. Shortly thereafter, Brannan developed some somatic symptoms, which led his pediatrician to refer him for psychological evaluation.

EXAMINER: Brannan, you're really been a big help this evening. Thank you for helping me get a picture of what your week was like. Now as I understand it, you usually get sick when you're staying with your dad.

BRANNAN: Sometimes.

EXAMINER: Right. The three times this past week were all at your dad's house.

BRANNAN: I like staying at my dad's house.

EXAMINER: Yes, you and your dad seem to have a good time when you stay there. (*Brannan nods.*) And you get your chores done. (*Brannan nods.*) And your homework done. (*Brannan squirms.*)

BRANNAN: Most of the time.

EXAMINER: Right, most of the time. You enjoy spending time with your dad, the two of you have fun and also get things done when you need to. (*Brannan nods.*) And you like being at your mom's house (*Brannan nods*) and doing things with her. (*Brannan nods.*) And your parents like coming to your activities and sharing special times with you. (*Brannan nods and smiles.*) I guess the one person I don't know much about yet is your father's fiancée.

BRANNAN: (*change of voice tone*) His girlfriend.

EXAMINER: Yes, his girlfriend. How long have you known her?

BRANNAN: I don't know. Always. She was never around much until last year. Now she comes to things and we have dinner with her.

EXAMINER: What do you call her?

BRANNAN: Dad's girlfriend. (*conspiratorial voice*) Mom calls her "your father's friend." Once I heard her call her a bad name when she was arguing with Dad on the telephone.

EXAMINER: Yes, sometimes adults get angry with one another. Sometimes they say things they shouldn't. Do you ever do that?

BRANNAN: (*cautiously*) Sometimes.

EXAMINER: Me, too. Sometimes I've said things and then later I feel bad about what I said.

BRANNAN: Why?

EXAMINER: Oh, different reasons. Often because I'm mad or my feelings have been hurt. Sometimes because I get jealous or cranky. Sometimes because I'm tired or don't feel well.

BRANNAN: Oh.

EXAMINER: What do you call *your father's friend* when you are talking to her?

BRANNAN: (*Smiles.*) She told me I could call her Rosemary. Dad says I should call her Ms. Ryner.

EXAMINER: Oh, that kind of sticks you in the middle, doesn't it?

BRANNAN: Yeah, she's pretty nice but I wish she wasn't around so much.

EXAMINER: What does she do that's nice?

BRANNAN: She's pretty good at listening to me, even when Dad's in the room. Sometimes he just talks to her, and she doesn't forget I'm there.

EXAMINER: That sounds pretty nice. What else?

BRANNAN: She's funny, and Dad laughs a lot when she's around. I like that.

EXAMINER: You really care a lot about both your parents.

BRANNAN: (*No reply.*)

EXAMINER: That's probably part of why it's so hard knowing what to do about Rosemary.

BRANNAN: Yeah.

EXAMINER: And Rosemary's working hard to stay out of the "evil stepmother" role.

BRANNAN: Yeah. (*Smiles.*)

EXAMINER: We could call her E.S. for short.

BRANNAN: We shouldn't do that. (*Laughs.*)

EXAMINER: I suppose not. What do you call Rosemary when you're talking to your mom?

BRANNAN: (*Shifts in chair.*) Dad's friend.

EXAMINER: I'm guessing you don't bring up Rosemary much when you're talking to your mom.

BRANNAN: Mom gets sad sometimes.

---

making friends. The schizoid child is usually relatively content with his or her limited interpersonal world and has little real interest in seeing things change.

## PROBLEMS IN MANAGING AND SUSTAINING RELATIONSHIPS

### Social Skill Deficits

Social skill difficulties are common across a wide range of cognitive, behavioral, and emotional problems of adjustment in youth. Any mental health problem that limits the child's social interaction with peers carries a risk of associated delays in social learning, because it is in the context of peer interactions that children's social skills are shaped. At least a portion of the morbidity associated with a quite disparate range of disorders, from ADHD to gender identity problems, appears to derive from the social skill difficulties associated with the disorders. Ignorance of social cues, mores, and patterns and ineptitude in dealing with common social situations can lead to negative interactions and peer rejection.

Not surprising given the complexity of the subject area, valid assessment of social skills is a challenging problem (Sheridan, Hungelmann, & Maughan, 1999). Much of the research literature on social skills derives from work with middle-class caucasian children (Feng & Cartledge, 1996). The work of Fantuzzo and colleagues (1995, 1998a, 1998b) provides a good model for developing ecologically valid measures of social competence for groups of children from diverse cultural and economic backgrounds, but a great deal more work needs to be done. The assessment of social skills in young females also raises challenging questions for the evaluator (Henning-Stout, 1998). Even in traditional populations (principally male) with high base-rate problems (conduct difficulties), the evaluation of social competence is a complex matter (Webster-Stratton & Lindsay, 1999).

The initial mental health assessment only begins the evaluation of a child or adolescent's social skills. It is important to view the youth's behavior in the context of his or her social competence in the mainstream culture and in the context of his or her social effectiveness within his or her own world. How the child responds to the examiner can be taken as a behavior sample of how this youth compares with the abstract "child" we interact with, but this sample can also be considered in the context of how caretakers interact with the mental health professional. We all bring our own backgrounds and cognitive filters to our interactions with the world. I have found that actively working to deliberately view behavior from multiple perspectives has been a more useful strategy than trying to eliminate all my potential biases.

## Problems in Emotional Regulation

Some children experience difficulty in sustaining their peer relationships because of their lability of emotions and inability to maintain consistency in their responses to friends. Their actions are contrary from day to day, their feelings run "hot and cold," and eventually they exhaust the patience of friends and potential friends. The child may be very distressed by the rejection he or she experiences from others, and older children and adolescents may even show some insight into the role they play in their own problems; but it remains very difficult for the child to maintain the equilibrium necessary for most relationships. These youths may have a long history of difficulty with regulation of emotional intensity and instability of affective response. Georgia DeGangi (2000) has discussed how difficulties in learning effective self-regulation of affect and behavior can contribute to problems with irritability, sleep, feeding, and attention in infants. She reviews a number of instruments useful in the assessment of very young children, including parent rating scales and observational instruments to assess parent–child interaction (DeGangi, 2000). An alternative conceptualization of these children would see them as manifesting either a cyclothymic or rapid cycling bipolar disorder (Levy, Harper, & Weinberg, 1992).

A variant pattern of difficulty in sustaining friendship is seen in the child described as "emotionally needy." These children appeared starved for close emotional relationships and tend to "smother" friends and potential friends. They may show social skill deficits, but the core difficulty is their tremendous need for seemingly constant interpersonal engagement. They are usually highly extroverted and actively seek attention and approval from others. Both dependency and jealousy may be additional difficulties that act to limit their relationships with others.

### Problems in Behavior Control

A final group of difficulties in supporting long-term relationships is shown in children who have trouble keeping their actions within appropriate boundaries. Some children repeatedly manifest highly exploitative or manipulative relationships that eventually tend to alienate friends. Many of these youths show other problems with acting out, such as were discussed in Chapter 6; a proportion are able to conform their behavior to the general rules of society but not to the expected reciprocal expectations of friendship. Their interpersonal behavior is selfish and reflects a degree of egocentricism and narcissism that is age-inappropriate. Their general personalities are usually extroverted and they may have few problems in making friends, but they tend to "burn out" these relationships relatively rapidly by their selfish and exploitative actions.

## TEMPERAMENT

Individual differences in children's temperaments can be recognized early in life and can contribute to development in both positive and negative ways. In the classic New York Longitudinal Study, early temperament was found to interact with parental style to place the child at greater or lesser risk for later emotional and behavioral problems (Thomas & Chess, 1977). Although most clinicians acknowledge the importance of individual differences in children's personalities, the technical difficulty in evaluating temperament in a reliable and valid manner has limited the applied use of these findings. Differences in child temperament are often not considered in diagnosis of youths (Burger & Lang, 1998), but recent developments appear to hold promise in this regard (Clarke-Stewart, Fitzpatrick, Allhusen, & Goldberg, 2000). A recent miniseries of articles on the implications of temperament for practice was published by the *School Psychology Review* (Carey, 1998; Eisenberg, Wentzel, & Harris, 1998; Henderson & Fox, 1998; Rothbart & Jones, 1998; Teglasi, 1998a, 1998b; Teglasi & Epstein, 1998; McClowry, 1998).

I have found in a few cases that it has been helpful to directly address the issue of an adolescent's temperament or "style" with the youth during an evaluation in an effort to gain a better understanding our how his or her personality interacts with the people and events in his or her world. This is often a topic of concern in ongoing psychotherapy with a youth but is less frequently addressed in an initial assessment. A useful exchange about another individual's basic perceptual, emotional, and behavior predispositions usually requires a history of interaction to establish the shared trust and evolved mutual understanding that allows for such a dialogue. In a few instances, however, it seems possible to move into this topic relatively rapidly and with productive results. I am more likely to do this if the case is known to be complicated, with an extensive history of problems and various intervention efforts; if the child appears relatively nondistressed during the initial contact; and if the child's interpersonal style appears to be one of active engagement in the situation.

Temperament may also be assessed in discussion with parents and other informants who have had extensive contact with the young person. The clinical evaluation of broad personality dispositions is often undertaken with general, open-ended inquires such as were previously illustrated for anxiety/behavioral inhibition and accommodation/ compliance traits (see Practice Notes 5.2 and 6.2).

## PERSONALITY DISORDERS

The practice of diagnosing personality disorders in youths is problematic due to a number of factors (House, 1999). Despite these difficulties, there may be underlying validity to addressing the possibility of stable and problematic personality factors in children and adolescents. Putative personality disorders in adolescence appear to identify youth at high risk for major emotional and behavioral disturbances (Axis I disorders), maladjustment, and suicidal behavior; and these risks continue into adult life (Johnson et al., 1999). Regardless of how the symptoms of personality disorders are conceptualized, the appearance of these features in children appears to be an important prognostic variable. A great deal of basic investigation needs to be done before the practicing clinician can ap-

### Interview Segment 7.2. Kari

Kari's mother reported that she was a "troubled child." Kari had been seeing counselors and physicians since she was 6 years old; she was now 15. Early referrals had been for oppositional behavior, aggression, rule breaking, and poor self-control. Later referrals were for continued conduct problems, as well as depression, mood swings, and possible dissociative symptoms. Kari had accumulated a wide range of psychiatric diagnoses, most of which had seemed to fit her at the time but none of which were sustained patterns of problems. The current referral had been precipitated by another suicide attempt following a family argument.

EXAMINER: So, you've really seen a lot of counselors before. How is this going to be any different?

KARI: Probably won't be. Didn't do any good before.

EXAMINER: Yeah, sounds like a waste of time.

KARI: Tell my mom. She dragged me here.

EXAMINER: Uh huh. But I thought your mom said it had been better for a while after the two of you saw Dr. Smiley last year.

KARI: Maybe for a while, but then everybody got stupid again. My family sucks.

EXAMINER: Yeah, it can be a pain dealing with people who care about you.

KARI: What do you mean?

EXAMINER: Kari, who are you most like in your family?

KARI: I'm not like any of them. They're all perfect and I'm fucked up.

EXAMINER: I'll bet you are pretty unique in your family. Everybody else sounds pretty predictable.

KARI: Boring.

EXAMINER: A lot of the time I bet. You're not like that.

KARI: No, I'm not.

EXAMINER: How are you?

KARI: What do you mean?

EXAMINER: What kind of a person are you? What is it like to live in a home with you?

KARI: I don't know. That's a stupid question.

EXAMINER: You know, your mother had a little problem remembering what the argument was about that led to the fight just before you took the pills last week and went into the hospital. Why do you think that was?

KARI: I don't know, it was a stupid argument.

EXAMINER: What was it about?

KARI: God, I don't want to talk about this.

EXAMINER: Can you remember what the fight was about?

KARI: Something about homework or curfew. What does it matter now?

EXAMINER: Sometimes does it just seem that the problems are because you're so different from everyone else in your family?

KARI: (*Pauses.*) Sometimes.

EXAMINER: Maybe that's what you and I should be talking about.

This exchange led into a discussion of how Kari's personality interacted with the other personalities in her family to exacerbate their difficulties. This discussion extended well beyond the initial assessment and became the main theme in a course of interpersonal psychotherapy, but it was initiated in our first evaluation session.

proach this topic with confidence. The core issue of prevalence, closely tied to method of identification, remains unclear (Bernstein et al., 1993; Lewinsohn et al., 1997). I have found that noting personality traits, which may interact with the child's other problems to affect his or her adjustment, can add valuable clarity to our understanding of a case.

Borderline personality disorder (BPD) in young people continues to receive a great deal of attention (Bleiberg, 2000; Meijer, 1995), due in part to its high prevalence in clinical populations, as well as the potential it has for disruption of the therapeutic relationship and poor treatment outcome. Known risk factors for BPD in children and adolescents are similar to those identified in adult populations—physical and sexual abuse, neglect, and parental maladjustment (Goldman, D'Angelo, De Maso, & Mezzacappa, 1992; Guzder, Paris, Zelkowitz, & Marchessault, 1996; Guzder, Paris, Zelkowitz, & Feldman, 1999). These risk factors, however, are neither necessary nor sufficient for the development of a personality disorder, and fundamental questions remain as to the essential pathway to this problematic pattern of human relationships. Because borderline traits overlap with some of the normal vicissitudes of adolescence and can be dramatically exacerbated during the experience of acute clinical syndromes, I have found it most prudent to identify borderline characteristics in youths descriptively and to defer making definite personality disorder diagnoses until there is a substantial historical record available. Some authors have attempted to clarify the diagnosis of "borderline symptoms" in children (Vela, Gottlieb, & Gottlieb, 1983). Kernberg, Weiner, and Bardenstein (2000) consider the use of different sources of assessment data in the diagnosis of personality disorders in youths, including the diagnosis of borderline personality disorder. In an interesting and ambitious approach, they discuss (1) the use of the Personality Assessment Interview (PAI) technique of injecting into the interview, at 5- to 10-minute intervals, questions that call for self-representation, object representation, ego observation, and empathy; and (2) looking at items in the Achenbach Child Behavior Checklist that possibly reflect characterological psychopathology (items 3, 12, 16, 18, 20, 33, 41, 57, 68, 87, 91, and 95 for borderline personality disorder; Kernberg et al., 2000). Guzder and colleagues (1999) have pointed out that "borderline pathology" in adolescents does not necessarily correspond to the entity "borderline personality disorder" as identified in DSM-IV. They note that some authors have used an alternative phrase, "multiple complex developmental disorder," to identify a syndrome that shows impairments in affect regulation, social behavior, and cognitive processing (Cohen, Paul, & Volkmar, 1987; Lincoln, Bloom, Katz, & Boksenbaum, 1998; Towbin, Dykens, Pearson, & Cohen, 1993; Van der Gaag et al., 1995). This general topic remains controversial and will undoubtedly receive a great deal of continuing empirical and theoretical attention. Lincoln and his coauthors (1998) believe that children with these characteristics, regardless of how they are labeled, makes up a significant portion of the child inpatient psychiatric population and is at risk for morbidity into adulthood.

Assessment of borderline characteristics in children, atypical pervasive developmental disorder, or multiple complex developmental disorder is complicated by the absence of agreement among authorities on defining characteristics or diagnostic criteria. Bleiberg (1994) discussed difficulties in the diagnosis of "borderline disorders" in children, including the overlap with developing narcissistic or histrionic personality disorders, and suggested adaptations of the diagnostic criteria for children. Goldman et al (1992) suggested modifications of the DSM-III-R criteria for BPD to increase the sensitivity for child cases. Towbin et al. (1993) have offered proposed diagnostic criteria for multiple complex developmental disorder (MCDD), as have Buitelaar and Van der Gaag (1998). Guevremont and Dinklage (as cited in Barkley, 1998a) have developed a behavior rating scale for the evaluation of multiplex developmental disorder, the Children's Atypical Development Scale (Barkley, 1998b), which I have found clinically useful. Barkley (1998a) discusses five domains of development—thinking, affect, social, sensory, and motor—that may help differentiate multiplex developmental disorder from ADHD and suggest that children with odd or atypical disturbances in three of these domains be viewed as showing multiplex developmental disorder. He also observes that extreme ratings on a majority of items endorsed by parents on broad-spectrum behavior rating scales, such as the Child Behavior Checklist, may be an indication that the possibility of multiplex developmental disorder should be considered. Finally, Barkley (1998a) notes that family members of children with multiplex developmental disorder show a much higher occurrence of major psychiatric disorders than those of normal or ADHD youth and suggests that a family history of schizophrenia, other psychoses, or major affective disorder may help identify cases in which this possibility should be entertained. The intriguing proposed category of CDD is discussed further in Chapter 8 in terms of its boundary with autistic disorder.

Grilo, Walker, Becker, Edell, and McGlashan (1997) brought to light a potentially important relationship between borderline personality disorders (BPD) in adolescents and comorbid diagnoses of major depression and substance use disorder. Although BPD, using modified personality disorder examination criteria, was frequently comorbid with major depression (31% of patients) and with substance use disorder (37% of patients), the combination of major depression and substance use disorder showed a remarkably high comorbidity with BPD (86%). The combination of serious depression and substance abuse in an adolescent's clinical picture may be a useful clue that possible personality trait disturbance should be carefully considered.

## PATHOLOGICAL PARENTING

The topic of harmful parental behavior and the short- and long-term consequences of this for children is of undeniable importance. Child neglect and abuse are major problems for society, for health care professionals, and for the individual children and their families who are affected. The issues involved in the detection and assessment of destructive parenting are complex and difficult. We are far from achieving professional unanimity as to what constitutes best practice. The difficulty is amplified by the broad range of family behavior that is represented within the subfield. Simple distinctions of neglect versus abuse are necessary but insufficient. Abuse is often subdivided into psychological, physical, and sexual, but each of these in turn encompasses highly heterogeneous populations. In the absence of better population discrimination, it is not surprising that the empirical findings are mixed and sometimes inconsistent.

Despite the difficulties, it is incumbent on all mental health professionals to remain vigilant regarding possible insufficient care of young people or harmful actions they have been exposed to or both. My experience has left me doubtful about the reliability of any simple listing of the "signs" of child abuse. The effects of destructive interaction with adults are highly varied and affected by many factors, including the age of the child; other cognitive and behavioral characteristics of the child; the nature of the family system; the nature, frequency, and pattern of damaging behavior; and responses made by other adults and authorities. I offer this one consideration: A clinical picture that "doesn't make sense" calls for explanation. One possible explanation is that the important data are not being made available to the examiner. This may represent a failure on someone's part to be forthright because the information is sensitive. Parents may be reluctant to discuss family strife and conflict, such as marital problems between the spouses, or embarrassing behavior of some family member, such as signs of dementia in a grandparent. Youths may be reluctant to incriminate themselves by admitting to drug experimentation or involvement with a delinquent gang. In some instances, the purpose of the dissimulation may be to hide behavior that reveals neglectful or abusive parenting. All members of the family may be in collusion with this deception, either willingly or because of fear or coercion. I do not believe that neglect and abuse is the most common explanation for our failure to be able to achieve a clear formulation of a child's difficulties, but while conceptual clarity continues to elude us, these possibilities need to stay in the differential diagnosis.

At the opposite extreme from the neglectful parent is the adult who expects too much of the child and is too caught up in the youth's life. The line between "encouraging" a child and "pushing" him, or "giving her space" and "neglecting" her, can be exceedingly thin and ill defined. It can be especially difficult to differentiate these actions with children who show potential talents and abilities that may need dedicated nurturing to fully manifest. Tofler, Knapp, and Drell (1999) discussed what they described as the "achievement by proxy" spectrum, which ranges from supportive to potentially pathological. Determining the child's best interests may not be possible with any real certainty. The situation will be even more difficult if there is conflict among the caretakers themselves over this issue. Problems with relationships and pseudomaturity are among the short-term negative sequelae feared for "pushed" children; risk of mood disorders and substance use problems rank among the more serious long-term concerns. These clinical formulations usually appear to be based on limited case experience, however, and an adequate empirical foundation for evaluation and intervention is not available.

Some specific events that may occur within family systems have received attention because of their potential harm for children. One variable that has received attention is violence between caretakers that is witnessed by the children of the family. Witnessing marital violence has been reported to be associated with adjustment problems during childhood (Cummings, Pepler, & Moore, 1999; Grych, Jouriles, Swank, McDonald, & Norwood, 2000) and problems of violence in later relationships (Jankowski et al., 1999). Witnessing parental aggression may also interact with other risk factors, such as mistreatment of the child (Feerick & Haugaard, 1999). Unfortunately, the interpretation of this literature is difficult because almost all studies have used either clinical or college population samples. The selection influence of such restricted samples may lead to an overestimation of the relationship between family violence and maladjustment in the clinical populations and to an underestimation of any such relationship in the college samples (Feerick & Haugaard, 1999).

Beyond the extremes of parental neglect and overinvolvement and the occurrence of specific deleterious experiences such as witnessing violence, there probably exist numerous patterns of family relationships that may be less than ideal for the optimal growth and development of some children within these family systems. Most children are highly adaptable and respond well to parenting styles and practices within a wide range of variation. A minority of youths show characteristics of temperament that place them at risk unless they are given the advantage of optimum parental consistency, support, and care. We continue to learn more about the effects of life stresses within family systems on children's development (Beardslee, Versage, & Gladstone, 1998; Drotar, 1997; Kelly, 2000; Lancaster, 1999), and this knowledge will eventually provide the basis for more helpful assessments of family functioning.

Human relationships are among the most complex phenomena ever to come to our attention. It should not be surprising, then, that relationship difficulties and the evaluation of these problems are highly challenging. Extreme cases are clear and easy to recognize and to defend our formulations of. But the behaviors discussed in this chapter uniformly occur along a continuum, and between the milder cases of problematic adjustment and the more severe instances of normal range adaptation, there is not a clear boundary or demarcation. For a fuller discussion of the many issues involved in the assessment and intervention of children exposed to destructive family relationships, the reader is referred to more in-depth treatment of this important topic (Horton & Cruise, 2001; Wekerle & Wolfe, 1996).

# 8  *Evaluating Pervasive Problems in Children*

$A$ most challenging area for the mental health professional is assessing children who show pervasive disorders. The concept of a *pervasive disorder* is commonly well understood but on closer inspection found to be somewhat difficult to articulate clearly. Many of the cognitive, emotional, and behavioral difficulties of children touch multiple aspects of their lives and have far-ranging repercussions in terms of their adjustment and functioning. The prognostic significance of conduct problems can be almost as severe as that of autism; mood disorders may disrupt efficient adaptive behavior as widely as mental retardation does; anxiety may lend to daily behavior the crippling mental pain and dread seen in schizophrenia. Despite these comparisons, there is something different about some patterns of mental health problems. The nature of this difference can be seen more clearly by considering the concept of a "usual and typical life."

Most children are able to live with their families. It may be a birth family, extended family, or a foster or adoptive family. The important notion here is that we expect a child to be able to live within a family setting. Even if an original family has been lost through parental death or other adversity, the child could live in a home-like environment if one were available. An important element of those disorders thought of as pervasive is that they call into question this usual assumption—that the child will live with a family. In the past, mental retardation, autism, and psychosis during childhood (as well as severe physical challenges) often lead to institutionalization. Today we find most children with these disorders living with their families or in a home-like setting, but the issue of placement is an issue for them in a way it never becomes for the majority of other children.

Pervasive disorders call into question the issue of what type of environment may be necessary for the child's and the family's best interests. I suggest that this question and the realities that have led to its being asked are like a Pandora's box; once considered, the issue of placement calls into question many other issues normally never considered by parents, siblings, or extended family. Although placement at home is almost always in the best interest of a child with a pervasive disorder, it is not necessarily in the best interests of other members of the family. The family functioning with a significantly compromised member faces trade-offs and costs that have only recently begun to be openly acknowledged. Issues of resentment, frustration, anger, guilt, shame, and remorse are background elements of a different character for families who struggle with the challenges of raising their very atypical member, along with all the usual business of being a family. Herein lie some of the differences for these children. It is the human perceptions that are critical here. A child with a conduct disorder, for instance, may be placed in a juvenile detention facility; this child has lost his or her family placement. Yet both family members and professionals tend to see this placement as a temporary departure from normal, which is the child living at home with his or her family. A child with autism may never need to be placed outside the home while growing up; the move outside the home is a goal to be achieved in young adulthood as a step toward independence. Yet, again, both family and professionals tend to experience this uninterrupted familial residence as an accomplishment; another, possibly unstated, goal that has been achieved: The child has been *able* to live at home with the family. My experience has been that pervasive disorders share this critical feature: At some level these are the problems that call into question whether the child will be able to live a typical life with respect to growing up at home or in a family-type setting.

I have been using the phrase *pervasive disorder* in a descriptive sense. In order to avoid confusion, it is important to note that one diagnostic grouping often discussed with regard to youth is typically titled "pervasive developmental disorders," the exemplar case here being autism. Another group of diagnoses, mental retardation, would usually be consider *pervasive* in a descriptive sense by most mental health professionals. This chapter also includes a discussion of evaluating psychotic disorders, such as schizophrenia, which not all authors would think of in this context. The decision to address schizophrenia and associated problems here reflects my view that these disorders can also call into question the issue of the child's long-term placement and threaten his or her status as a family member. Although severe cases of traumatic brain injury and other neurological disorders can certainly constitute "pervasive" conditions in the sense in which I use the term, these problems were considered previously in the chapter on cognitive disorders.

## MENTAL RETARDATION

Children with tested IQs below 50 (moderate, severe, and profound ranges) usually first come to attention during infancy and early childhood. General intellectual capacity 3 standard deviations below the mean is associated with major developmental lags and behavior deficits, and often with serious physical, sensory, and medical conditions that also set the child apart from age peers. The correlation between IQ and adaptive behavior tends to be strong in the group of highly compromised children. Psychological assessment with this population may serve to document their levels of intellectual handicap and establish eligibility for services. When this documentation is one objective of evaluation, it is important to use the most appropriate cognitive instruments available for intellectual assessment. The mental health examiner must consider not only the standard issues of reliability and validity of potential test instruments but also legal standards that may apply in his or her state. The age-appropriate version of the Wechsler scales is probably the most frequently used and acceptable measure of general intellectual functioning in the United States. The dominant practical issues of assessment for these children tend to involve evaluation of adaptive behavior.

A variety of assessment tools have been developed for the formal assessment of adaptive behavior. Informal assessment typically relies on clinical or semistructured interview of caretakers, usually in combination with informal observations of the child in the office setting. For diagnostic assessment, this procedure is adequate and necessary. All modern definitions of mental retardation are structured on the tripartite criterion advocated by the American Association on Mental Deficiency (AAMD), now known as the American Association on Mental Retardation (AAMR), in its historic 1959 publication (Heber, 1959,

1961). Both the DSM and ICD definitions of mental retardation require evidence of an impairment in adaptive behavior as one of the necessary criteria to establish a diagnosis of mental retardation. Although administration of formal assessment tools such as the Vineland Adaptive Behavior Scales or Scales of Independent Behavior may seldom be necessary, at least a brief inquiry into the areas of adaptive behavior delineated in DSM and ICD and by the AAMR (Luckasson et al., 1992) would seem good practice (see Table 8.1). Educational districts, state and federal statutes, and preadmission screening regulations in force in a particular locale may impose specific requirements and should be reviewed if the assessment involves issues of entitlement or eligibility establishment. Because most assessments of adaptive ability rely on parents and other caretakers as informants, it is valuable for the evaluator to remain sensitive to how caretakers' views of competence can vary across diverse cultures and subcultures (Durbrow, 1999).

Evaluating and documenting areas of strength and competency is another important area of assessment for severely compromised children. The general correlation seen between cognitive abilities and behaviors that have a cognitive aspect tends to pull from all of us the expectation and perception that a severely handicapped child will be limited in all ways and areas. A brief period spent with a number of profoundly disabled youths will illustrate the inaccuracy of this conclu-

---

**TABLE 8.1  Categories of Adaptive Behavior from AAMR and DSM-IV**

Adaptive skill areas identified in the 1992 definition of mental retardation published by the American Association on Mental Retardation (Luckasson et al., 1992)

| | |
|---|---|
| Communication | Self-direction |
| Self-care | Health and safety |
| Home living | Functional academics |
| Social skills | Leisure and work |
| Community use | |

Adaptive functioning areas identified in DSM-IV (American Psychiatric Association, 1994, 2000)

| | |
|---|---|
| Communication | Functional academic skills |
| Self-care | Work |
| Home living | Leisure |
| Social/interpersonal skills | Health |
| Use of community resources | Safety |
| Self-direction | |

sion. The correlation between areas of mental ability, although high in this population, is not perfect; and even slight differences of relative cognitive strengths and weaknesses can have important meaning to family, caretakers, and friends. Even more powerful is the effect of "personality" variables—trait-like attributes reflected in prevailing mood, adaptability to change, regularity of biological rhythm, and intensity of emotional response. A positive demeanor, social gregariousness, and a sense of humor can make a profound difference in the life of a child with disabilities, as well as in the lives of those who care for the youth. Inquires as simple as asking the caretakers to tell you the child's most positive features can be very informative.

The evaluation of behavior problems associated with the child's mental retardation is another important task of psychological assessment with seriously retarded youths. Diagnosed mental retardation is a risk factor for behavior and adjustment difficulty (Dykens, 2000; Szymanski, 1994). In addition to the problems directly associated with the intellectual retardation, there is a high reported comorbidity of other mental disorders in young people diagnosed with mental retardation (Bregman, 1991; Campbell & Malone, 1991; King, State, Shah, Davanzo, & Dykens, 1997; State, King, & Dykens, 1997). Missed diagnoses of potentially treatable mental disorders is a serious problem in serving developmentally disabled youths; these comorbid conditions can have serious effects on the child's overall adjustment and functioning. Unfortunately, this is probably not a rare error (Fuller & Sabatino, 1998). The examiner of these children needs to make a deliberate review of the child's performance and situation before concluding that a single diagnosis of mental retardation adequately captures all the relevant clinical information available in the case. Matson and his colleagues have worked to develop reliable rating instruments for the assessment of other mental disorders in individuals with known mental retardation (Matson & Bamburg, 1998; Matson, Gardner, Coe, & Sovner, 1991; Matson & Smiroldo, 1997; Matson, Smiroldo, & Hastings, 1998).

Inquiry into any occurrences of self-injurious behavior and aggression is almost always warranted. These problem behaviors can be associated with significant retardation and are often threats to the child's social acceptance and even residential stability. Although infrequent and mild self-injurious behavior is developmentally unremarkable in the general population of infants and very young children, it is important to ascertain if this behavior is or has been an adjustment problem with retarded youth. The same general statement holds true for aggression. Caretakers of all children need to learn effective and acceptable methods of suppressing aggressive actions and helping the child to learn behavioral self-control. This is no less necessary with impaired children, and it is valuable to establish how much progress the family has made in addressing this important developmental need.

It can be extremely difficult to establish the child's prevailing mood and emotional adjustment, especially with nonverbal children and those with very limited communicative behavior. Nonetheless, the examiner must be sensitive to the possibility of mood or anxiety disorders in disabled children. Mental retardation does not confer any protection against other mental health problems. If anything, the overall available data strongly suggest that most mental disorders are a risk factor for other mental disorders and that comorbidity is more the rule than the exception. Given the high base-rate occurrence of mood and anxiety disorders in the general population, it is inevitable that many children and adolescents who are mentally retarded also manifest emotional disorders that are often unrecognized and untreated. The examiner should be especially alert to reports of acutely developing behavior problems and behavioral regressions. The general developmental path of mentally retarded children is positive, albeit at a significantly lower slope than for children with normal cognitive abilities. A loss of performance requires an explanation; this is not consistent with our general expectation. Also, "natural" behavior problems of either externalizing or internalizing symptoms, for example, oppositional behavior or social difficulties, usually develop gradually over repeated interaction with the environment. The "sudden" appearance of acting out or emotional problems should occasion a high index of suspicion for the possibility of an acute mood or anxiety disorder.

Assessment of youths with tested IQs in the mild or borderline range of cognitive limitations is challenging because of the wide variability between different aspects of the child's cognitive functioning and adaptive behavior. Establishment of areas of relative strength and weakness is important because these have significant implications for adjustment, growth and development, and prognosis for functional independence, social adjustment, and competitive community employment. Much of the time and attention in a comprehensive psychological evaluation of a youth with mild intellectual limitations may be directed toward profiling these areas of success and challenge, documenting progress, and formulating recommendations for continuing personal, social, and academic education. Bucy, Smith, and Landau

(1999) discuss practical considerations in the assessment of preschool children who show mental retardation and other developmental disabilities.

Just as with the more compromised youths, determination of areas of strength and positive success can be very important in the overall evaluation of youths with mild cognitive limitations. In addition to the important functional information elicited by such inquiry, there is an associated emotional benefit to assessing the child's strengths for both the youth and any collateral caretakers interviewed. Too often, psychological assessments for children with mental challenges consist only of being asked questions they do not know the answer to and of being asked to perform tasks that are beyond their capabilities. Needless to say, this is not a particularly pleasant experience. Intellectual assessment can be somewhat frustrating for a child with average abilities, given the usual strategy of discontinuing testing only after the child has begun to repetitively fail in an area. For youths with mild mental limitations, this experience only confirms what they have already begun to know about themselves—that they are limited in ways their peers are not. In my experience only a few retarded youths recognize that the nature of IQ tests is to continue until failure *and that this applies to all children*. I have known a few young people with mild mental handicaps who were visibly startled and somewhat incredulous at my revelation that all the children I saw began "failing" the test at some point. Communicating, by question and attention, that you are also interested in what the child can do well and where his or her joy and competencies lie can help dispel the burden of being asked again to show how "dumb" one is.

For the parents of an exceptional child, a psychological assessment can also be a rather grim experience of another concrete demonstration, with little clear benefit, of how their child is failing and behind in one area after another. The ameliorative effects of being asked to describe the areas in which the child has shown the greatest gains and the positive features and strengths the child has cannot be overstated. The best assessments of children, whether initial screenings or comprehensive evaluations, need to establish what is right, as well as what is wrong.

As in the case of the most limited children, with mildly impaired youths it is important to determine any associated difficulties and comorbid disorders. Lags in social skills development, inadequate coping responses, and inappropriate actions are probably more critical determinants of social acceptance than mental retardation per se. These are the real potential barriers to community acceptance, competitive employment, and maximum integration into our society. We should never be content with an explanation for behavior problems that begins with the premise, "He is like that because he's retarded." Brief and simple behavior report forms can be useful in screening for behavior and adaptive problems and strengths. I have used various versions of a Behavior Report Form (Figure 8.1) for a number of years as a device for eliciting information from informants about developmentally disabled clients.

## PERVASIVE DEVELOPMENTAL DISORDERS

The broad category of pervasive developmental disorders evolved out of Leo Kanner's early infantile autism syndrome. These children show a combination of severe behavioral deficits, such as might be seen in serious mental retardation, along with "abnormal" behaviors such as stereotypic motor movements or object play, gaze avoidance, or self-injurious behavior. The DSM-IV classification system identifies the core features as impairments in social interaction, communication, and breadth of repertoire of behavior. Autism must be differentiated from mental retardation on one boundary and from schizophrenia on another. With increasing attention to this severe behavior disorder of childhood came growing recognition that autism was but one presentation of a group of severe behavior disorder patterns arising early in life and challenging almost all areas of a child's adaptation to life. Although full syndrome autism was probably historically misdiagnosed as mental retardation, there are probably few cases of classical, full presentation that are misclassified today. The regressive courses of Rett's disorder and childhood disintegrative disorder very likely aid our discrimination of these patterns. The greatest challenges in detection and evaluation are probably represented by atypical autism (which would be classified as pervasive developmental disorder not otherwise specified) and Asperger's syndrome, with its essentially normal language performance. Then there are the many different presentations of problems seen in the remaining pervasive developmental disorders not otherwise specified. Shriver, Allen, and Mathews (1999) provides a good overview of assessment instruments that can assist in the evaluation of autism.

Behavior deficits are not unique to pervasive developmental disorders, but the combination of impairments in skills and abilities, in com-

Client _____     Date _____

Person completing form _____

Position _____

Based primarily on observations at:   Home   ____

                                                  Work   ____

                                                  School ____

                                                  Other  ____ : _____

Based on your observations and knowledge of the client, has he or she had problems with any of the following over the past 12 months? Please circle any problems, estimate how often this problem has occurred in the past 2 weeks, and indicate if the problem is getting worse.

| Circle any problem | How often in the past 2 weeks? | Getting worse? |
|---|---|---|
| Unprovoked physical aggression | ____ | Yes / No |
| Unprovoked verbal aggression | ____ | Yes / No |
| Reactive (defensive) aggression | ____ | Yes / No |
| Social withdrawal / isolation | ____ | Yes / No |
| Fearfulness / anxiety | ____ | Yes / No |
| Depression / sadness / crying | ____ | Yes / No |
| Overactive / excessive talking | ____ | Yes / No |
| Destruction of property | ____ | Yes / No |
| Stealing | ____ | Yes / No |
| Poor personal hygiene | ____ | Yes / No |
| Physically self-injurious actions | ____ | Yes / No |
| Sexual misbehavior | ____ | Yes / No |
| Alcohol or drug abuse<br>  What? _____ | ____ | Yes / No |
| Bizarre behavior<br>  What? _____ | ____ | Yes / No |
| Legal problems / criminal behavior<br>  What? _____ | ____ | Yes / No |

(continued)

**FIGURE 8.1** Behavior Report Form.

What are the client's major/greatest behavior problems right now?

None / _____

_____

_____

Over the past 12 months have these:    increased    decreased    stayed the same

What are the client's major/greatest strengths or positive features at this time?

_____

_____

_____

Over the past 12 months have these:    increased    decreased    stayed the same

Does the client take behavior control or seizure control medications?

   No    Yes:  Doctor _____

                    Medications _____

Does the client actively socialize with others?            Yes     No

Does the client seek out activities or work when unoccupied?    Yes     No

Did the client finish high school?                       Yes     No

  Regular classes    Special education    GED

What are the client's living circumstances?

  Parents'/family home ____

  Apartment/house: ____ Alone     Roommate(s)

  HIP home ____

  Group home ____

  Homeless/mission/institution ____

  Other: _____

What is the client's employment situation?

  Competitive community employment _____ where: _____

  Supported employment ____ where: _____

  Sheltered workshop ____ where: _____

  Unemployed ____ where: _____

Does the client have any health/medical problems? What? _____

_____

_____

**FIGURE 8.1**  *(continued)*

bination with problems in reciprocal communication, interactive social behavior, or a varied repertoire of behavior, should raise a concern in the examiner's mind. A lack of social responsiveness is highly suspicious, as is high-frequency stereotypic behavior or self-injurious behavior. It is useful to inquire of both child and parent as to the child's relationships with other children and his or her usual activities when self-occupied. Special interest in stereotypic behavior in children is supported by the interference of high-frequency stereotypies with a variety of appropriate and desirable behavior (Willemsen-Swinkels, Buitelaar, Dekker, & van Engeland, 1998).

Given the high comorbidity of pervasive developmental disorders with language disorders, you should inquire into and compare the obtained reports with your own experience of the child's receptive and expressive skills. It is also valuable to ascertain whether the family is using signing or other alternative communication approaches to augment oral communication with the child. Communication failure and the attendant frustration is often a precipitating stimulus for tantrums or aggressive behavior, and this possibility should be explored.

Given the high risk of adolescent onset seizure disorders in autism and related pervasive developmental disorders (Mouridsen, Rich, & Isager, 1999), it is well to inquire into possible epilepsy with teenagers who have a history of developmental disorders. If the youth has a history of seizures, you should determine what the current medications are, how effectively seizures are being controlled, the frequency of breakthrough seizures, and the date of the child's last seizure. As mentioned previously, I usually defer the evaluation of a child who has had a seizure within the previous 72 hours. I have also found it useful to take a few minutes to review with the parent or guardian the child's overall physical health, any problems being treated, and any medications being taken.

Especially with very young children, with whom diagnostic certainty can be very limited, it can be quite useful to observe the child interacting with age peers if an opportunity can be arranged. Qualitative difficulties in the child's social interaction, especially his or her modeling and observational learning, can be quite helpful in prompting a more thorough diagnostic evaluation. Adequate clinician diagnostic reliability for autism can be demonstrated with 2-year-old children (Stone et al., 1999). Baron-Cohen, Allen, and Gillberg (1992) identify behavior items that may allow for the discrimination of autism as early as 18 months. Behavior rating scales for caretakers, such as the Autism

| Interview Segment 8.1.  John |
| --- |

The mental health evaluation of a youth with a pervasive developmental disorder is often based on observations of his or her presentation and ongoing behavior, interviews with informants, and review of available records. The documentation in school reports, Individualized Education Plans, psychological testing, developmental and medical studies, and other permanent product records can provide valuable information and a developmental perspective. The verbal reports of parents, teachers, caseworkers, and others who know and have experience with the child can be invaluable in establishing the youth's patterns of actions and problems. But the final source of data is the behavior of the children themselves. Careful observation, informed analysis, and detailed recording of this material provides a compelling foundation for the final diagnosis assessment.

John was a 14-year-old boy brought to the evaluation by a house parent. He lived in a group home for developmentally disabled youths, and an assessment was sought for documentation and treatment planning. When approached in the waiting area, he was sitting next to the staff person, gazing in the direction of the secretarial pool. As I approached I greeted him by name:

EXAMINER: You must be John.

JOHN: (*No response, continues to gaze to side.*)

HOUSE PARENT: John, here's the doctor. Go talk to him now.

EXAMINER: Could you come visit with me?

JOHN: (*No verbal response; covers eyes with right forearm.*)

HOUSE PARENT: John, get up and go with the doctor.

EXAMINER: Come with me, John, let's visit a little while.

JOHN: (*No verbal response; rises and accompanies examiner to office.*)

John followed me into the office and took an offered chair. His gait had appeared unremarkable. His posture was erect and relaxed. He avoided eye contact and made no verbal responses during the evaluation. He initially sat and raised his right arm to cover his eyes. I continued to "converse" with him as if engaging in an interaction.

EXAMINER: Do you like to draw, John?

JOHN: (*No response, but slight rocking.*)

EXAMINER: John, here is a pencil and some paper. Why don't you draw something?

JOHN: (*Drops arm and takes pencil. Begins to scribble systematically over surface of paper–left to right, top to bottom of page, very rapidly. The sheet is soon filled. Turns sheet over and begins on the other side. No marks are made on the desk.*)

This very brief sample yielded some important observations that were eventually supportive of a diagnosis of autism. Even more important, several areas of behavioral strengths and ability were identified: fair oral comprehension, compliance with simple directions, and participation in nonverbal activities. Observations of John's hands, arms, and face showed no lacerations or scars that might indicate problems with self-injurious behavior. He was able to deal with the stress of meeting the examiner and separating from the familiar staff person reasonably. This was of especial importance because one of the reasons for the evaluation was the plan to move John into a work activities program through his school. His tolerance for dealing with new situations and people would be critical for success in this anticipated shift in programming during the day.

---

Behavior Checklist (Krug, Arick, & Almond, 1980); standardized interview protocols, such as the Autism Diagnostic Interview—Revised (Le Couteur et al., 1989; Lord, Rutter, & Le Couteur, 1994); and direct observation instruments, such as the Autism Diagnostic Observation Schedule (Lord et al., 1989) or the Childhood Autism Rating Scale (Mesibov, Schopler, Schaffer, & Michal, 1989), can all contribute to a definitive diagnosis of autism. In my experience the key factor in diagnostic confidence is the adequacy of interview data obtained from early caretakers of the child. Children with pervasive developmental disorders show characteristic patterns of disturbance in bonding and social responsiveness, in developing repertoire, and in behavioral regulation over the first few years of life. The retrospective reports of caretakers can be invaluable in documenting the child's early deviations from normal development.

The more valid and useful subclassifications of pervasive developmental disorders will continue to be the subject of debate and discussion for some time to come. Increasingly, this debate is based on empirical findings, and this fact holds promise for future efforts to help these most disabled youths (cf. Mazzocco et al., 1998; Volkmar, Klin, & Pauls, 1998; Zappella, Gillberg, & Ehlers, 1998). Volkmar, Klin, Marans, and McDougle (1996) provide a useful review of differential diagnostic features of the various pervasive developmental disorders (see Table 8.2). The heterogeneity of the residual cases that do not fit into current specific classifications will continue to be a major challenge for evaluation. Buitelaar and Van der Gaag (1998) have recently articulated some proposed decision rules for diagnosis of pervasive developmental disorder not otherwise specified and a proposed category of multiple complex developmental disorder (MCDD). Van der Gaag and colleagues (1995) used chart review to determine variables that best discriminated between children showing autism and children showing multiple complex developmental disorder (see the previous discussion of MCDD in Chapter 7).

**TABLE 8.2   Differential Diagnostic Features: Autistic and Nonautistic Pervasive Developmental Disorders**

| | | Disorder | | | |
|---|---|---|---|---|---|
| Feature | Autism | Asperger's disorder | Rett's syndrome | Childhood disintegrative disorder | PDD NOS |
| Age at recognition (months) | 0–36 | Usually > 24 | 5–30 | > 24 | Variable |
| Sex ratio | M > F | M > F | F | M > F | M > F |
| Loss of skills | Usually not | Usually not | Marked | Marked | Usually not |
| Social skills | Very poor | Poor | Varies with age | Very poor | Variable |
| Communication skills | Usually poor | Poor to fair | Very poor | Very poor | Fair to good |
| Circumscribed interests | Variable | Marked | NA | NA | Variable |
| Family history of similar problems | Uncommon | Frequent | No | No | Unknown |
| Seizure disorder | Common | Uncommon | Frequent | Common | Uncommon |
| Head growth decelerates | No | No | Yes | No | No |
| IQ range | Severe MR to normal | Mild MR to normal | Severe MR | Severe MR | Mild MR to normal |
| Outcome | Poor | Fair to poor | Very poor | Very poor | Fair to good |

*Note.* PDD NOS, pervasive developmental disorder not otherwise specified; MR, mental retardation; M, males; F, females. From Volkmar and Cohen (1996). Copyright 1996 by Lippincott Williams & Wilkins. Reprinted by permission.

Mental retardation is frequently associated with pervasive developmental disorders. A formal evaluation of IQ with a widely accepted measure of general intellectual functioning (for instance, the age-appropriate Wechsler scale) is worthwhile in most children with autistic disorder and may be usefully supplemented by the addition of one of the nonverbal intelligence tests. An interesting controversy that has not yet been satisfactory resolved is whether the diagnosis of autism should be precluded by IQ scores below a certain level, for instance, 30 (cf. Rapoport & Ismond, 1996). Intelligence testing of children with pervasive developmental disorders also offers the opportunity for observation of their behavior and interaction under somewhat standardized conditions.

## PSYCHOTIC DISORDERS

Psychotic disorders are diagnosed on the basis of so-called characteristic symptoms: hallucinations, delusions, or acute disorganization of behavior. Their impact on adjustment is usually pervasive, and the emergence of psychotic symptoms often threatens the stability of many areas of a child's life and performance. The long-term disabling aspects of schizophrenic spectrum disorders seem to be strongly associated with the negative symptoms: anhedonia, little apparent motivation, limited spontaneous activity and speech. The emergence of pronounced negative symptoms after an initial psychotic episode of positive symptoms (hallucinations and delusions) carries a much more guarded prognosis than the simple occurrence of even florid symptoms of cognitive and perceptual distortions. Indeed, hallucinations and delusions in isolation have limited diagnostic significance because a variety of psychiatric conditions can show psychotic behavior: schizophrenia, delusional disorders, severe depression, mania, posttraumatic stress disorder, atypical dissociative disorders, borderline personality disorders, severe adjustment disorders. More narrowly defined psychotic distortions can be seen in eating disorders, obsessive–compulsive disorder, parasomnic sleep disorders, and unusual sexual disorders. Psychotic symptoms can occur during the context of acute substance intoxication or withdrawal, dementia, brain trauma, and a variety of medical illnesses. Impaired reality testing is a defining feature of delirium. The differentiating aspect among disorders showing psychosis is often the course of the disturbance. Schizophrenia shows long periods of acute symptoms; schizophreniform patterns show identical psychosis but are more limited in duration; brief reactive psychoses are quite short lived; psychoses in mood disorders follow the periodicity of the affective disturbance; drug-induced psychoses and other organic conditions follow on biological causes; and clear associations with triggering stimuli are seen in PTSD and other adjustment phenomena.

Childhood-onset schizophrenia can be effectively diagnosed using DSM criteria (Jacobsen & Rapoport, 1998), but diagnostic errors are unfortunately frequent (Rapoport & Ismond, 1996). Childhood-onset schizophrenia must be differentiated from both pervasive developmental disorders and psychotic mood disorders. Careful data collection and systematic review of findings are important precautions to make in cases of suspected early-onset schizophrenia. Kronenberger and Meyer (1996) discuss interviewing, behavior rating, and formal testing techniques that may contribute to the assessment of schizophrenia in children. The available literature suggests that children who develop early-onset schizophrenia have often experienced language, social, and cognitive difficulties for long periods prior to the diagnosis of obvious psychotic symptoms (Alaghband-Rad et al., 1995). Premorbid adjustment is a major prognostic factor in schizophrenia and should be carefully evaluated in childhood-onset cases. Some youths will have clear histories suggesting schizotypal characteristics and, in rare cases, a premorbid diagnosis of schizotypal personality disorder may be indicated; but other patterns of personality trait disturbance have been noted (Werry, 1996). A history of nonspecific problems in pragmatic communication, of difficulty forming and maintaining reciprocal social relationships, of occasional problems with behavioral acting out, and of unusual ideas and interests has been common in the small number of children I have know who were diagnosed with early-onset schizophrenia. These associated characteristics contribute greatly to the morbidity of this disorder.

Given the frequent comorbidities between mental disorders commonly observed and frequently cited in this book, it is interesting to note those psychiatric disorders that do not associate beyond chance frequencies. A good deal of evidence now exists to support the absence of association between autistic disorder and schizophrenia in children, beyond the overlap expected between independent conditions (Rapoport & Ismond, 1996). The development of prominent hallucinations or delusions in the clinical picture of a child with a history of pervasive developmental disorder does justify the additional diagnosis of schizo-phrenia if the symptoms persist for more than a month.

In adults and older adolescents who have hallucinations, a useful differentiation can be made on the basis of whether the client recog-nizes the unreality of the perceptual experience. Good insight tends to lead to a better prognosis for psychotic disorders, and such disorders tend to be more closely associated with discrete biological etiologies. In children it is more problematic to establish such recognition and its clinical meaning is not as clear. Children are highly suggestible to inter-nal, as well as external, communications. I have found it worthwhile to attempt to explore how strongly a child believes in the reality of dis-torted perceptions, as well as his or her own efforts to deal with these experiences.

Subtyping of schizophrenia with onset during childhood is often more problematic than subclassifications of older adolescents and adults. Rapoport and Ismond (1996) note the literature suggesting less differentiation among subtypes of schizophrenia in cases with early on-set. This problem continues to occasion some discussion of features in schizophrenia that are specific to age of onset, but the overall literature is clear in supporting the essential similarity of schizophrenia from childhood through adult initial manifestation. As is the case with most low-incidence disorders, for which most clinicians will have limited per-sonal experience with affected children, care should be taken to avoid over- and underinclusion of cases. Rapoport and Ismond (1996) discuss the risk of diagnostic errors and note the problem of missing alterna-tive classifications that may be more descriptive of the particular case under review. They suggest that diagnoses such as mood disorder with psychotic features are often missed in children. A careful review of differential diagnoses is probably very desirable when dealing with childhood-onset cases of psychosis.

I conclude this chapter with some comment on the fact that tran-sient and nonpervasive hallucinations do not appear to be necessarily rare or pathognomic in young children (Berenson, 1998). Rapoport and Ismond (1996) note that "brief hallucinations and delusions under stress without further deterioration are more common than is recog-nized in children, especially those with other handicaps" (1996, p. 120). Thought disorder, despite its deemphasis in current formal diagnosis systems, remains a relatively sensitive sign of schizophrenia in children (Caplan, Guthrie, Tang, Komo, & Asarnow, 2000). Attention to characteristics of formal thought disorder (Caplan, Guthrie, Fish, Tanguay, & David-Lando, 1989) and language deficits (Abu-Akel, Caplan, Guthrie, & Komo, 2000) may be very helpful in enhancing diagnostic acuity. Berenson (1998) comments on the greater than commonly expected frequency of hallucinations in trauma spectrum disorders. She suggests that hallucinations associated with dissociative phenomena in particular should prompt a consideration of possible traumatic syndromes.

# 9 Evaluating Substance Use and Other Impulse Problems in Children and Adolescents

## CHEMICAL INFLUENCE OVER MOOD

Few topics arouse more concern or anxiety within our society than that of child and teenage drug use and abuse, and few topics have shown greater resistance to conceptual and methodological clarity. Identifying the boundary between adolescent experimentation with chemicals and adolescent abuse of chemicals is often a difficult task and frequently challenging to defend even to oneself. Although adolescence tends to predict drug "use," it does not predict drug "abuse" or "dependence." Drug use, even heavy drug use, during adolescence does not predict continuing problems with substance use in adolescents at an impressive level of confidence. Also, similar to studies with adults, relatively poor diagnostic agreement has been found for the assessment of substance abuse across different major diagnostic systems (Pollock, Martin, & Langenbucher, 2000). A number of years ago Blum (1987, p. 527) commented on the tendency of health professionals to "over-pathologize adolescent behaviors," including drug use; this appears to be a continuing difficulty.

There are, nonetheless, real reasons to be concerned. Drug abuse does tend to be associated with comorbid diagnoses and does tend to worsen the prognosis of adjustment expected from other disorders (Federman, Costello, Angold, Farmer, & Erkanli, 1997). Substance use and abuse also interacts with other potentially risky behavior during adolescence (Langer & Tubman, 1997). Newcomb and Bentler (1989) sketched out a number of issues that should be considered in making the differential between adolescent use and abuse of drugs. Age of first use has been consistently reported to be a predictor of problematic use during adolescence (Blum, 1987; Zarek, Hawkins, & Rogers, 1987). Frequency and magnitude of use and associated adjustment consequences related to the substance use both appear to be critical in determining the degree of risk associated with problematic drug use (Blum, 1987; Zarek et al., 1987). Colder and Chassin (1999) found that level of family disruption and poor psychological functioning were correlates of problem alcohol use in adolescents, which differentiated this sample from teenagers who showed moderate alcohol use. At the conclusion of any discussion is the reality that drug abuse and dependence have been found to be among the most frequently occurring mental disorders in our society (Anthony, Warner, & Kessler, 1994) and is among the most frequently missed diagnoses (Berenson, 1998). O'Malley, Johnston, and Bachman (1998) provide a review of current alcohol use patterns in American adolescents. Moolchan, Ernst, and Henningfield (2000) provide a review of the recent clinical literature on tobacco smoking in youths. The research review by Weinberg, Rahdert, Colliver, and Glantz (1998) gives an overview of the literature published during the past 10 years on substance abuse in adolescence, including screening and assessment instruments.

## Assessment of Chemical Use

Creating the circumstances in which useful data regarding a young person's chemical use can be obtained is not fundamentally different from the process of asking about any other socially sensitive topic. The majority of teenagers, confronted with questions about drug use from an adult, operate on the basis of: "Deny everything; minimize if you get caught." The initial response is often that the young person has never tried drugs: "When was the last time you drank alcohol?" "I have never drunk." Any reports of drug use are treated as mistaken: "I was holding the cigarette for a friend"; "There were other kids smoking grass and the odor hung on my sweater"; or as an overreaction: "I only did it once; it was no big deal"; "Everyone tries a little marijuana; it wasn't as if I were using drugs or something." A history of known drug use is claimed to have been exaggerated: "It [the drinking] wasn't a problem, except for my being on probation." "Everyone knows that CDU [Chemical Dependency Unit] programs always think you have a drinking problem." Finally, even if there have been problems in the past, there is almost never any suggestion or possibility that there are still problems now:

YOUTH: I used to have a problem with drinking but I quit.

EXAMINER: I'm glad to hear that. When did you quit?

YOUTH: Yesterday.

At the other extreme of dissimulation is the rebellious or manipulative youth who deliberately exaggerates his or her history of substance involvement to either enhance a delinquent image or "mess with your head."

Even given the probable negative reporting bias of most youths, there is some indication that useful information can be obtained through interviews with many young people. I have found that it seems to help if an effort is made at the onset of the interview to clearly establish the purposes of the assessment, exactly what information will be disclosed, and who will have access to the disclosures. I find occasion to point out my access to prior information, such as court-ordered drug screening or blood tests from emergency room treatment, as well as my intention to ask similar questions to other informants such as parents, counselors, or teachers. Especially with respect to chemical use, it is useful not only to have access to more than one source of data but also to ensure that everyone involved knows that multiple sources of information will be consulted.

The available literature suggests that more objective questions pertaining to patterns of use may yield the most reliable data: "When was the last time you drank? What did you drink? How much did you drink? When was the time before that? What did you drink then? How much did you drink on that occasion?" It may be useful, as with adult interviews on sensitive topics, to phrase questions in an affirmative manner: "How many times have you fallen asleep in class because you were drinking during school hours?" as opposed to "Have you ever . . . ?" "What kinds of problems has your drinking caused for you?" versus "Has drinking ever caused problems for you?" Weinberg and colleagues (Weinberg et al., 1998) note that formulating a careful history of drug use continues to be the pivotal component of assessment; they review briefly the use of screening instruments for the detection of substance abuse. Martin and Winters (1998) provide a good discussion

**Interview Segment 9.1. Inquiring about Alcohol Use: Martha**

Martha was a 17-year-old high school senior referred for evaluation of mood problems by her pastor. This segment followed an initial discussion of symptoms of depression and associated events in her life. Martha lived with her parents, earned mostly Bs in regular classes, had a driver's license, and had no prior history of behavior or learning problems. She lived in a middle-class neighborhood in a university community.

EXAMINER: Now I would like to ask you some questions about your habits and about things you have tried. Some of these questions may not pertain to you—I ask most young people pretty much the same questions and cover the same ground with their parents. OK?

MARTHA: Sure. Are you going to tell my parents everything I tell you?

EXAMINER: That depends on what you and I decide. As the four of us discussed at the beginning, your parents don't really need to know any of the details of what you and I talk about. They're interested more in my conclusions and recommendations. You and I will talk about those before anything gets said to anyone else; anyway, you will probably be the one doing the talking when we call your parents back in.

MARTHA: Oh.

EXAMINER: In any event, you will always know what I'm going to tell your parents and have a chance to talk to me about it first. That was our deal, remember?

MARTHA: Yeah. That's OK.

EXAMINER: And you remember the exceptions?

MARTHA: Yeah! If I say I'm going to kill myself or hurt somebody or I've been abused.

EXAMINER: That's right. Now, how often do you smoke cigarettes?

MARTHA: Oh, I never smoke. That is so gross. My friend Sara smokes and everything she has stinks of cigarettes.

EXAMINER: You never tried it, even once?

MARTHA: No! Sara tried to get me to once but I told her to put it away. It just smells so bad, I can't imagine anyone wanting to smoke. I'm trying to get Sara to quit. She has some of the patches but doesn't use them all the time.

EXAMINER: OK, I'm glad to know you don't smoke. I hope your friend can stop. Let me ask you about some other things. When was the last time you drank alcohol?

MARTHA: Well, Maybe a few weeks ago. I was at a party.

EXAMINER: What were you drinking at the party?

MARTHA: Just beer.

EXAMINER: How many beers did you drink?

MARTHA: Not even one. They had a keg and you brought these cups. I drank about half of mine and carried it around the rest of the night.

EXAMINER: How did you get to the party?

MARTHA: I rode with my friend, Sara; but I had to drive home because she was pretty wasted. I spent the night at her house.*

EXAMINER: How did the two of you get into the party?

MARTHA: Sara has some I.D.s, but you can usually get in if you dress hot. The cops are usually there at the beginning and after midnight; if you go in between it's not hard to get in.

EXAMINER: How about the last time you were drinking, before the party on Saturday, can you tell me about that?

MARTHA: Oh, that was when we were at Sara's while her parents were out of town. Jeannie and Sara and a couple of other girls and me. There were some boys for a while, but we got rid of them after a while.

EXAMINER: What were you drinking?

MARTHA: We had two cases of beer and there was some wine.

EXAMINER: Anything else?

MARTHA: One of the boys had some pills. And there was a pint that some-one passed around. It was gross.

EXAMINER: How many of the pills did you take?

MARTHA: Just two. I don't like taking pills.*

EXAMINER: What were they?

MARTHA: I'm not sure. Jay said they were good with booze.*

EXAMINER: How much beer did you drink?

MARTHA: A lot, but I puked most of it up because I drank from the pint.

EXAMINER: How many beers did you drink?

MARTHA: I don't know. Maybe eight or nine.

EXAMINER: What else did you drink?

MARTHA: Some wine, maybe a glass.

EXAMINER: How many times have you drunk alcohol during the past three months?

MARTHA: Just a couple, well, maybe once a week. Once or twice a week.

EXAMINER: What's the worst thing that's happened while you were drinking?

MARTHA: At Sara's party. I passed out and they said one of the boys tried to mess with me. But they wouldn't let him and that's when they made the boys go home. Then I woke up and started throwing up. I think I felt pretty bad. I didn't wake up again until the next afternoon. That was why I didn't drink very much at the frat party.*

EXAMINER: How old were you the first time you drank alcohol?

MARTHA: Well, we always drank a little at holiday dinners. Mom has these little glasses she pours just a thimbleful of wine in. Dad will give a toast and we all have a sip. I never liked it very much.

EXAMINER: How about the first time you drank on your own, away from your parents?

MARTHA: After I started going out, my sophomore year; I drank a beer once in a while at a friend's or in a car. I never drank more than one beer at a time until last year, when we started going to house parties.

EXAMINER: House parties?

MARTHA: At the school. People give these "parties." They charge admission and you can drink. You know, couple college guys and their 200 or 300 close personal friends. Some of us started going last year on the weekends.*

EXAMINER: How often do you go to house parties?

MARTHA: Well, pretty much every weekend, to one anyway. Unless we have our own party at someone's home. But I don't know if I want to go to any more house parties. They're not much fun unless you drink a lot.

EXAMINER: Other young people have told me that. Let me ask you some questions about other drugs you have tried. . . .

In this segment of the interview the examiner begins to establish some basic information regarding Martha's drinking behavior and its consequences in her life. There were several choice points (*) at which additional topics or information could have been developed on associated themes, such as driving under the influence of alcohol or risky sexual behavior. Most areas could have been explored in much greater detail. The examiner stayed focused for the moment on alcohol use—the frequency, amount, kind, and consequences of alcohol consumption. An effort was made to be largely nonjudgmental but to support wise decisions whenever possible. Notice how the information on frequency of use from near the end of the segment compares with the earlier report of frequency of use.

of diagnostic interviewing and screening tools useful in the assessment of adolescent alcohol use disorders.

Assessing chemical use in children and teenagers is as important in initial evaluations as is assessing problematic chemical use. Almost any appreciable level of use of mood-altering chemicals in children is of concern, in part due to the status of early use as a significant risk factor for problematic use and prognosis. In adolescence, however, some level of chemical use is likely. In our society adolescence tends to predict some level of substance experimentation in many children, most of whom do not have mental health problems and are at low risk for continuing substance abuse problems. Despite this common view, substance use is always a potentially complicating factor in a youth's life, especially if it places him or her in association with criminals. It is an error to assume that any use of alcohol by a teenager is alcohol abuse; it is also an error to assume that the teen does not drink outside his or her parents' supervision. The examiner needs to actively assess the nature, extent, and consequences of any substance use by the young person.

This issue is further complicated by our existing diagnostic categories, which remain highly problematic for substance abuse and substance dependence in adolescents. Pollock and Martin (1999) point out that a teenager may show one or two of the DSM-IV symptoms of alcohol dependence (a diagnosis that requires at least three of seven symptoms) while not showing any of the four symptoms of alcohol abuse (a diagnosis that requires at least one of the four symptoms). This youth is manifesting meaningful evidence of problematic drinking but does not quality for classification with either of the two primary DSM-IV alcohol use disorders. Pollock and Martin (1999) suggest the phrase "diagnostic orphans" to refer to such young people and present data that this is actually a common developmental pattern in youthful drinkers, a pat-

tern that tends to be missed by a focus on the most commonly used diagnostic system.

Although alcohol and nicotine are the chemicals most commonly
abused by children and adolescents, other drug use is an ongoing social
problem and a frequent contributor to adjustment problems. It is wise
to make at least an initial survey of overall chemical involvement during the initial evaluation. I have also found it useful to return to this
topic as a potential explanation whenever an assessment or treatment
program fails unexpectedly or for reasons that are not clear. Bailey
(1994) comments on the reality that youths seldom identify substance
use or abuse as a major presenting concern. My professional experience has been that undetected or underappreciated chemical use is
among the most frequent reasons for discovery that my previous evaluations have been incorrect or unproductive. Although many adolescents and the majority of children do not use or abuse mood-altering
chemicals, many others do. Failure to take this possibility seriously into
account is a risky position from which to attempt useful evaluations of
adjustment and functioning in youth.

It may be helpful to explore with the young person his or her perceived reasons for drinking or using drugs. Although the role of peer
influences is often discussed, it is also possible that adolescents, especially those with behavior disorders, may be using chemicals, much as
adults do, to control negative moods and stress (Segal, Hobfoll, & Cromer, 1984). Adolescents at risk for alcohol abuse may show cognitive
distortions regarding expected positive facilitation of cognitive and
motor functioning from substance use (Christiansen, Smith, Roehling,
& Goldman, 1989). Productive ideas for intervention strategies may develop from a careful assessment of the perceived reasons for chemical
use.

It is worthwhile for the mental health counselor to recognize the
limitations of urine drug screens in evaluating the chemical use of
youths. Jaffe (1998) points out that most substances are eliminated
from the body in 24 to 36 hours. An exception is THC (the active agent
in marijuana and hemp), which is fat soluble and may remain in the
body and show up in urine for 2 to 3 weeks after use. Jaffe also points
out that many adolescents may be aware that drinking large amounts of
water (hydration) may dilute their urine to the point of producing a
negative drug screen. Whereas a positive drug screen can be a relatively reliable indicator of use, a negative drug screen is often not a reliable assurance of the absence of any substance use. Jaffe suggests that a

teenager's refusal to cooperate with a drug screening is highly suggestive of his or her need to hide some activity.

## Areas for Evaluation

The young person's current and historical chemical use behavior should be assesed. I attempt to determine, with as much objectivity as possible, the following: the specific circumstances, chemicals used, amount used, source, and consequences of the past few instances of use; the pattern of use over the past several months and if it has changed; lifetime experiences with various substances; and the ages at which various substances began to be used. It is also very valuable to assess the family's history of substance use and abuse. The age at which alcohol use begins is a significant predictor of problematic use (Grant, 1998). Children who first drink at a younger age than their peers appear to be at greater risk for problematic involvement with alcohol, as well as for movement into other areas of chemical involvement. We need to evaluate the social context in which drug use occurs, the frequency of drug use, and how drug use has affected the youth's life. Ask young people to share what they see as the positive and the negative consequences of chemical use. Discuss with them any efforts they have made to limit or stop smoking, drinking, or using other chemicals. Finally, determine their history of formal cessation efforts (Alcoholics Anonymous, chemical dependency units, counseling for substance use) and of societal responses to their chemical use (expulsion from school, juvenile court). I have found it productive to ask the young person what their plans for future chemical use are and what they believe the consequences of these plans are likely to be.

Evaluation of substance use attitudes and behavior in the youth's peer group is another area worth exploring in the assessment of substance use problems in children and adolescents. Although child characteristics may predispose the youth to early experimentation with chemicals and contribute to association with more deviant peer groups, peer use appears to be the proximal factor in initiating adolescent substance use (Wills & Cleary, 1999). In discussing substance use with young people, work at gaining an understanding of how much alcohol, cigarette, and marijuana use takes place within their peer group(s), as well as the occurrence of other substance abuse. After establishing a rough working estimate of the number of youths the client regularly associates with, inquire along the following lines: How many of your

**Practice Note 9.1. An Interview Protocol for Reviewing Chemical Use in Youths**

As with other topics, questions about substance use are interactive—the answers given determine to some extent the subsequent questions. Certain topics and areas, however, should be addressed irrespective of the previous responses. In the sample questions below, those marked with an asterisk should always be asked.

"Now I'd like to ask you about your experience with cigarettes, alcohol, and other drugs."

*"When was the last time you smoked tobacco?"

"Have you ever smoked? Tell me about that."

"How old were you when you first smoked a cigarette?"

"How many cigarettes do you smoke a day now?"
  "How long have you smoked this much?"

"Where do you usually do your smoking?"

"Where do you usually get your cigarettes from?"

"What kind of problems has smoking caused for you?"
  "How do your parents feel about your smoking?"
  "Have you gotten into trouble at school for smoking?"
  "Have you lost any friends or had problems with friends over smoking?"

*"What other tobacco products have you used?"

*"When was the last time you drank any alcohol?"
  "How much alcohol did you drink? What kinds of alcohol were you drinking? What happened afterward?"
  "Who was with you the last time you were drinking? What happened?"
  "How about the time before that? Tell me about that."

"What is the most alcohol you have ever drunk? What happened?"

"How do you get alcohol?"

"What kinds of problems have drinking caused for you?"
  "How do your parents feel about your drinking?"
  "Have you ever gotten into problems at school due to drinking?"
  "Have you ever gotten into legal problems due to drinking?"
  "Have you had problems with your friends because of drinking?"
  "What is the worst thing that has happened while you were drinking?"

"How old were you the first time you drank alcohol? When did most of your friends start drinking? How does your drinking compare with other kids in your classes at school or other kids your age?"

"How has your drinking changed over the past year?"

*"When was the last time you used any marijuana?"

"How old were you when you first tried marijuana?"

"How often have you used marijuana in the past month?"

"What's usually going on when you use marijuana?"

*"What other drugs have you used?

"When was the first time you used _____?"

"When was the last time you used _____?"

"How many times have you used _____?"

"Where did you get the _____? How did you know that's what it was?"

"How did the _____ affect you?"

"What other drugs have you used?"

"What has been the biggest effect you have gotten using _____?"

"What has been the worst thing about using _____?"

*"Have you ever 'huffed' or inhaled something to get high? Tell me about that."

*"Have you ever used another person's prescription medications? Tell me about that."

*"How many people do you regularly do things with—hang out, party with, talk to?"

"How many of your friends smoke tobacco occasionally?"

"How many of your friends smoke tobacco regularly?"

"How many of your friends drink alcohol occasionally?"

"How many of your friends drink alcohol regularly?"

"How many of your friends smoke marijuana occasionally?"

"How many of your friends smoke marijuana regularly?"

"What other drugs do your friends use?"

"How has drug use affected your friends?"

---

friends smoke occasionally, regularly? How many of your friends drink occasionally, regularly? How many of your friends use marijuana? What other drugs has the group you associate with used?

Counselors often discover that questioning a youth about friends' substance use is one of the more sensitive topics that comes up with children and adolescents. Young people may be relatively open and forthright about their own chemical experimentation but reluctant to report on their knowledge of friends' activities and experiences. A brief review of whatever standards of confidentiality are in play for the session may be a useful prologue to any questions about smoking, drinking, and drug use in a youth's peer group. I find it helpful to remind my client that his or her friends' chemical use is not really my principal concern—I am interested in learning more about the world in which my client functions. Limiting conversations to first names or even allowing the youth to use aliases for his or her companions may help relieve some of the anxiety over "ratting out your group."

## Comorbidities with Chemical Use

Child and adolescent abuse of drugs is more common in youths with a history of behavior problems (Weinberg et al., 1998), and drug use is a risk factor for other behavior problems, including family problems and delinquency (McGarvey, Canterbury, & Waite, 1996), psychiatric diagnosis (Federman et al., 1997), and dropping out of school and precocious sexual activity (Newcomb & Bentler, 1989). Early conduct problems, as well as early substance abuse, is a risk factors for adult alcohol use disorders (Harford & Muthen, 2000). Careful review of substance use history in adolescents and older children who present with disruptive behavior disorder pattern problems is warranted. Children with a known history of substance use should be carefully evaluated for substance use problems.

Use of one substance of abuse is a risk factor for use of other substances. There does appear to be at least a rough hierarchical relationship among substances. Alcohol and nicotine do tend to serve as "gateway drugs," and it is unusual, though not unknown, to find youths abusing cannabis and other illicit substances who have not previously used at least tobacco or alcohol. Similarly, most individuals who abuse "more serious" substances, such as stimulants, barbiturates, analgesics, or hallucinogens, have used marijuana previously or currently. It is productive to determine how extensive a range of chemicals has been experimented with and regularly used. My typical protocol is to ask about nicotine, alcohol, marijuana, "other drugs," and "What other drugs?" until the domain of drug use or the client's willingness to reveal this information is well defined.

In addition to illicit drugs, the youth's exposure to over-the-counter and prescription drugs—both as used under adult direction and for recreational effects—needs to be evaluated. Many teenagers do not view utilization of legal and adult-sanctioned chemicals to be "drug use." For instance, a youngster may be fully aware of the fact that she has used her asthma inhaler at times to obtain a "high" and may realize that this is an inappropriate and dangerous activity. Nevertheless, she may not think of this as "drug use" and may not report this activity when asked about "drug use." As many parents can attest, adolescents are sometimes expert at making literal responses to inquiries. We tend to get the answer to exactly and only the question we asked. At times compulsive questioning is necessary in order to obtain a full understanding of a youth's chemical use. In some cases I have found it valuable for my understanding of clients to have a teenager keep track for a week of his or her consumption of coffee, caffeinated beverages, over-the-counter medications, prescriptions, and any illicit drugs. This may bring to light unrealized or unappreciated chemical contributions to stress, interpersonal conflict, and fluctuations of mood, energy, and alertness.

## Comorbidities with Other Behavior Problems

In addition to the reality that use of one drug tends to be associated with use of other drugs, the relationship between chemical use and behavior problems must be evaluated. Substance use is a risk factor for exacerbation of behavior and conduct problems, and substance abuse is often associated with severe emotional disturbance in adolescents (Greenbaum, Prange, Friedman, & Singer, 1991). Multiple clinical concerns are commonly seen in youths with substance use problems. Weiner, Abraham, and Lyons (2001) reported that youths with dual diagnoses of substance use problems and serious emotional disorders are significantly more likely to be at risk for suicide, elopement from residential placement, and delinquent behavior than youths with serious emotional disturbance without associated substance use problems. Among other concerns are reports of risky sexual behavior among substance-abusing adolescents (Langer & Tubman, 1997). Health and safety factors associated with being sexually active need to be carefully reviewed with teenagers who are also actively abusing chemicals. As noted previously in the discussion of emotional disorders, adolescents who are chemically dependent tend to be exposed to a differentially high frequency of traumatic experiences and show high prevalence of posttraumatic stress disorder (Deykin & Buka, 1997; Clark, Lesnick, & Hegedus, 1997). This was especially the case with female adolescents, in part due to the risk of rape. This is an area of risk that is probably frequently underreported and underevaluated in female adolescents who abuse substances.

## EATING DISORDERS AND OBESITY

The most common eating disorders of children and adolescents are discussed in the next chapter, but some aspects of eating problems can certainly seem similar to substance abuse problems. There is the obvious compulsive quality to the binge-eating episodes seen in bulimia nervosa. Less dramatic, but possibly much more widespread, low-intensity compulsive eating may play a significant role in the obesity seen in too many children and teenagers. The cultural obsessions of current U.S. society with physical appearance and youth, immediate gratification, and individualism at all costs may well contribute to our ongoing difficulties with developing reasonable feeding practices in our youth. Obesity carries physical, social, and psychological risks for children (Wicks-Nelson & Israel, 2000). Unfortunately, the most common attempted solution, dieting, is often of limited effectiveness and frequently plays a role in the onset and maintenance of eating disorders (Wilson, Heffernan, & Black, 1996). Eating, body weight and appearance, and dieting can be tremendously explosive emotional issues for a family.

There is no easy to deal with presentation of weight-control problems within a family. If one or both parents are obese, it may be very difficult for them to deal with concerns that their child is overweight—questions of genetics and of accepting people for who they are and their own, likely failed, experiences with diets and social intolerance all contribute to conflicted emotions about addressing the problem. If both parents are unremarkable in weight and appearance, problems of guilt and/or conflict often appear over assignment of blame for the child's obesity. Family therapy is usually indicated, and an assessment of the entire family system is necessary to gain a full appreciation of the multiple determinants of eating behavior. Family efforts to regulate eating behavior in youths can occasion major power struggles within the family, and the absolute amount of control the parents are likely to achieve is limited by the nature of our society. The child usually spends large amounts of time outside the immediate presence of his or her parents, often in settings in which a variety of foodstuffs are available. The difficulties are simply multiplied when there are major health issues, such as diabetes or phenylketonuria (PKU) that require strict adherence to special diets. Thinking of food as a "substance" that may be abused can remind us how sensitive this topic is likely to be for both the youth and his or her caretakers and can prompt an interview approach that takes into account how difficult these issues are for many of us.

I have also witnessed cases in which children's weight and weight control strategies became major issues of contention among divorced parents. Although the medical, social, and psychological consequences of obesity in children demand that every effort be made to help youth who are seriously overweight, this problem also requires the cooperation of the child's extended social environment if real gains are to be made and maintained. There are few more destructive interpersonal situations than that of having two parents fighting over the weight problems of their child. Again, great sensitivity and prudence is necessary in bringing these problems to the table in a manner that promotes rather than inhibits the possibility of change.

## OTHER IMPULSE CONTROL PROBLEMS

### Stealing

Serious stealing by youths is usually a manifestation of a conduct problem and covaries with other externalizing symptoms. There is a subpopulation, however, of "pure stealers" who, in many respects, do not resemble the general population of antisocial children (Patterson, Reid, & Dishion, 1992). Some of these children may be showing an early manifestation of compulsive impulse stealing—kleptomania. This is a relatively rare problem and can be difficult to accurately evaluate in youths. The efforts by the failed shoplifter to reduce his or her culpability can sometimes be expected to take the tack of the "irresistible impulse" defense: "I don't know what made me do it; it was like I wasn't myself." Differentiating feigned attempts to diffuse guilt from genuine experiences of an impulse control disorder can be quite challenging. At a minimum, you need to get a careful history from several different informants to establish with confidence the absence of any general pattern of acting out.

## Gambling

Gambling is another area of growing concern regarding the adjustment of youths. The excitement and intermittent reinforcement produced by gambling produces a pattern of gratification that is very difficult for many adults to effectively regulate. We may well underappreciate the degree to which this has become a social problem for U.S. society, especially in subtler presentations such as Pog and "games" played with collectible cards. Shaffer, La Brie, Scanlan, and Cummings (1994) have developed a short screening questionnaire, the Massachusetts Gambling Screen (MAGS), to help assess problematic gambling in youth. I believe gambling is an area of youth adjustment in serious need of continued study.

## Video Game and Internet Addictions

The similarities between some aspects of video game playing and excessive time spent "surfing the net" and gambling have been noted by a number of clinicians (Griffiths, 1991; Gupta & Derevensky, 1996). Fisher (1994) adapted the criterion set used to assess maladaptive gambling in DSM-IV to form a scale for evaluating pathological gaming. A similar approach can be used to help evaluate possible excessive involvement with the Internet among youths. We as evaluators need to know if there is a computer in the home, if Internet access is available, and what the family's procedures are for monitoring time and activity on such devices.

## Self-Injurious Behavior

Deliberate self-harm is a behavior problem of concern in a number of distressed adolescents. The variety of self-injurious behavior that has been reported is remarkable. Common manifestations are cutting oneself, either with a knife or some other sharp object; picking at the skin until damage is done; burning oneself with cigarettes, cigarette lighters, candles, curling irons, and other devices; hitting walls or other objects; banging the head into an object; cutting off the circulation to parts of the body; grinding glass or other material into the flesh; and a variety of other destructive acts. There is one essential difference between self-injurious behavior and suicidal behavior—self-injurious behavior is not intended to produce death. The motivation is to produce pain or damage to the body. Self-injurious behavior is commonly reported in adults with borderline personality disorder and is seen in some individuals with autistic disorder, in individuals with profound mental retardation in institutional settings, and in some biological syndromes, such as Lesch–Nyhan disease. Self-injurious behavior is also sometimes seen in association with eating disorders, especially bulimia nervosa; in adolescents with conduct disorders; and occasionally with schizophrenia. Low-intensity self-injurious behavior may sometimes be seen as an apparently temporary disturbance in a wide variety of distressed adolescents. In some settings the report of self-injurious behavior is treated as tantamount to a diagnosis of borderline personality disorder; I caution against any such reflexive classification with teenagers. I have seen self-injurious behavior occur in too wide a range of clinical presentations with adolescents to support such simplistic conceptualizations.

An illustration of the conceptual issues involved in the topic of self-injurious behavior is seen in the current popularity of body piercing and tattooing among youth and young adults in many areas of the United States. Neither body piercing nor tattooing would usually be considered clinical instances of deliberate self-harm (except probably by parents). These activities are quasi-legitimate opportunities to defy the norm, the status quo, the authorities of family and society. The pain and risk attendant to these activities is largely secondary to the social meaning of the act; the primary motivation is to make a statement. With self-injurious behavior, the pain and damage is the primary motivation; many or most acts of self-harm are kept secret.

Self-injurious behavior certainly can assume an addictive-like quality for adolescents. These youths describe urges, temptations, resistance, giving in, satisfaction, and guilt and remorse in essentially the same language that a client struggling with a drinking or drug problem would use. The phenomenology of self-injurious behavior is often described as a building sense of "pressure" or some other negative affective state, often poorly articulated. This pressure is relieved by the pain or the sight of blood running from the wound. There may be some fantasizing prior to a self-injurious incident and some rumination afterward. Careful assessment of the phenomenological experience leading to and following from the incidents may be very useful in helping the young person develop effective control strategies.

Given suggestions of a disturbing, but not reliably known, prevalence for self-injurious behavior in adolescents, I have found it worthwhile to routinely inquire of teenagers if they have any experience in deliberately harming themselves. It is important to differentiate this topic from that of suicide. The majority of young people have no such experiences and have no difficulty expressing this. A subset of the adolescents I see do have a history of self-injurious behavior, and direct inquiry seems the most effective and efficient means to learn about this. Obviously, the youth who is committed to keeping this information from you will in all likelihood be successful. Most adolescents who struggle with deliberate self-harm, however, appear to be in some conflict over it and often respond readily to any opportunity to discuss it openly with a sympathetic consultant. As with many sensitive topics, judgment and clinical "diagnosis" should be reserved until you possess a comprehensive perspective on the behavior in question and the effects these actions are having on the youth.

# 10 Evaluating Highly Focused Problems in Children and Adolescents

The high-prevalence problems of youths—disruptive behavior disorders and negative affective state disturbances—are, by definition, frequent presenting concerns for children and adolescents. These easily identified and commonly presenting concerns of young people, however, often coexist with other difficulties. The majority picture of frequently comorbid externalizing and internalizing syndromes notwithstanding, a significant proportion of our clients come into offices and clinics with relatively specific concerns. Focused and specific problems of adjustment may occur in isolation and against the context of generally normal development and satisfactory adjustment or in combination with other difficulties and syndromes. Most highly specific problems of youths will have lower base rates than major syndromes in a clinical population, and can sometimes be missed in our assessments because of failure to inquire into any other difficulties than the pressing need that brings the child into counseling. I have found it very helpful to review, either in interview with the caretakers or by means of general child behavior checklists, at least some of the more frequent problem areas that sometime show up as isolated problems.

## TIC DISORDERS

Tics are stereotyped responses that are nonpurposeful and are characterized as "sudden, rapid, recurrent, nonrhythmic, stereotyped motor movement or vocalization" (American Psychiatric Association, 2000, p. 108). Tics may be simple or complex and involve motor or vocal productions. Occasional simple motor tics such as eye blinking or facial grimacing can be frequently observed in children, especially under conditions of fatigue or stress, and have little diagnostic significance. Tic behavior becomes of clinical significance when the frequency and intrusiveness of the responses causes the child distress and interferes with his or her adjustment and functioning. The most well-known tic disorder shows a combination of complex motor and vocal tic behavior and is usually referred to as Tourette's disorder. This pattern tends to be thought of in terms of the dramatic symptom of coprolalia (the sudden spewing forth of socially inappropriate language—obscene expressions, racial or ethnic slurs, cursing), although this form of vocal tic occurs in only a minority of individuals with Tourette's disorder (American Psychiatric Association, 2000; Bruun, Cohen, & Leckman, 1990).

Tourette's disorder or Gilles de la Tourette's syndrome, is coming to be recognized as a more prevalent clinical problem than was previously believed. Even without coprolalia, the disorder can be disruptive in a classroom, can interfere with the child's attention to tasks, and can create significant social problems for the young person (Walter & Carter, 1997). The clinical impact of this pattern of motor and vocal tics is magnified by its high comorbidity with other psychiatric problems (Olson, 1996; Walter & Carter, 1997). Commonly reported associations include ADHD, obsessive–compulsive symptoms and disorder, learning disabilities, and what some have referred to as "empathy/autism spectrum problems" (Kadesjo & Gillberg, 2000). Many children who suffer with Tourette's disorder also have problems with social interaction and relationships (Dykens, Sparrow, Cohen, Scahill, & Leckman, 1999). Academic learning problems also seem to be overrepresented in children with Tourette's disorder (Walter & Carter, 1997). Although our current understanding of the causal associations between these difficulties is limited, the significance for the lives of affected children is clear—much of the morbidity and distress seen in Tourette's disorder is associated with the comorbid conditions (Kadesjo & Gillberg, 2000). Beyond sensitivity to the occurrence and diagnosis of tic syndromes in children, one of the major tasks in evaluation is often to assess and therapeutically address comorbid emotional and behavioral difficulties. A positive development for youth with Tourette's disorder and related neurobehavioral syndromes is the availability of a steadily increasing pool of educational and support materials to aid families and teachers (Carter et al., 1999; Robertson & Baron-Cohen, 1998).

Walter and Carter (1997) astutely point out that the assessment of possible Tourette's disorder is complicated because of several interrelated features of the problem: (1) the symptoms often fluctuate in topography, frequency, and severity; (2) children may be able to suppress tics for periods of time; and (3) tic behavior may reduce during tasks that require attention and concentration. These characteristics can make accurate evaluation of possible Tourette's disorder difficult in a highly focused clinic or office visit. Careful observation of the youth over extended periods may be necessary for a confident diagnosis.

## IDENTITY PROBLEMS

Identity problems are possibly most commonly discussed in the context of borderline personality disorder, as they have been identified as a symptom of the syndrome (Wilkinson-Ryan & Westen, 2000); but identity disturbances in adolescents can be commonly seen as more isolated and transitional facets of the move into adult status. In DSM-III and DSM-III-R identity disorder was identified as a mental disorder usually first diagnosed in infancy, childhood, or adolescence. In DSM-IV identity disturbance has become a V code, indicating a condition that may be the focus of clinical attention but does not meet the DSM-IV criteria for a mental disorder. Despite this changing diagnostic status, concerns over one's place in the world and questions about goals, careers, religious belief, moral values, sexual attitudes, friendships, and groups remain perennial areas of conflict and turmoil for many teenagers. In my experience, these concerns are not usually the reasons the young person has been referred for evaluation or counseling, but they may be among the personal issues that weigh heavily on the adolescent's mind. Significant conflict in identity and social role issues can affect the presentation and dynamics of other mental health issues—anxiety, depression, or interpersonal conflict. Inquiry into these areas, often of central concern to the youth, can help capture his or her involvement in the evaluation and counseling and help build rapport between the examiner and the client.

Issues of identity confusion and conflict probably seldom come to attention in the initial evaluation of adolescents and have rarely been the presenting concerns in my experience. It may nonetheless be productive to make a passing inquiry into this area in the course of an assessment of teenage clients. At the point at which the examiner judges that maximum rapport has likely been achieved, a broad, open-ended question can be placed before the youth: "Overall, how do you see your life going now?" This type of inquiry allows the young person a great deal of freedom in choosing how to respond. He or she may emphasize external circumstances, such as grades, making the senior team, or being able to drive; interpersonal events, such as a first serious romantic relationship or pattern of friendships; or he or she may take the opportunity to speak of his or her own sense of self. Some youths are "hungry" for the opportunity to speak of the ambiguities and confusions of finding their way and place in the world. The more talented may pour themselves into verse or art or dance. The highly motivated submerge their doubts in driven service to an ambition or a cause, earning impressive accomplishments or performing commendable service. Some youths choose, early in life, a career direction that serves, for them, to define their identity (physician, mother) and seem never to question it. Each of these potential resolutions can be functional or dysfunctional, depending on many aspects of circumstance and execution. The seductive appeal of ideological, religious, and political extremist groups to some youths is probably a manifestation of these coping responses.

A particular case of identity challenge is faced by the youth who is beginning to experience a gay or lesbian sexual orientation. As Ryan and Futterman (2000) observe, most lesbian (and gay) adolescents will not disclose their sexual identity or confusion about sexual orientation in an initial interview. By working to create a nonjudgmental and supportive relationship, by not assuming that all adolescents are heterosexual, and by not equating sexual behavior with sexual identity, examiners can provide the type of environment in which young clients will eventually feel safe discussing these concerns. They recommend using a modification of the HEADS questionnaire (Goldenring & Cohen, 1988) as a good guide to assessment of risk behavior in youths who may be lesbian, gay, or bisexual (Ryan & Futterman, 1998, 2000). This provides a set of interview questions reviewing the adolescent's circumstances with respect to <u>H</u>ome, <u>E</u>ducation, <u>A</u>ctivities, <u>D</u>rugs, <u>S</u>exual activity/identity, <u>S</u>uicide/depression.

Although I have seldom encountered identity conflict as the primary problem bringing an adolescent into psychotherapy, it has been my experience that this is a common area of some uncertainty and turmoil for many young people. Providing a setting in which these uncertainties can be addressed, even without perfect resolution, can reduce the youth's overall level of distress. This, in turn, may reduce the intensity of the other concerns that did lead to therapy.

## EATING DISORDERS

The major issue in assessing focused behavioral problems, such as eating disorders, is to become aware of their existence. As with the highly prevalent but often underappreciated substance abuse difficulties, the key to finding out about eating problems is to *ask* (Perkins et al., 1997). A general inquiry, at least, about eating problems is a prudent addition to any initial interview with older children and adolescents. Becker, Grinspoon, Klibanski, and Herzog (1999) provide a list of behavioral and emotional problems that may indicate an undisclosed eating disorder. Inquiries of parents about the child's difficulties in eating while in public settings and changes in eating habits may be useful. Although often a phenomenon of adolescent females and young women, eating disorders occur in children and males also (Becker et al., 1999; Bryant-Waugh & Lask, 1995). Given the risk of morbidity and mortality, as well as the guarded prognosis (Herzog et al., 1999), early detection and intervention is very important. Finally, given the many medical complications possible with medical disorders (Palla & Litt, 1988), ongoing medical monitoring appears prudent in children and adolescents being treated for eating disorders.

Distortions of body image are common in youth with eating disorders. Clients with anorexia nervosa may perceive themselves as overweight even though they are objectively severely underweight. Katzman and Davis (2000) offer some useful screening questions to assess the adolescent female's body image. They begin with the basic inquiry: "Is there anything about your body that you wish you could change?" (p. 45). Responses that suggest possible undue concern over body image are followed up with further questions:

"How important is your body size to how you feel about yourself as a person?"
"Do you spend a lot of time thinking about your body?"
"Are there things you intentionally avoid because of the way you feel about your body?"

"Do you try to do something about your weight?"
"Are you trying now?"
"What are you doing to control your weight?"
(Katzman & Davis, 2000, pp. 45–46)

Evaluators need to be aware that both ethnicity and socioeconomic status influence adolescent female body image (Katzman & Davis, 2000).

Bulimia nervosa appears to be the most common general pattern
of disturbed eating behavior (Herzog et al., 1999). Whereas the long-
term prognosis may be somewhat better than for other eating disorders, the short-term risks are frightening. A further complication is
that, in contrast to anorexia nervosa, in which the youth's physical state
is obviously of concern, clients with bulimia can appear healthy. In a
casual discussion, their lifestyle may sound exemplary—regular exercise, attention to diet, ambitious, goal-directed, and positive. Unless the
referral is for an eating problem or spontaneous self-disclosure reveals
it, the examiner may know of bulimia only if there is a deliberate inquiry. If there is evidence of bulimia, further inquiry into possible associated depression, substance abuse, and impulse control difficulties is
important given the association of these problems with binge–purge
eating patterns (Keel, Mitchell, Miller, Davis, & Crow, 2000).

The experience of "binge" eating, a perception of loss of control
and associated overeating, may be a clinically important dynamic even
in the absence of a formal mental disorder. In reviewing data on the
proposed category of binge-eating disorder in DSM-IV, Wilson, Heffernan, and Black (1996) note a consistent finding of greater psychopathology in obese binge eaters than in obese individuals who do not show
binge eating. Given the clinical significance of "bingeing," as well as
the high frequency of subclinical binge eating episodes in some populations of youth, routine inquiry about binge episodes seems appropriate as part of a general review of adjustment.

The practitioner should realize that a large number of children with
eating problems do not present with a well-defined "eating disorder" that
fits neatly into one of the DSM-IV categories. Bryant-Waugh and Lask
(1995) provide a useful discussion of atypical presentations of eating
problems in youths. As is often the case, comorbidity with other mental health problems is very common with eating disorders. Obsessive-
compulsive disorder has been found to be a frequent co-occurrence with
eating disorders, and obsessive traits have been reported as premorbid
features in cases of dysfunctional dieting and eating disturbance (Thorn-

### Interview Segment 10.1. Inquiring about Eating Symptoms

Eating disorders and subclinical patterns of disturbed eating patterns are disturbingly frequent in our society and probably go underdetected in mental health assessments. Females appear to be at greater risk than males for disturbed eating patterns. Female college students and other women in high-achievement situations may be at especial risk. Alice was a high school senior who was coerced into seeing a counselor by her younger sister with threats of telling their parents about Alice's "ritual."

EXAMINER: Now let's talk about why you are at the clinic. On the intake sheet you wrote that you are bothered by "rituals" when you eat. Would you tell me about those?

ALICE: (*Appears uncomfortable.*) Well, I didn't really want to come in. I don't feel it's a problem, but Zoe began to notice and got all wigged out about it.

EXAMINER: Zoe—that's your 14-year-old sister?

ALICE: Right. She's a sophomore with me at our high school.

EXAMINER: How do you and Zoe get along?

ALICE: Usually pretty good. We talk and everything. It's just this that she's so . . . about.

EXAMINER: What is it that concerns Zoe?

ALICE: Well, sometimes after I eat, I do this thing.

EXAMINER: Tell me about that.

ALICE: Well, sometimes, not all the time, just sometimes, you know how if you eat too much you feel all stuffed out and achy?

EXAMINER: Yes.

ALICE: Yeah. And I hate it when I feel like that, so bloated. God. Sometimes I feel I'm going to pop, like a zit.

EXAMINER: What do you do?

ALICE: I throw up.

EXAMINER: Do you do anything to help yourself throw up?

ALICE: Yeah, do you know what Ipecac is?

EXAMINER: Yes, it's called an emetic—it can be used to induce vomiting.

ALICE: Right, I found some in back of the medicine cabinet once. The bottle looked as old as I am.

EXAMINER: It might have been. There was a time when hospitals would send home a kind of care package with a new mom, and sometimes an emetic was included for use in cases of poisoning.

ALICE: No kidding? Huh. Well, maybe that's where it came from. Anyway, it looked like no one had touched it in years. Only Zoe and I use that bathroom.

EXAMINER: When did you try the Ipecac?

ALICE: The first time was last fall. I followed the directions on the label, and it worked pretty good.

EXAMINER: Had you ever made yourself throw up before?

ALICE: A few times, usually just sticking my fingers down my throat, but that was pretty bad.

EXAMINER: When was the first time you caused yourself to vomit?

ALICE: About a year and a half ago, just after I turned 15. I had eaten a lot and saw myself in the mirror. I looked so big, and I felt so stuffed. I couldn't stand it. I went into the bathroom and did it.

EXAMINER: Put your fingers down your throat?

ALICE: Yeah.

EXAMINER: How did you feel afterward?

ALICE: Well, the throwing up part was gross but afterward I felt a lot better. My stomach didn't seem to stick out so much.

EXAMINER: Alice, about how many times do you think you made yourself throw up by sticking your fingers down your throat?

ALICE: I don't know. I would just use it when I ate too much. It was getting harder to do, actually. Then I found the Ipecac.

EXAMINER: Harder how?

ALICE: Harder to make myself throw up. I had to reach down further, it seemed, or put something down my throat.

EXAMINER: What did you try using?

ALICE: The eraser end of a pencil once. This little plastic thingee for hair braiding once. But those hurt more. The Ipecac seemed a really good way to do it.

EXAMINER: Alice, how may times have you taken Ipecac in the past week?

ALICE: I don't know.

EXAMINER: Every day?

ALICE: Maybe most days.

EXAMINER: Can you remember any day you didn't use Ipecac?

ALICE: No.

EXAMINER: Do you make yourself throw up pretty much every day?

ALICE: Pretty much.

Alice had a severe and very dangerous problem with self-induced vomiting. Further data indicated that she had actually begun to develop a tolerance to the emetic she was using and had had to increase her use to continue to induce vomiting. She was buying the emetic from several stores in town so as to avoid arousing suspicion in the pharmacy personnel. Continued persistent and very focused questioning was necessary to obtain a complete picture of her situation and behavior.

In other cases, the young person may present the eating pattern very openly. Even with these more informative cases, a systematic inquiry is valuable due to the high comorbidity of eating disorders with other emotional and behavioral disturbances. This case was seen in a 17-year-old girl, Alexandra.

EXAMINER: OK, thanks for listening to all that. Alexandra, you said you wanted to talk with someone about an eating problem you have.

ALEXANDRA: That's right. I've been worried about my weight for as long as I can remember. I was a chunky kid, and in junior high I decided I was never going to be fat. I starved myself and worked out and counted calories. I got into a size 6 and am still wearing that size.

EXAMINER: Feeling in control of your eating and your body was really important to you.

ALEXANDRA: It was everything. I did well in school and was pretty popular, but nothing mattered like my weight. If I ate anything, I would jump on the exercise bike. I must have ridden around the world five times.

EXAMINER: How were your parents about your weight and the exercise and dieting?

ALEXANDRA: As long as I was doing well in school and seemed happy, they didn't pay much attention. My mom has always been a little heavy, and I'm sure she was happy I was staying slim. My dad never really knew what was up with me.

EXAMINER: So, you've controlled your weight, and you certainly look healthy. What's the rest of the story?

ALEXANDRA: Every so often, I just can't stand it any more. I've got to eat. I really pig out until I just feel bloated. And then I purge.

EXAMINER: "Purge"?

ALEXANDRA: Yeah, that's what the magazine article called it. Bulimia, bingeing and purging. It sounded just like me.

Over several minutes, with minimal prompting from the evaluator, Alexander gave a detailed account of bulimic behavior extending back over 4 years. She provided a complete description of the onset, methods, frequencies, and course of her problem. She reported difficulties with her self-esteem, as well as subclinical mood swings. She was an intelligent, well-informed client, with a fairly accurate understanding of eating symptoms. My job was simply to frantically take notes and try to keep up with her. It would have been easy to conclude that she had an eating disorder, which she did, and draw the assessment to a close. Doing so would have missed an additional important concern.

EXAMINER: Alex, you've really helped me understand the problem you've been having with eating. I appreciate how open you've been. I know some of this was difficult to discuss. Before we begin to talk about our next steps, I want to make sure I haven't missed anything. Are there any other problems that have been bothering you?

ALEXANDRA: Mhhh. We talked about how I get to feeling.

EXAMINER: Yes, anything else?

ALEXANDRA: And how I feel about myself.

EXAMINER: Yes, anything else?

ALEXANDRA: Isn't that enough?

EXAMINER: It certainly is. It's a lot for anyone to deal with. I just want to be sure I haven't missed anything that troubles you. Is there anything else?

ALEXANDRA: It's hard for me to talk about this.

EXAMINER: I've been really impressed with how open and honest you've been with me.

ALEXANDRA: Sometimes I cut myself.

EXAMINER: Can you tell me about that?

ALEXANDRA: It's hard to describe. I get this feeling inside. It won't go away until I do something to myself. I cut my arm a few times, but the scars were showing, and I was scared someone would notice. I had to wear long-sleeved blouses all the time. Then I found I could cut the soles of my feet and no one could see it.

EXAMINER: Cutting yourself makes the feeling go away.

ALEXANDRA: When I start to see the blood.

The association between bulimia and self-injurious behavior is high enough that inquiry into possible deliberate self-harm is probably a good standard practice in cases of purging.

---

ton & Russell, 1997). Other mood, anxiety, impulse control, substance abuse, and personality difficulties have been frequently found in association with eating disorders (House, 1999; Wiederman & Pryor, 1996). A careful general review of adjustment and functioning is necessary for a proper evaluation of youths presenting with eating disorder symptoms. Particular attention should be given to the assessment of suicide risk, as well as to any history of self-injurious behavior.

In evaluating youths who show indications of using inappropriate weight control behaviors, you should give special attention to their social competence and functioning. Whereas poor self-esteem, feelings of inadequacy, and self-doubt have been implicated as risk factors for eating problems in adolescent females, personal competence has been found to be a protective factor (Phelps, Johnston, & Augustyniak, 1999). Thus, along with reviewing possible areas of dysfunctional eating behavior, you should learn about contexts and activities in which the young person feels successful, accomplished, and validated. This information assists in both a comprehensive conceptualization of the problem(s) and development of intervention plans.

Eating disorders in infants may present in the aftermath of a history of medical problems involving structural abnormalities or trauma. Chatoor, Conley, and Dickson (1988) introduced the concept of "posttraumatic eating disorder" to describe children whose food refusal followed episodes of choking or severe gagging. More recently, she has offered diagnostic criteria for a number of patterns of eating disorder (Chatoor et al., 2000, 2001). Current and historical anatomical or mechanical problems involving body systems affect the prognosis of therapeutic work with eating disorders (Benoit & Coolbear, 1998). In the absence of known organic causes, concepts such as "nonorganic failure to thrive" and "reactive attachment disorder" tend to be introduced. Care is needed in carefully assessing individual cases with a minimum of preconceptions as to the causal pathways. Although insecure attachment probably exacerbates feeding disorders, feeding problems can arise in the context of secure attachment and normal parental behavior (Chatoor, Ganiban, Colin, Plummer, & Harmon, 1998). We can usually serve our clients best in the context of a careful and objective evaluation of their problems and the circumstances of their lives.

The area of eating disorders in children and adolescents continues to be an actively investigated subfield of the helping disciplines. Steiner and Lock (1998) provide a good review of recent clinical findings, and Kerwin and Berkowitz (1996) provide a critique of current diagnostic conceptualizations. The most useful conceptualizations and boundaries of diagnostic categories of eating disorders continue to be investigated (Bulik, Sullivan, & Kendler, 2000). Comorbidity with other psychiatric disorders is very high for eating disorders, and a careful review of cognitive, emotional, behavioral, social, and occupational adjustment is usually warranted. Given the difficulty of relapses reported in eating disorder clients who have improved with treatment, a planned, long-term monitoring of continued progress and adjustment is a worthwhile component of discharge planning.

## HABIT PROBLEMS

"Habit disorder" is a phrase that has fallen out of the current vernacular of behavior problems. In DSM-II (American Psychiatric Association, 1968) the difficulties traditionally labeled habit problems were grouped under the category of "special symptoms." Since DSM-III (American Psychiatric Association, 1980) the majority of the diagnoses have simply been included among those problems that usually show a developmental onset or have been grouped thematically with similar difficulties. The concept of a habit problem, however, remains useful. Habit problems were defined as highly focused patterns of difficulty, restricted to a single area of the youth's life and having little implication for his or her overall adjustment and functioning. It is this aspect that remains particularly useful—many children have very delimited emotional or behavioral disturbances. Although not all technically involve "habits," these patterns do tend to show a narrow range of associated features beyond the identified difficulty. Further, the most frequent subtypes typically show a decreasing prevalence over the developmental years. Although one would hardly use the term "benign" to describe problems that often cause anxiety, embarrassment, shame, and/or actual danger, nevertheless, these problems are relatively benign in the sense that there is very little associated risk for the young person's long-term adjustment.

Assessment of a habit problem is occasioned by two circumstances: First, it may be the principal reason for the child's contact with a mental health professional. Second, it may come to light incidentally in the course of an evaluation of some other problem. The first case is quite straightforward and involves a thorough interview and associated assessments to serve as a basis for baseline measurements and treatment planning. The details of this assessment will follow from our current state of knowledge regarding the behavior pattern. For enuresis, for instance, we must determine whether possible medical factors have been ruled out; whether the history of wetting is continuous or discontinuous; whether wetting occurs at night, day, or both; what the recent frequency of wetting has been, and so forth. This information contributes to a treatment plan, helps establish anticipation of how rapidly the child will respond to treatment, and sets the standard against which change will be measured. As our knowledge of the empirical patterns and associations of behavior problems continues to grow, inquiry will become more and more refined. For some habit problems our current level of understanding is relatively advanced, and for others it is still woefully inadequate. We hope that the near future will see significant advances in our knowledge base regarding most of these phenomena.

Habit problems that come to light during the course of evaluating other adjustment problems are more of challenge. In the course of a general review of systems, the evaluator may discover that the child has a habit problem. Because habit problems are usually highly focused and compartmentalized, it is quite possible that the evaluator may know nothing about this aspect of a youth's life until "stumbling across it" almost by accident. The press for highly problem-focused initial assessment in much managed care works against the type of broad-spectrum interview that would be more likely to eventually spotlight such an area of concern. Some evaluators address this by using problem lists completed by youths or their parents to supplement the clinical interview. Low-frequency items can be efficiently surveyed in this manner and only "hits" followed up on in the interview. Broad, nonspecific interview questions can also be used: "Are there any other problems in your son's or daughter's life that we haven't discussed yet?"

When a secondary issue of concern does come to light, the underlying challenge is always: "What concern is this in the context of serving my client?" There may well be no functional association between the habit problem and the primary focus of treatment. Many habit problems seem to have little relationship with other aspects of the child's life and situation. Several have come to be recognized as having subtle biological etiologies, and more will probably be so characterized in the near future. Children can, and often do, have more than one problem at a time. The two problems do not necessarily have anything to do with each other. Yet any problem taxes the family system to some degree. Resources (time, energy, attention) are or are not brought to bear on the difficulty; sometimes the family ignores a problem because there is just too much to deal with. Any and all of these considerations have consequences for how the primary difficulty is perceived, responded to, and dealt with. Such "economic" considerations have implications for treatment planning. Sometimes a therapist may want to deal with a secondary difficulty first; for instance, when a highly effective treatment is available. A "quick fix" of even a minor problem may help family morale, increase motivation for counseling, and strengthen the working relationship between mental health professional and family members. Sometimes very little treatment is available but information can be provided that relieves the concerns a family has (e.g., night terrors).

## Elimination Problems

Occasional incidents of urinary incontinence without associated disease or biological etiology are common in children, decrease with age, and allow for reasonably direct evaluation. Soiling accidents unrelated to a general medical condition are markedly less common but also decrease with age and are straightforward to assess. One important aspect of the psychological evaluation of enuresis and encopresis is to ensure that the case actually involves a mental disorder and not a general medical condition. "Apparent enuresis" may be an early objective sign of juvenile-onset diabetes, sickle cell disease, or other illnesses. Fecal incontinence can be a symptom of serious illness and require rapid medical treatment. An initial and comprehensive pediatric evaluation to rule out organic factors should be a standard of care. Beyond this, a careful assessment of prior history of continence, frequency of events, and settings associated with incidents (nocturnal, diurnal, mixed) establish the basic functional and diagnostic subgroupings. The examiner needs to use some care is assuming that a family's private terminology for personal events corresponds closely to the clinician's conceptual categories. I have found that, in addition to retrospective accounts of events, at least a brief period of behavior recording is vital in the evaluation of children's elimination problems.

## Sleep Problems

Sleep problems in youth may represent management problems for caretakers but are not usually reliable signs of generalized maladjustment, nor do they carry significant negative prognostic implications for future adjustment. Although arousal parasomnias (night terrors, sleepwalking, and confusional arousal) may be associated with mental disorder in adults (Ohayon, Guilleminault, & Priest, 1999), these phenomena are much more common in children and do not have strong clinical significance. It is probably more accurate to say that those children whose sleep problems are meaningfully associated with other adjustment disturbances are embedded within a much larger group of children showing the same patterns of sleep problems as isolated, developmental phenomena. Anders and Eiben (1997) provide a nice review of the recent literature on pediatric sleep disorders.

I have seen very few children with primary sleep disorders in my practice. A careful behavioral analysis of the child's sleep patterns, as well as of the expectations of the family with respect to sleep and wakefulness, is usually a good basis on which to develop intervention plans. Behavioral treatment programs and emotionally supportive counseling are the interventions that have the greatest empirical support at this time (Anders & Eiben, 1997). In complicated or refractory cases I recommend more comprehensive evaluation by a sleep study in an accredited sleep laboratory.

## GENDER DISORDERS

Gender disorders, in my experience, are seldom "discovered" by the evaluators; these problems, when they come to our attention, are usually brought in by concerned caretakers or other adults. Evaluation can be relatively straightforward, although intervention decisions remain somewhat controversial (Cohen-Kettenis & Van Goozen, 1997). Lothstein (1992) has called attention to a potential concern: He believes that the symptom of genital mutilation may often be missed if it is not specifically inquired into. Bradley and Zucker (1997) review the recent literature on gender identity disorders in youths and their discussion serves as a good introduction to this problem area.

Children with gender identity disturbances often experience a great deal of external and internal conflict. Problems with peers, school personnel, and usually at least one parent are common. Comorbid internalizing problems are reported to be common (Bradley & Zucker, 1997). A careful review for possible comorbid depression and an assessment of the child's social skills and peer relationships is advisable in these cases. Social skills deficits due to peer rejection and isolation may have the greatest impact on long-term morbidity.

## CHILD SEXUAL ABUSE

The topic of child abuse and sexual abuse is a tremendous social problem that goes beyond the purposes of this book. Although the empirical basis for this area is still developing, several recent publications offer sound advice for the evaluator (Horton & Cruise, 2001; Hamby & Finkelhor, 2000). In offering only a few general comments, I echo the statements of Babiker and Herbert (1998): " 'Sexual abuse' is not a diagnosis; it is an event or a series of events that occurs in a relationship in which the child is involved" (p. 233). The major task of the mental health evaluator is understanding the consequences this event has had on the feelings and actions of the child who was victimized. Establishing a safe and supportive environment within the evaluation setting, allowing the youth to set the pace of exploration, and recognizing the tremendous variety of human adaptations to trauma are essential elements of assessing childhood sexual abuse without further assaulting the child's sense of self. The evaluator is further burdened by the need to be cognizant of the forensic implications of assessment decisions made. Methodological differences in interview technique affect both the information produced and the acceptability of any disclosure in a court hearing (Cantlon, Payne, & Erbaugh, 1996). The American Academy of Child and Adolescent Psychiatry (1997) offers practice guidelines for the evaluation of children who may have been abused.

A basic knowledge of what sexual behavior is typical and what is unusual in both population and clinic samples of children is tremendously helpful in evaluating children who may have been sexually abused (Friedrich et al., 1992). Johnson (1993a) provides a good review of the development of childhood sexuality, and Gil (1993a) discusses the differentiation of age-appropriate sex play from problematic sexual behavior. One major concern is the association between a history of sexual abuse and subsequent behavior that has been characterized as "eroticized" (Yates, 1987), "sexually preoccupied" (Johnson, 1993b), or "sexualized" (Gil, 1993b). Gil uses the term "sexualized children" to refer to "young children who appear to be overly focused and compulsively drawn toward sexual matters when most of their peers do not seem to exhibit similar interest." (1993b, p. 91). Such behavior can both interfere with the child's subsequent peer relationships and social development and expose him or her to risk of further abuse or exploitation.

Rape and sexual assault are unfortunately common crimes, often directed against young females (Silverman, 2000). Adolescent victims of sexual assault are more likely than adult female victims to know their assailant (Silverman, 2000). Major risk factors for adolescent rape include alcohol and drug use, interactions with strangers in unsupervised settings, interactions with older males, staying out late, coping limitations (physical, emotional, or intellectual challenges), and homelessness (Holmes, 1998). We need to be particularly concerned that the most commonly reported psychological symptom following rape is denial (Felice et al., 1978). Adolescent women may have ambivalent thoughts about forced sex, especially acquaintance rape (Parrot, 1989). Date rape victims may experience feelings of guilt, shame, and self-blame and they may be concerned over the loss of virginity (Silverman,

2000). All of these reactions may make it difficult for the young woman to acknowledge, sometimes even to herself, that she has been raped. The mental health evaluation may be in response to the psychological symptoms that often develop following rape—fears, psychosomatic complaints, insomnia, depression, school problems, or suicide attempts (Felice et al., 1978). Silverman (2000) recommends that questions about sexual activity, including unwanted sexual contacts, be routinely incorporated into medical evaluations of adolescents; an equally compelling case could be made for addressing these issues in psychological assessments.

The evaluation of the adolescent perpetrator of sexual assault is an increasingly frequent assignment for the child mental health specialist. Despite the pressing need, the assessment and typology of youthful sex offenders has a limited empirical basis at this time (Morenz & Becker, 1995). Denial and minimization are common among individuals who commit sexual offenses, and no specific pattern of test results reliably identifies those youths most likely to reoffend (Morenz & Becker, 1995). This is an especially difficult area of professional work because many of the children who abuse other children have themselves been victimized in the past, it can be very challenging for therapists to maintain their emotional balance in the face of such human suffering (Ryan & Lane, 1997a). Lane (1997) and Hudson and Ward (2001) provide good discussions of the issues involved in assessment of juveniles who have participated in sexual abuse against others. Ryan (1997a, 1997b, 1997c, 1997d, 1997e; Ryan & Lane, 1997b) and Johnson and Gil (Gil, 1993a, 1993b; Johnson, 1993a, 1993b) have written extensively on the epidemiology, conceptualization, treatment, and prevention of sexually abusive behavior in youths.

Another consideration in terms of a youth's sexual behavior is his or her exposure to adverse consequences from this activity. These can include sexually transmitted infections and diseases (STDs), unwanted pregnancy, and reduced self-esteem. An adolescent's risk of STD reflects his or her history and current level of sexual activity. Early onset of sexual intercourse, greater number of lifetime partners, use of alcohol or drugs, and poor judgment in partner selection all increase the risk of an adolescent acquiring an STD (Bonny & Biro, 1998). A more subtle risk factor is ignorance, on the part of both the adolescent and the mental health or primary care practitioner. By age 19 approximately 80% of young women have become sexually active (Rosenfeld &

Coupey, 2000). Of the approximately 1 million pregnancies among adolescents in the United States each year, about 85% are unintended (Gold, 2000). In the face of statistics such as these, it becomes incumbent on all practitioners who interact with adolescents to make reasonable inquiry into their sexual practices and to encourage safe and responsible behavior. Surveys clearly indicate that adolescents accept in a positive manner professionals' direct address of sensitive topics (Rosenthal et al., 1999). It is vital to the well-being of our clients that these critical areas of health be brought up and explored.

*Data and Integration*
Diagnosis, Recommendations,
and Records

## A GENERAL INITIAL EVALUATION SESSION PROTOCOL

As an evaluator, you have a tremendous amount of ground to cover and
material to elicit and consider in your initial mental health evaluation
of a young client. Although the nature of this work calls for flexibility
and the ability to adapt to unique situations, you need to have at least a
general framework in mind for how the assessment will begin and proceed. This outline can be adjusted to the particular circumstances of a
case, but it provides a beginning point and helps you make the most efficient use of the available time. Each practitioner will evolve his or her
own individual formation of the initial session over time, shaped by his
or her training and experience and by the agencies and populations he
or she serves. What follows is my own basic protocol for the mental
health assessment of a child or adolescent (see Practice Note 11.1).

### Before the First Meeting

In my private practice, I usually make at least one telephone contact
with a parent prior to any initial session. During this telephone contact
I establish in brief overview the parent's perceptions of the problems
and usually obtain some basic information about age, developmental
history, school placement, health and any current medication, and
prior problems and treatments. This information allows me to make at
least an initial decision as to whether I will accept this case. I also take

## Practice Note 11.1. Outline of a General Protocol for the Mental Health Evaluation of a Minor

**Preliminary meeting**—usually jointly with youth and caretakers

1. Review and clarify purpose of session.
2. Communicate policy and regulations covering confidentiality and the limits of privilege.
3. Obtain releases of information and permission to evaluate or treat (from parents and client, depending on youth's age and state laws).
4. Assign behavior rating scales for parents to complete while you are meeting with youth.

**Meet with child or adolescent**

1. Conduct mental status assessment.
2. Obtain child's perception of presenting problems.
3. Review emotional, behavioral, relationship, (substance use), and highly focused syndromes, possibly with the assistance of symptom report forms.
4. Summarize for youth your perspective and any communications you plan to make to the parents.

**Meet with parents**

1. Review presenting concerns and situation, including behavioral description, history of problem, course, and response to interventions.
2. Briefly review child's developmental history.
   a. Birth and health, current medication.
   b. Social developments, peer relationships, (dating).
   c. Academic progress and adjustment.

   (d. Work history).

   (e. Tobacco, alcohol, and drug use).
3. Inquire about other problems.

**Meet jointly with youth and parents**

1. Review and summarize situation.
2. Give initial impression and recommendations.
3. Make immediate decisions regarding further sessions, referral, and follow-up.
(4. Schedule next session and make any homework assignments.)

this opportunity to communicate to the parent some basic information about my practice and expectations for clients and their families. I often ask the parent to obtain school records and any other relevant records and either forward these to me or bring them to the initial session.

In other cases, a child is being referred for evaluation by an agency or other mental health professional. This contact with a third party usually begins to provide some of the same basic data about the child and his or her family, as well as about the nature of the referral questions to be addressed. Arrangements regarding the referral of the family to me can be settled, and these often result in a telephone contact with a parent. In other cases, an initial appointment is made directly with the referring professional, and there may not be a telephone contact with the family prior to our first meeting.

Within an agency practice, the evaluator may be working in an intake service in which the family is met without any prior contacts or possibly with only an initial contact with a receptionist. There may be no information at all available prior to your first face-to-face meeting with the family, or the information may be limited to demographic, insurance, and "face sheet" data filled out in the waiting area prior to the family's appointment.

My preferred method of practice is to have as much information as possible available prior to my first actual meeting with the youth and his or her family. My experience is that this maximizes my productivity in the initial session and facilitates the most efficient use of the available time. The direct benefit to the family is to keep the time, and hence the expense of the initial evaluation as low as reasonably possible. I explain these points in the typical initial telephone contact, when I am asking the parent to "run around" and acquire as many records as possible for me to review prior to our first appointment. When these records can be obtained, the family benefits, and I am provided with another kind of data on their ability to follow directions and complete an assignment.

## Preliminary Meeting

In most settings there is a need for some initial interaction with the family as a whole prior to the beginning of the formal assessment. Beyond the matter of introductions and familiarizing everyone with the facilities and immediate procedures—where everyone is going to be or go, where the rest rooms are—at least a few essential issues require attention. The primary one is a discussion of the confidentiality of any information discussed, as well as the legal limits of this privilege in the state you are practicing in. All individuals you are dealing with need to understand what rights to privacy they have with you and under what circumstances these rights would be superseded by other legal mandates. There may also be a need for you to review with the family the policies of your agency regarding emergencies and what actions would be taken under various circumstances (a health emergency, a natural disaster, a parent leaving the child at the clinic and failing to return to pick him up on time, etc.). Whether in a clinic or a private practice situation, practical questions of fees, billing, and insurance policies need to be attended to, if they have not already been settled in prior contacts.

Often an aspect of this "business" portion of the session is the reviewing and signing of various forms. These could include your written policy on confidentiality, consent for evaluation and/or treatment forms that outline the basic practice policies of your agency or private practice, and release-of-information forms for other individuals you would need to communicate with (for instance, a teacher or the child's pediatrician or a grandparent). This paperwork can be a tedious and time-consuming process. "Informed consent" means that the parties are sufficiently informed that their consent is meaningful, and this often requires more than a cursory, "Sound OK?" on the way to getting a hastily scribbled signature. I usually plan on a 90-minute period in order to obtain 60 minutes of clinical interaction in an initial session, and I find that a 2-hour block is often necessary for a first clinical contact.

As a final element of this beginning to my contact with the family I usually request some time alone with the young person. The parents are typically left with additional paperwork tasks to complete—usually several behavior rating scales and a child and family history form. If more than one adult has come in with the youth, each of them is given a copy of the behavior rating scales and asked to complete them without consulting the partner. They are told they can compare perceptions afterward if they wish but are specifically asked not to change any response—even if one of them believes their initial answer was mistaken. They are reassured that there will be an opportunity to discuss any responses that they might want to modify. If a child or family history form is used and more than one adult is available the form is usually offered as a collaborative project. At this point the youth and I leave the parents and meet alone for a period.

## Meeting with Child or Adolescent

As was discussed in Chapter 3, my initial one-on-one interactions with the youth focus for a few minutes on collecting some basic mental status data and background information regarding his or her school and neighborhood situations. For most youngsters this conversation is a relatively nonstressful series of exchanges, and it gives the evaluator the opportunity to observe the child and to begin establishing a working relationship. From this beginning the discussion proceeds to the child's perceptions of the situation that has led to the evaluation and then to a review of associated emotional, behavioral, and relationship difficulties. With older children and all adolescents, questions of substance use are addressed. Finally, an effort is made to briefly question the possibility of any focused syndromes that have not already come to light. This meeting concludes with a discussion of what information I will be sharing with the parents when I meet next with them. The child is sometimes left with a self-report questionnaire to complete or is asked to occupy him- or herself with the waiting room materials while I meet with the parents.

## Meeting with Parents

The period spent alone with the parent or parents typically begins with a review of the difficulties that have brought them into my office, including the history of the problem: its onset, course, and response to previous efforts to help. This is a time to try to be very sensitive to the possibility of associated or comorbid problems. The critical and sensitive topics of possible suicidal and self-injurious behavior, substance abuse, and/or eating disorders need to be directly addressed. A brief developmental and health history must be obtained, including any history of or current use of psychotropic medication. Although there will be insufficient time to address any of these topics fully, you should inquire about the child's social and academic development and the adolescent's dating and vocational development.

## Meeting Jointly with Youth and Parents

At this point the parents, the youth, and I meet together again. I give an overview of my understanding of their situation and seek any clarification that is necessary. I offer my working impression and what recommendations seem appropriate to me at that time. If these suggestions include the possibility of meeting again with me for further evaluation, treatment or both, I usually leave the family alone for a least a few minutes to discuss the recommendation in private. Finally, with all of us together again, we jointly arrive at the immediate decisions regarding further actions to be taken. Future appointments, if indicated, are made and any homework assignments arranged.

This is a terribly ambitious program for the initial contact with a youth and his or her family, but it is a framework that I have found productive. Sometimes it can be concluded in a single session, and sometimes more than one session is needed. It gives the examiner an opportunity to meet with several of the functional subsystems within the family. It gives the youth and his or her parents an opportunity to be fully heard, both alone and in the context of the family. My experience has been that this framework for the evaluation "makes sense" to most families, and they readily cooperate with it. I have enjoyed sufficient opportunity to proceed in this manner so that when a family does have difficulty conforming to it—for instance, being uncomfortable with my seeing the child alone—I recognize this difficulty as clinically meaningful. This family is unusual among the great majority of families seeking mental health services for their children, and caution is necessary to understand other ways in which they may be atypical. There are many other possible ways to structure the initial evaluation, and I am sure than any number would be just as satisfactory as this protocol, but I have found this framework useful in my practice and usually proceed with it unless there is some clear indication to do otherwise.

## RECORDING DATA AND DOCUMENTATION

Assessment of emotional and behavioral difficulties in children and adolescents requires not only the accurate and comprehensive evaluation of the youth and his or her situation but also the accurate recording of these data for later use. Psychological records are the responsibility of the clinician, and care needs to be taken so that the meaningful data about our clients are effectively gathered and accurately preserved.

### A Simple Aid for Prompting Recording of Mental Status and General Observations

Our contact with clients is a rich source of information, through both their verbal responses and our observations of behavior and presentation. In order to make the most efficient use of this information, it must be systematically sampled and recorded for later use. A variety of protocols for mental status examinations have been developed for different purposes. Some of these have evolved into highly structured activities, with the use of prepared forms for either stimulus or recording functions or both (Strub & Black, 1993). Prepared forms have the advantage of being highly convenient, and they can ensure systematic collection of data. Disadvantages of prepared forms are cost and, more important, availability. In a multisite practice involving assessments, consultations, and therapy sessions at more than one location, it can develop that you and your client are in one office and the form you want is in another office, building, or city. Relying on memory to note and record the desired information is common clinical practice. This practice has the advantage of no financial expense and the flexibility of constructing a completely unique tailored evaluation of each client. The disadvantage of constructing a novel record on each occasion is the real possibility that areas of inquiry are forgotten, relevant observations missed, and an incomplete record generated. The nature of mental status information is usually such that few or no permanent product records are generated beyond the notes of the examiner. If the observations are not made or made and not recorded, then the information is lost. At the time of report preparation, there may be little opportunity to fill in the gaps in the clinical record.

An alternative to preprinted forms in guiding the collection of mental status data and general clinical observations can be the use of a generated visual cue, which can be easily constructed using the layout of the standard 8.5″ × 11″, lined pad of paper often used by evaluators. Hospital progress notes, legal pad sheets, and other routinely used paper can also be employed in the same manner. My evaluation of a new client begins with taking notes on a pad of paper as we interact. I collect the information in a fairly routine manner and record it on the paper in a fixed structure. As we exchange initial pleasantries, I write the following letters vertically down the left margin of the paper: V, H, S, M, line skip, O, M, J, C, I, line skip, VF, VC, line skip, A, M, T, line skip, line skip, g, p, line skip, med, s, a, d (see Figure 11.1). These letters are reminders of the categories of observations that need to be made (see Figure 11.2).

I stress that both these categories and the abbreviations are somewhat idiosyncratic to my background and training, but they do sample the major domains of mental functioning and behavioral pre-

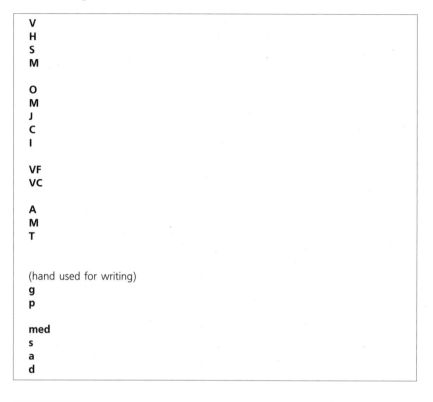

V
H
S
M

O
M
J
C
I

VF
VC

A
M
T


(hand used for writing)
g
p

med
s
a
d

**FIGURE 11.1**   Cues for the observation and recording of behavioral data.

sentation developed in initial mental health evaluations. Each evaluator would probably find him- or herself over time developing his or
her own unique list to fit his or her position, population, and needs.
The key to the advantage of this approach is that with repeated use
the very length of the left-hand column of abbreviations becomes a
reliable prompt for the recognition and recall of forgotten elements
of data. Many clinicians find it useful, for instance, to note which
hand the client uses for writing and drawing. Many of us, I suspect,
have also had the privately embarrassing experience, when writing an
evaluation or reviewing our notes, of realizing that the child's handedness had not been recorded. Then begins the mental deliberation:
Can we reliably recall which hand the youth used? Did the child actually write with his or her right hand, or is this a "high base rate" recall? Today I seldom miss noting data on handedness because, before
terminating an evaluation, I routinely scan my left column to ensure

| | |
|---|---|
| **V**ISION: | wearing glasses, report of contact lenses; apparent visual acuity |
| **H**EARING: | gross registration of conversational speech |
| **S**PEECH: | articulation; rating on MAE Speech Articulation scale |
| **M**OTOR COORDINATION: | gross motor, fine motor |
| | |
| **O**RIENTATION: | within normal limits, poor, impaired; error score on Benton Orientation Test |
| **M**EMORY: | normal, fair, poor, impaired |
| **J**UDGMENT: | normal, fair, poor, impaired |
| **C**ONCENTRATION: | normal, distractible, attention deficit |
| **I**NTELLECTUAL FUNCTIONING: | normal, low average–borderline, impaired |
| | |
| **V**ERBAL **F**LUENCY: | normal, word-finding problems, aphasic |
| **V**ERBAL **C**OMPREHENSION: | normal, receptive language problems |
| **A**FFECT: | appropriate/inappropriate; labile, blunted, flat |
| **M**OOD: | normal, depressed, anxious, angry |
| **T**HOUGHT PROCESSES: | normal, concrete, confused, psychotic |
| | |
| (hand used for writing): | right, left, no predominant |
| **g**rip: | used for writing: standard, typical variations, fist, variable; good, adequate, poor control |
| **p**lacement: | of hand on pencil shaft: normal, low, high |
| | |
| **med**ication: | current prescriptions and over-the-counter medications |
| **s**moke: | cigarettes smoked per day and other tobacco use |
| **a**lcohol: | frequency and amount of alcohol use reported |
| **d**rugs: | report of any illicit drug use |

**FIGURE 11.2**  Categories for observation during the session.

that information is entered for all categories. I have almost never forgotten to jot down the cues—a blank line to note whether the right or left hand is used to hold a pencil, a "g" for grip, and a "p" for placement—because leaving these out causes the column to be the wrong height, prompting a focused review of what is missing.

My initial interview typically begins with asking the client to spell his or her full name for me. Very young children are asked to tell me their names. Either way, I record this information at the top of the page, in the middle. Questions about the child's name are followed by asking for the date of birth, age, and grade in school. I ask adolescents about their employment status. This information is abbreviated and recorded in a column beneath the child's name, to the right of the column of mental status abbreviations (see Figure 11.3).

Underneath the child's name goes his or her report of the date, month, year, and day of the week. Older children and adolescents may be asked the approximate time of day (followed by the actual time). If any errors are made on temporal orientation, the correct data are recorded under the client's responses. The youth is asked his or her address and telephone number (this is checked against the client's records); the city and state we are in, the state capital, and the largest city in the state; and the name of the current president (and, for older children and adolescents, a few immediate past presidents).

As the preceding information is being obtained, I am gaining another set of data by observation: whether the client was on time, who accompanied him or her, how easily the child separated from his or her caretaker, the child's gait and posture, dress and grooming, compliance

*Jason S. Goodfellow*

| | | |
|---|---|---|
| **V** | OK | Jason Goodfellow |
| **H** | OK | J a s o n nr (no response) |
| **S** | OK | 5 |
| **M** | OK | bd: May (+) (?) nr |
| | | |
| **O** | OK | (address) nr |
| **M** | OK | (ph) 555-1212 (+) |
| **J** | OK | (name) comb + |
| **C** | OK | keys + |
| **I** | OK | (emergency) call (?) Mom (how) call Mom |
| | | (# eyes) 2 |
| **VF** | OK | (# fingers) 6 (?) 5; (# fingers) 5 |
| **VC** | OK | (# pencils) 3 (+) (# pencils) 6 (−) |
| | | (1 + 1) 2 (2 + 2) 4 (1 + 2) 2 (2 + 1) 4 |
| | | (red) + (blue) + (green) + (red) + (yellow) + |
| **A** | OK | (blue) + (brown) + (green) + (yellow) + |
| **M** | OK | (teacher) Mrs. Wood (+) |
| **T** | OK | (school) KG (?) school |
| | | (after) day care (+) (teacher) teacher |
| | | |
| | rt. | |
| **g** | immature | |
| **p** | ok | |
| | | |
| **med** | none | |
| **s** | na | |
| **a** | na | |
| **d** | na | |

**FIGURE 11.3**   Initial mental status data on Jason (see Interview Segment 4.1).

with questions and directions, and cooperation with the interviewer are all evaluated. His or her social skills and presentation are judged to be age appropriate, advanced, or immature. If formal testing is undertaken at some point, a note as to the child's apparent task motivation is added to the information. These observations on presentation and behavior are made in a column to the right of their responses to basic questions (see Figure 11.4). The final routine question concerns the child's understanding of why we are meeting: the reason or circumstances of the evaluation. From this point forward, the recording of content data for the interview follows the particular features of the case, but the preceding information is routinely collected, or at least attempted, from almost all clients in an essentially identical sequence. With repetition the process becomes routine, the questions flow naturally, and attention is somewhat freed for observations and careful attention to the visual and vocal presentation of the youth. The area of paper consumed by notation of these initial exchanges can also come to serve as a cue as to whether some major category of data has been missed. The interaction between the interviewer and the youth and the youth's responses to questions and requests provide a sample of behavior to consider in responding to the mental status categories on the left side of the paper. Initial impressions can be noted and either altered or reinforced by subsequent observations. Most important is that you observe systematically and record your impressions.

When formal psychological testing is a part of the evaluation, the far right column of the paper is used to note the sequence of test administration (and duration of each test, when this is useful to note). Most of my initial clinical records would show on the right edge, from the top down: "MS," "interview," followed by any other testing I had conducted.

This general format has proved highly valuable to me over the years. Any number of individual modifications can be made to fit the circumstances of an agency, type of assessment, or particular client. For instance, in a rehabilitation setting or with youths who struggle with acute or chronic pain, a left column prompt of "pain," followed by the client's subjective rating of his or her discomfort on a 0 ("no pain") to 10 ("as bad as it could be") scale and the time the rating was made can be a valuable addition. The basic structure given here, however, is almost always kept intact, and modifications are almost always add ons that are attached at the bottom of the page. This procedure preserves the fundamental purpose of the format—to ensure that essential obser-

Jason S. Goodfellow

7-7-01    page 1 of 2

Birthdate:  4-20-96      arrived on time with mother

| | | | |
|---|---|---|---|
| **V** | OK | "Jason Goodfellow" | separates easily |
| **H** | OK | "J, a, s, o, n" nr (no response) | gait OK |
| **S** | OK | 5 | posture erect & relaxed |
| **M** | OK | bd: May (+) (?) nr | cooperative & compliant; friendly |
| | | | |
| **O** | OK | (address) nr | |
| **M** | OK | (ph) 555-1212 (+) | |
| **J** | OK | (name) comb + C | |
| | OK | keys + | |
| **I** | OK | (emergency) call (?) Mom (how) call Mom | |
| | | (# eyes) 2 | |
| **VF** | OK | (# fingers) 6 (?) 5; (# fingers) 5 | |
| **VC** | OK | (# pencils) 3 (+)  (# pencils) 6 (−) | |
| | | (1 + 1) 2    (2 + 2) 4    (1 + 2) 2    (2 + 1) 4 | |
| | | (red) + (blue) + (green) + (red) + (yellow) + | |
| **A** | OK | (blue) + (brown) + (green) + (yellow) + | |
| **M** | OK | (teacher) Mrs. Wood (+) | |
| **T** | OK | (school) KG (?) school | |
| | | (after) day care (+) (teacher) teacher | |
| | rt. | | |
| **g** | immature | | |
| **p** | OK | | |
| | | | |
| **med** | none | | |
| **s** | na | | |
| **a** | na | | |
| **d** | na | | |

**FIGURE 11.4** Observations of Jason (see Interview Segment 4.1).

vations are made, vital questions asked, *and* the data recorded. The format becomes very comfortable with routine use, use prompts learning of the pattern, the act of noting the abbreviations acts as a prompt, and the configuration of the space and writing on the paper acts as a visual–spatial prompt.

A final, useful step is to conclude note taking at the end of any session by recording the client's name or initials, the date, and the page number on each separate page. I note both the page number and the total number of pages from that session's record (e.g., "3 of 4"). This makes it easy to reassemble a session that may have occurred several years ago, possibly after the data have been reviewed several times for different purposes.

## CONCLUSIONS AND INTEGRATION

The end result of the initial psychological evaluation of the child is a working conceptualization of the case, a provisional diagnosis, and initial plans for disposition of the case. This disposition may involve scheduling additional sessions for continued assessment, referral to another service, proposing the beginning of counseling, or taking other actions as indicated. Arriving at these conclusions requires integrating the data that have been gained in the initial evaluation, along with other information that is available regarding the youth's situation, into as complete and functional a working hypothesis as possible. This process is seldom complete after the first session but usually can be brought to a "working" resolution.

The diagnostic formulation is usually made in terms of a formal system of classification—DSM-IV, ICD-9-CM, ICD-10, IDEA, or a similar taxonomy. My perspective on psychological diagnosis is that it involves capturing the most important features of the child's adjustment, problems, and situation so that the most comprehensive picture can be communicated within the diagnostic system being used. Sometimes the communication is only to ourselves; we use the framework of diagnosis as an exercise that forces us to think through the case in a formal manner. This kind of exercise can help to clarify missing pieces of information or understanding, prompt us to test our hypotheses, and justify our next set of plans for the case. At other times the communication is directed to other people involved in the child's life—her or his parents, the school, pediatrician, guidance counselor, juvenile probation office, or social worker. In my own practice, which specializes to a large extent in assessment, the evaluation may have been carried out at the request of another therapist who would be in the position of acting or not acting on any recommendations I might make.

The critical point here is that evaluations lead to communications, even if only to ourselves. For a communication to be effective, it must be clear, well organized, and in the language of the receiver. Any recommendations must also be clear and persuasive to be effective. Psychological evaluations are ultimately a process of social influence. If we recognize and act on this understanding, our evaluations will become more effective in assisting our clients.

Psychiatric diagnosis is an interesting and often controversial topic in the service of children and adolescents, and it will not be addressed here beyond the issue of diagnostic uncertainty. Sometimes our understanding of a case seems complete and satisfactory. The child is wetting the bed; this is the only problem noted by anyone who knows the child, the potentially complicating factors have been ruled out, and there seems no question as to what the difficulty is or what should be done. A diagnosis of "enuresis, primary type, nocturnal" is made, and the parents are counseled on how to use a urine alarm to help their child learn to stay dry at night. Assuming the treatment program goes well, there is no reason to revisit the evaluation.

In other cases, the initial evaluation leads to a working formulation and tentative diagnosis. An initial set of treatment recommendations is formulated, possibly with backup plans that depend on the results of the first efforts. The difference is that the examiner does not have full confidence that his or her first approximation of a case conceptualization is either complete or accurate. The working formulation is a "conclusion in progress." The DSM-IV diagnostic system gives professionals a variety of mechanisms by which to indicate their degree of confidence regarding the diagnostic conclusions reached (American Psychiatric Association, 2000; House, 1999). In complex or difficult cases, giving a clear indication of how sure you are of your appraisal is of great value, especially when the readers of your findings do not have immediate access to you for consultation. The careful use of "provisional" and "not otherwise specified" diagnoses can help inform the report reader of both what is known and what remains to be demonstrated in the case under consideration. The clinical value of expressions of the clinician's level of confidence in assessments has been demonstrated in such difficult areas as violence prediction (McNiel, Sandberg, & Binder, 1998).

## EFFECTIVE COMMUNICATION OF RECOMMENDATIONS

The goal of an initial evaluation is usually not only to understand a child's situation and difficulties but also to affect his or her adjustment in some way. The case formulation is developed into a treatment plan, recommendations are made, resources are accessed, and therapeutic dispositions are arranged. This final stage of the initial assessment may be informal, such as a conference with the family to discuss your impressions and recommendations, or formal, as in a written report. Attending to a few basic principles helps increase the likelihood that your effort yields productive results.

In oral conferences with parents, I have found it very useful either to leave them with a written summary of my main points and recommendations or to prepare a summary afterward to send to them. Sometimes I have written out my main points, either to give them to follow along while I am presenting my findings or as a review after we have finished talking. My overall experience is that it is usually more helpful to hold the summary back without discussion until we are finished. If additional points, needs, or recommendations have evolved out of the session, they can be written in, and modifications to the printed recommendations can be noted. Thus the parents are not struggling to listen to you and read the summary at the same time. An alternative is to follow up the oral review session with a letter to the family summarizing the main points and recommendations. This can be especially helpful if your relationship with the family is terminating. With either method, the family has a printed list of your suggestions and directions, and I have found that this greatly increases the chances of their following through on the recommendations.

More research needs to be done on how to help families make the best use of the information produced by psychological evaluations. The analysis of feedback sessions by Abrams and Goodman (1998) suggests that parents may have difficulty dealing with ambiguous statements regarding their child's condition and that trying to protect parents by withholding complete information may limit the family's ability to move on to other issues. They offer an interesting alternative to "optimistic" versus "pessimistic" feedback—involving the parents in the negotiation over the most appropriate label for their child. Their analysis of feedback sessions suggests that professionals already do this to some extent—varying the bluntness of remarks to the parents in terms of how realistic the parents' attitudes appeared to be. This and other alternative strategies need ultimately to be empirically evaluated in terms of how helpful to families such variations are.

In writing recommendations I find it very helpful to clearly separate out each different suggestion. Recommendations are often enumerated to stress that there are three or seven or however many courses of action being suggested. In general, providing as much concrete information as possible to aid the follow-through on recommendations also seems to increase compliance. To suggest that the family see a therapist for family counseling, for instance, might be a general recommendation, and perhaps the parents have the motivation, energy, and sophistication to seek out and select a family counselor who is well prepared to help them. Alternatively, suggesting they contact either "Dr. Allan at the Public Health Outpatient Clinic, 111 Main Street, Oldtown, (000) 111-2222"; or "Dr. Brown at the Family Center, 222 Cross Lane, Oldtown, (000) 111-3333" provides the parents with the specific information needed to reach two professionals who are accepting new cases, who have experience working with problems like theirs, and who may be a good match for the family. It is your judgment, of course, that the therapists are good matches for the family, and you or your secretary made sure that there were currently openings in their schedules. You have invested more time and effort into this second recommendation, but it is more likely that it will be followed up on, especially if you build in feedback; for instance, asking the parents to call and let you know when an appointment has been set up. Some approaches to recommendations emphasize having the client take as much responsibility for his or her own therapy as possible, and there is certainly an important principle at work in proceeding in this manner. Most clients, however, are looking to us for expert help and guidance, and easing the obstacles to following your instructions tends to yield better compliance.

## REEVALUATION: THE NEED FOR ONGOING EVALUATION AND ASSESSMENT

The focus of this book has been on the *initial* evaluation and assessment of children and adolescents with mental health difficulties. This evaluation is, of course, often the prelude to providing intervention services for the youth, consultation for caretakers and teachers, and other types of counseling services. The initial evaluation often serves both to document the need for services and to form the basis for initial treatment planning. The original assessment also provides the baseline against which change can be assessed for treatment evaluation. In this age of increasing need for accountability, an objective basis on which to base program reviews is usually essential. A thorough beginning evaluation provides the basis for carefully reviewing service delivery efforts.

Beneficial programs can be retained and supported, and less effective efforts can be corrected or discontinued. With continuing attention to empirically verified treatments in most of the helping professions, such review will doubtlessly become an increasingly important aspect of evaluation.

The Global Assessment of Functioning (GAF) rating made as part of the standard DSM-IV (American Psychiatric Association, 2000) diagnosis can provide a simple and easy basis for the evaluation of program effectiveness. The GAF represents "the clinician's judgment of the individual's overall level of functioning" (American Psychiatric Association, 2000, p. 32). The rating is to be made by considering the individual's psychological, social, and occupational (or school) functioning. The use of GAF ratings to track treatment progress is one of the applications noted with DSM-IV, and I have found that it can function well for this purpose. The new text revision of DSM-IV (American Psychiatric Association, 2000) includes more explicit discussion of making GAF ratings. Additional consideration can be found in House (1999) and Rapoport and Ismond (1996). Shaffer and colleagues (1983) propose a Children's Global Assessment Scale for use with children and adolescents and provide relevant examples of its use.

## MENTAL HEALTH RECORDS

The results of our evaluations of children and adolescents lead to therapeutic decisions and treatment planning. This process and the data supporting this process need to be documented in the youth's records. Referral and intake data, copies of session notes, any assessment results obtained, releases, treatment contracts, billing information, and records of incidental contacts and actions all are entered into the client's file. This record provides the database for treatment planning and evaluation and also provides documentation of case management. Most mental health practitioners with any extent of experience are well aware of the changes in expectations within the field over the past few decades regarding what constitutes "good practice." Well-managed therapeutic records serve the client by supporting the provision of good care and serve the counselor by documenting acceptable levels of care.

In today's world few mental health professionals act in complete independence and isolation, and consideration of the standards of practice in your agency or practice group is a good initial step in setting up a record-management practice. The practitioner needs to be aware of federal, state, and local statutes regulating mental health records. The American Psychological Association (1992, 1993) has drafted guidelines pertaining to professional records. Other professional groups, as well as state and local organizations, frequently have recommendations and position papers on these topics. All of this can serve as a useful starting point to designing your practice procedures. An annual review of record keeping and office practice with respect to any issues that have arisen over the past 12 months can be very productive. Taking a few minutes to deliberately consider records that have been flagged as having questions has led to several beneficial changes in my standard practice and has helped ensure that my procedures are consistent with current guidelines and standards. This process of ongoing review and evaluation is a positive stimulus to development of better assessment and treatment practices. Similar effects can be seen in other areas involving the evaluation of youths (Demers & Fiorello, 1999).

# 12 *Concluding Thoughts*
## The Professional Practice
## of Mental Health Evaluations

$O$ver my professional career as a psychologist I have found working with children and adolescents to be among the most demanding and the most rewarding aspects of my clinical practice. To influence the life of a young person is to touch the face of tomorrow. As my own journey through life proceeds, this lesson becomes ever more salient and powerful for me. The uniqueness, vitality, and "realness" of human life is seldom more directly experienced than in interactions with youth. It is difficult to imagine how the initial evaluation of a child or adolescent could become routine. The format, the procedures, the questions, the rating scales or questionnaires might be standard; but from the moment the young person enters the room, everything becomes original. This is the first encounter with this human being. Every human is unique in a multitude of ways, and certainly every child is unique in obvious and dramatic ways. Yet our services are based on commonalities—our knowledge base is the nomothetic, the general, the shared. Within this inherent tension is the exciting dynamic that drives the psychological evaluation of our clients: how to best understand the particularities of their lives in the context of constant human variation. It makes every day exciting and every case another lesson to benefit from.

The initial mental health evaluation of children and adolescents presented and presenting for psychological services is a challenging enterprise. Our clients deserve our best preparation and efforts. Effective diagnosis in the original meaning of the term—a full "knowing" of the problem—requires a solid background in the areas of psychopathology, development, and family and social relationships. Conducting an evaluation session depends on interviewing skills, managing several relationships, and formulating a plan for the assessment. To link our "knowing" with effective intervention requires awareness of the resources available, skill with consultation and therapeutic procedures, and organizational practice. In this book I have attempted to provide some assistance along these lines.

Yet, as important as all these topics are, there are still other dimensions of vital significance for the effective and efficient initial evaluation of youths. A recurrent theme in this book has been the critical role in the assessment process of the evaluator's attitudes and beliefs. In my own experience I have found that when we approach each person, young or old, whom we encounter in our professional practice with an attitude of respect, with an awareness that his or her life has been wrestled from the pushes and pulls of experience, and with an acknowledgment that all lives are a compromise between the aspiration and the possible—then a tremendous amount can be accomplished. The vast majority of professionals in the social service field are bright, motivated, and hardworking. They approach their caseloads with dedication and their clients with dignity, and they rise to the challenges of a demanding vocation. Over the years I have been consistently impressed with the knowledge, insight, compassion, and empathy that colleagues have brought to bear on consultation work. In making sense of our client's lives we can help them begin to see the sense in things. This understanding can be the first step toward a greater sense of autonomy, of personal power, of self-determination. I have actively enjoyed my work in mental health evaluations, both for the intellectual curiosity and challenge that is stimulated and for the emotional satisfaction of helping another person take the first steps toward a more satisfying, pleasant, or effective adjustment. For a child, this may be the first step in a new direction; for the adolescent, the first step toward eventual maturity. Regardless of the issue, the particulars, the current solution—we were there, we walked beside our clients, our presence mattered.

It is a profoundly affecting experience to share in another person's life. It is difficult to truly engage another in a meaningful exploration of his or her actions and how these actions have been shaped by events without being touched in multiple ways. If we deny this by allowing our work to become routine or labored, we do so at the cost of closing ourselves off from some of the most important data available in coming to understand another individual's life. Ablow, in his moving essays on how patients have taught and touched him, makes this point repeatedly (Ablow, 1992). The behavior, the responses, the attitudes of another show us how a human life has been formed though the interactions of temperament, chance, and experience. In youths this process is fresh and acutely ongoing, and the shared participation in it is unlike any other activity. To use this understanding in the service of another gives us both satisfaction and appreciation for our fortune. It is this sense of accomplishment that ultimately makes counseling a uniquely fulfilling vocation.

In these brief parting words I have tried to convey to you, the reader, some of the excitement and pleasure I have found in what has been my principal applied professional activity over the past quarter century. The major thrust of my practice of applied psychology has been in mental health assessments and evaluations, a good number with children and teenagers. I am deeply committed as a professional to efforts to develop a sound empirical knowledge base for psychological practice. Good psychological assessment requires reliable and valid knowledge, meaningful conceptualizations, learned skills, and effective instruments. Good psychological assessment also requires good evaluators, who work diligently at their craft and at their own lives. If this book has been of value to your efforts in these areas, then I am well pleased. Now, your client is waiting to see you.

# References

Ablow, K. R. (1992). *To wrestle with demons: A psychiatrist struggles to understand his patients and himself.* New York: Carroll & Graf.

Abrams, E. Z., & Goodman, J. G. (1998). Diagnosing developmental problems in children: Parents and professionals negotiate bad news. *Journal of Pediatric Psychology, 23,* 87–98.

Abu-Akel, A., Caplan, R., Guthrie, D., & Komo, S. (2000). Childhood schizophrenia: Responsiveness to questions during conversation. *Journal of the American Academy of Child and Adolescent Psychiatry, 39,* 779–786.

Achenbach, T. M. (1991). *Manual for the Youth Self-Report and 1991 Profile.* Burlington: University of Vermont, Department of Psychiatry.

Adams, R. A., Stanczak, D. E., Leutzinger, M. R., Waters, M. D., & Brown, T. (2001). The impact of psychological disturbances on immediate memory. *Archives of Clinical Neuropsychology, 16,* 605–618.

Alaghband-Rad, J., McKenna, K., Gordon, C. T., Albus, K. E., Hamburger, S. D., Rumsey, J. M., et al. (1995). Childhood-onset schizophrenia: The severity of premordid course. *Journal of the American Academy of Child and Adolescent Psychiatry, 34,* 1273–1283.

Albano, A. M., Chorpita, B. F., & Barlow, D. H. (1996). Childhood anxiety disorders. In E. J. Mash & R. A. Barkley (Eds.), *Child psychopathology.* New York: Guilford Press.

Alderman, E. M. (2000). Negotiating confidentiality. In S. M. Coupey (Ed.), *Primary care of adolescent girls.* Philadelphia: Hanley & Belfus.

Allan, W. D., Kashani, J. H., Dahlmeier, J. M., Beck, N., & Reid, J. C. (1998). "Anxious suicidality": A new subtype of childhood suicide ideation? *Suicide and Life-Threatening Behavior, 28,* 251–260.

Aman, M. G., Pejeau, C., Osborne, P., & Rojahn, J. (1996). Four-year follow-up of children with low intelligence and ADHD. *Research in Developmental Disabilities, 17,* 417–432.

Ambrosini, P. J. (2000). Historical development and present status of the Schedule for Affective Disorders and Schizophrenia for School-Age Children (K-SADS). *Journal of the American Academy of Child and Adolescent Psychiatry, 39,* 49–58.

American Academy of Child and Adolescent Psychiatry. (1997). Practice parameters for the forensic evaluation of children and adolescents who may have been physically or sexually abused. *Journal of the American Academy of Child and Adolescent Psychiatry, 36*(10, Suppl.), 37S–56S.

American Academy of Child and Adolescent Psychiatry. (1998). Practice parameters for the assessment and treatment of children and adolescents with obsessive–compulsive disorder. *Journal of the American Academy of Child and Adolescent Psychiatry, 37*(10, Suppl.), 27S–45S.

American Psychological Association. (1992). Ethical principles of psychologists and code of conduct. *American Psychologist, 47*, 1597–1611.

American Psychological Association. (1993). Record keeping guidelines. *American Psychologist, 48*, 984–986.

American Psychiatric Association. (1968). *Diagnostic and statistical manual of mental disorders* (2nd ed.). Washington, DC: Author.

American Psychiatric Association. (1980). *Diagnostic and statistical manual of mental disorders* (3rd ed.). Washington, DC: Author.

American Psychiatric Association. (1994). *Diagnostic and statistical manual of mental disorders* (4th ed.). Washington, DC: Author.

American Psychiatric Association. (2000). *Diagnostic and statistical manual of mental disorders* (4th ed., text rev.). Washington, DC: Author.

Anders, T. F., & Eiben, L. A. (1997). Pediatric sleep disorders: A review of the past 10 years. *Journal of the American Academy of Child and Adolescent Psychiatry, 36*, 9–20.

Anderson, R. M., Jr. (1994). *Practitioner's guide to clinical neuropsychology.* New York: Plenum Press.

Angold, A., & Costello, E. J. (1996). Toward establishing an empirical basis for the diagnosis of oppositional defiant disorder. *Journal of the American Academy of Child and Adolescent Psychiatry, 35*, 1205–1212.

Angold, A., & Costello, E. J. (2000). The Child and Adolescent Psychiatric Assessment (CAPA). *Journal of the American Academy of Child and Adolescent Psychiatry, 39*, 39–48.

Anthony, J. C., Warner, L. A., & Kessler, R. C. (1994). Comparative epidemiology of dependence on tobacco, alcohol, controlled substances, and inhalants: Basic findings from the National Comorbidity Survey. *Experimental and Clinical Psychopharmacology, 2*, 244–268.

Aronen, E. T., & Soininen, M. (2000). Childhood depressive symptoms predict psychiatric problems in young adults. *Canadian Journal of Psychiatry, 45*, 465–470.

Aylward, G. P. (1997). *Infant and early childhood neuropsychology.* New York: Plenum.

Babiker, G., & Herbert, M. (1998). Critical issues in the assessment of child sexual abuse. *Clinical Child and Family Psychology Review, 1*, 231–252.

Babinski, L. M., Hartsough, C. S., & Lambert, N. M. (1999). Childhood conduct problems, hyperactivity-impulsivity, and inattention as predictors of adult criminal activity. *Journal of Child Psychology, Psychiatry, and Allied Disciplines, 40*, 347–355.

Bacharach, V. R., & Bandmaster, A. A. (1998). Effects of maternal intelligence, marital status, income, and home environment on cognitive development of low birthweight infants. *Journal of Pediatric Psychology, 23*, 197–205.

Bailey, G. W. (1994). Alcohol and substance abuse. In K. S. Robson (Ed.), *Manual of clinical child and adolescent psychiatry*. Washington, DC: American Psychiatric Press.

Barkley, R. A. (1997a). *Defiant children: A clinician's manual for assessment and parent training* (2nd ed.). New York: Guilford Press.

Barkley, R. A. (1997b). Behavioral inhibition, sustained attention, and executive functions: Constructing a unifying theory of ADHD. *Psychological Bulletin, 121,* 65–94.

Barkley, R. A. (1998a). *Attention-deficit/hyperactivity disorder: A handbook for diagnosis and treatment* (2nd ed.). New York: Guilford Press.

Barkley, R. A. (1998b). *Attention-deficit/hyperactivity disorder: A clinical workbook* (2nd ed.). New York: Guilford Press.

Barkley, R. A. (2000). Genetics of childhood disorders: 17. ADHD: Part 1. The executive functions and ADHD. *Journal of the American Academy of Child and Adolescent Psychiatry, 39,* 1064–1068.

Barkley, R. A., Guevremont, D. C., Anastopoulos, A. D., DuPaul, G. J., & Shelton, T. L. (1993). Driving-related risks and outcomes of attention-deficit/hyperactivity disorder in adolescents and young adults: A 3- to 5-year follow-up survey. *Pediatrics, 92,* 212–218.

Baron-Cohen, S., Allen, J., & Gillberg, C. (1992). Can autism be detected at 18 months? The needle, the haystack, and the CHAT. *British Journal of Psychiatry, 161,* 839–843.

Bartlett, E. E. (1996). *The Hatherleigh Guide to Child and Adolescent Therapy*. New York: Hatherleigh Press.

Beardslee, W. R., Versage, E. M., & Gladstone, T. R. G. (1998). Children of affectively ill parents: A review of the past 10 years. *Journal of the American Academy of Child and Adolescent Psychiatry, 37,* 1134–1141.

Becker, A. E., Grinspoon, S. K., Klibanski, A., & Herzog, D. B. (1999). Eating disorders. *New England Journal of Medicine, 340,* 1092–1098.

Beidel, D. C., Turner, S. M., & Morris, T. L. (1999). Psychopathology of childhood social phobia. *Journal of the American Academy of Child and Adolescent Psychiatry, 38,* 643–650.

Beitchman, J. H., & Young, A. R. (1997). Learning disorders with a special emphasis on reading disorders: A review of the past 10 years. *Journal of the American Academy of Child and Adolescent Psychiatry, 36,* 1020–1032.

Benjamin, A. E. (1987). *The helping interview* (3rd ed.). Boston: Houghton Mifflin.

Benoit, D., & Coolbear, J. (1998). Post-traumatic feeding disorders in infancy: Behaviors predicting treatment outcome. *Infant Mental Health Journal, 19,* 409–421.

Benton, A. L., & Hamsher, K. deS. (1989). *Multilingual Aphasia Examination* (2nd ed.). Iowa City, IA: AJA Associates.

Benton, A. L., Hamsher, K. deS., & Sivan, A. B. (1994). *Multilingual Aphasia Examination* (3rd ed.). Iowa City, IA: AJA Associates.

Benton, A. L., Sivan, A. B., Hamsher, K. deS., Varney, N. R., & Spreen, O. (1994). *Contributions to neuropsychological assessment: A clinical manual* (2nd ed.). New York: Oxford University Press.

Berenson, C. K. (1998). Frequently missed diagnoses in adolescent psychiatry. *Psychiatric Clinics of North America, 21,* 917–926.

Berg, R. A., Franzen, M., & Wedding, D. (1994). *Screening for brain impairment: A manual for mental health practice* (2nd ed.). New York: Springer.

Berman, A. L., & Jobes, D. A. (1992). *Adolescent suicide: Assessment and intervention.* Washington, DC: American Psychological Association.

Bernstein, D. P., Cohen, P., Velez, C. N., Schwab-Stone, M., Siever, L. J., & Shinsato, L. (1993). Prevalence and stability of the DSM-III-R personality disorders in a community-based survey of adolescents. *American Journal of Psychiatry, 150,* 1237–1243.

Bernstein, G. A., & Borchardt, C. M. (1991). Anxiety disorders of childhood and adolescence: A critical review. *Journal of the American Academy of Child and Adolescent Psychiatry, 30,* 519–532.

Besson, P. S., & Labbe, E. E. (1997). Use of the Modified Mini-Mental State Examination with children. *Journal of Child Neurology, 12,* 455–460.

Biederman, J., Faraone, S. V., Chu, M. P., & Wozniak, J. (1999a). Further evidence of a bidirectional overlap between juvenile mania and conduct disorder in children. *Journal of the American Academy of Child and Adolescent Psychiatry, 38,* 468–476.

Biederman, J., Faraone, S. V., Doyle, A., Lehman, B. K., Kraus, I., Perrin, J., & Tsuang, M. T. (1993). Convergence of the Child Behavior Checklist with structured interview-based psychiatric diagnoses of ADHD children with and without comorbidity. *Journal of Child Psychology, Psychiatry, and Allied Disciplines, 34,* 1241–1251.

Biederman, J., Faraone, S. V., Marrs, A., Moore, P., Garcia, J., Ablon, S., Mick, E., Gershon, J., & Kearns, M. E. (1997). Panic disorder and agoraphobia in consecutively referred children and adolescents. *Journal of the American Academy of Child and Adolescent Psychiatry, 36,* 214–223.

Biederman, J., Faraone, S. V., Mick, E., Williamson, S., Wilens, T. E., Spencer, T. J., Weber, W., Jetton, J., Kraus, I., Pert, J., & Zallen, B. (1999b). Clinical correlates of ADHD in females: Findings from a large group of girls ascertained from pediatric and psychiatric referral sources. *Journal of the American Academy of Child and Adolescent Psychiatry, 38,* 966–975.

Bishop, D. V. M. (1998). Development of the Children's Communication Checklist (CCC): A method for assessing qualitative aspects of communicative impairment in children. *Journal of Child Psychology, Psychiatry, and Allied Disciplines, 39,* 879–891.

Bleiberg, E. (1994). Borderline disorders in children and adolescents: The concepts, the diagnosis, and the controversies. *Bulletin of the Menninger Clinic, 58,* 169–196.

Bleiberg, E. (2000). Borderline personality disorder in children and adolescents. In T. Lubbe (Ed.), *The borderline psychotic child.* London: Routledge.

Bloom, D. R., Levin, H. S., Ewing-Cobbs, L., Saunders, A. E., Song, J., Fletcher, J. M., & Kowatch, R. A. (2001). Lifetime and novel psychiatric disorders after pediatric traumatic brain injury. *Journal of the American Academy of Child and Adolescent Psychiatry, 40,* 572–579.

Blum, R. W. (1987). Adolescent substance abuse: Diagnostic and treatment issues. *Pediatric Clinics of North America, 34,* 523–537.

Blume, S. B. (1997). Women: Clinical aspects. In J. H. Lowinson, P. Ruiz, R. B. Millman, & J. G. Langrod (Eds.), *Substance abuse: A comprehensive textbook* (3rd ed.). Baltimore: Williams & Wilkins.

Bohnert, A. M., Parker, J. G., & Warschausky, S. A. (1997). Friendship and social adjustment of children following traumatic brain injury: An exploratory investigation. *Developmental Neuropsychology, 13,* 477–486.

Bonner, M. J., Schumacher, E., Gustafson, K. E., & Thompson, R. J., Jr. (1999). The impact of sickle cell disease on cognitive functioning and learning. *School Psychology Review, 28,* 182–193.

Bonny, A. E., & Biro, F. M. (1998). Recognizing and treating STDs in adolescent girls. *Contemporary Pediatrics, 15,* 119–143.

Bowman, M. L. (1999). Individual differences in posttraumatic distress: Problems with the DSM-IV model. *Canadian Journal of Psychiatry, 44,* 21–33.

Boyle, M. H., & Pickles, A. R. (1997). Influence of maternal depressive symptoms on rating of childhood behavior. *Journal of Abnormal Child Psychology, 25,* 399–412.

Bradley, S. J., & Zucker, K. J. (1997). Gender identity disorder: A review of the past 10 years. *Journal of the American Academy of Child and Adolescent Psychiatry, 36,* 872–880.

Bregman, J. D. (1991). Current developments in the understanding of mental retardation: Part II. Psychopathology. *Journal of the American Academy of Child and Adolescent Psychiatry, 30,* 861–872.

Brown, G., Chadwick, O., Shaffer, D., Rutter, M., & Traub, M. (1981). A prospective study of children with head injuries: III. Psychiatric sequelae. *Psychological Medicine, 11,* 63–78.

Brown, L. K., Lescano, C. M., & Lourie, K. J. (2001). Children and adolescents with HIV infection. *Psychiatric Annals, 31,* 63–68.

Bruun, R. D., Cohen, D. J., & Leckman, J. (1990). *Guide to the diagnosis and treatment of Tourette syndrome.* New York: Tourette Syndrome Association.

Bryant-Waugh, R., & Lask, B. (1995). Eating disorders in children [Annotation]. *Journal of Child Psychology, Psychiatry, and Allied Disciplines, 36,* 191–202.

Bucy, J. E., Smith, T., & Landau, S. (1999). Assessment of preschool children with developmental disabilities and at-risk conditions. In E. V. Nuttall, I. Romero, & J. Kalesnik (Eds.), *Assessing and screening preschoolers: Psychological and educational dimensions* (2nd ed.). Boston: Allyn & Bacon.

Buitelaar, J. K & van der Gaag, R. J. (1998). Diagnostic rules for children with PDD-NOS and Multiple Complex Developmental Disorder. *Journal of Child Psychology, Psychiatry, and Allied Disciplines, 39,* 911–919.

Bulik, C. M., Sullivan, P. F., & Kendler, K. S. (2000). An empirical study of the classification of eating disorders. *American Journal of Psychiatry, 157,* 886–895.

Burger, F. L., & Lang, C. M. (1998). Diagnoses commonly missed in childhood: Long-term outcome and implications for treatment. In D. A. Tomb (Ed.),

*The psychiatric clinics of North America, Diagnostic dilemmas, Part II.* Philadelphia: Saunders.

Callahan, S. A., Panichelli-Mindel, S. M., & Kendall, P. C. (1996). DSM-IV and internalizing disorders: Modifications, limitations, and utility. *School Psychology Review, 25,* 297–307.

Campbell, M., & Malone, R. P. (1991). Mental retardation and psychiatric disorders. *Hospital and Community Psychiatry, 42,* 374–379.

Campo, J. V., & Fritsch, S. L. (1994). Somatization in children and adolescents. *Journal of the American Academy of Child and Adolescent Psychiatry, 33,* 1223–1235.

Campo, J. V., Jansen-McWilliams, L., Comer, D. M., & Kelleher, K. J. (1999). Somatization in pediatric primary care: Association with psychopathology, Functional Impairment, and use of services. *Journal of the American Academy of Child and Adolescent Psychiatry, 38,* 1093–1101.

Cantlon, J., Payne, G., & Erbaugh, C. (1996). Outcome-based practice: Disclosure rates of child sexual abuse comparing allegation blind and allegation informed structured interviews. *Child Abuse and Neglect, 20,* 1113–1120.

Caplan, R., Guthrie, D., Fish, B., Tanguay, P. E., & David-Lando, G. (1989). The Kiddie Formal Thought Disorder Rating Scale (K-FTDS): Clinical assessment, reliability, and validity. *Journal of the American Academy of Child and Adolescent Psychiatry, 28,* 408–416.

Caplan, R., Guthrie, D., Tang, B., Komo, S., & Asarnow, R. F. (2000). Thought disorder in childhood schizophrenia: Replication and update of concept. *Journal of the American Academy of Child and Adolescent Psychiatry, 39,* 771–778.

Carey, W. B. (1998). Temperament and behavior problems in the classroom. *School Psychology Review, 27,* 522–531.

Carrion, V. G., & Steiner, H. (2000). Trauma and dissociation in delinquent adolescents. *Journal of the American Academy of Child and Adolescent Psychiatry, 39,* 353–359.

Carson, D. K., Klee, T., Perry, C. K., Muskina, G., & Donaghy, T. (1998). Comparisons of children with delayed and normal language at 24 months of age on measures of behavioral difficulties, social and cognitive development. *Infant Mental Health Journal, 19,* 59–75.

Carter, A. S., Fredine, N. J., Findley, D., Scahill, L., Zimmerman, L., & Sparrow, S. S. (1999). Recommendations for teachers. In J. F. Leckman & D. J. Cohen (Eds.), *Tourette's Syndrome–Tics, obsessions, compulsions: Developmental psychopathology and clinical care.* New York: Wiley.

Caspi, A., Lynam, D., Moffitt, T. E., & Silva, P. A. (1993). Unraveling girls' delinquency: Biological, dispositional, and contextual contributions to adolescent misbehavior. *Developmental Psychology, 29,* 19–30.

Cauffman, E., Feldman, S. S., Waterman, J., & Steiner, H. (1998). Posttraumatic stress disorder among female juvenile offenders. *Journal of the American Academy of Child and Adolescent Psychiatry, 37,* 1209–1216.

Cepeda, C. (2000). *Concise guide to the Psychiatric Interview of Children and Adolescents.* Washington, DC: American Psychiatric Press.

Cervantes, R. C., & Arroyo, W. (1994). DSM-IV: Implications for Hispanic children and adolescents. *Hispanic Journal of Behavioral Sciences, 16,* 8–27.

Chatoor, I., Conley, C., & Dickson, L. (1988). Food refusal after an incident of choking: A posttraumatic eating disorder. *Journal of the American Academy of Child and Adolescent Psychiatry, 27,* 105–110.

Chatoor, I., Ganiban, J., Colin, V., Plummer, N., & Harmon, R. J. (1998). Attachment and feeding problems: A reexamination of nonorganic failure to thrive and attachment insecurity. *Journal of the American Academy of Child and Adolescent Psychiatry, 37,* 1217–1224.

Chatoor, I., Ganiban, J., Harrison, J., & Hirsch, R. (2001). Observation of feeding in the diagnosis of posttraumatic feeding disorder of infancy. *Journal of the American Academy of Child and Adolescent Psychiatry, 40,* 595–602.

Chatoor, I., Harrison, J., Ganiban, J., & Hirsch, R. (2000, November). A diagnostic classification of feeding disorders of infancy and early childhood. Paper presented at the annual conference of the Society for Research on Eating Disorders, Prien, Germany.

Christiansen, B. A., Smith, G. T., Roehling, P. V., & Goldman, M. S. (1989). Using alcohol expectancies to predict adolescent drinking behavior after one year. *Journal of Consulting and Clinical Psychology, 57,* 93–99.

Clarizio, H. F. (1997). Conduct disorder: Developmental considerations. *Psychology in the Schools, 34,* 253–265.

Clark, A., & Harrington, R. (1999). On diagnosing rare disorders rarely: Appropriate use of screening instruments. *Journal of Child Psychology, Psychiatry, and Allied Disciplines, 40,* 287–290.

Clark, B. (1997). *Growing up gifted* (5th ed.). Columbus, OH: Merrill.

Clark, D. B., Lesnick, L., & Hegedus, A. M. (1997). Traumas and other adverse life events in adolescents with alcohol abuse and dependence. *Journal of the American Academy of Child and Adolescent Psychiatry, 36,* 1744–1751.

Clark, E., Russman, S., & Orme, S. (1999). Traumatic brain injury: Effects on school functioning and intervention strategies. *School Psychology Review, 28,* 242–250.

Clarke-Stewart, K. A., Fitzpatrick, M. J., Allhusen, V. D., & Goldberg, W. A. (2000). Measuring difficult temperament the easy way. *Developmental and Behavioral Pediatrics, 21,* 207–220.

Cohen, D. J., Paul, R., & Volkmar, F. (1987). Issues in the classification of pervasive developmental disorder and associated conditions. In D. J. Cohen & A. M. Donnellan (Eds.), *Handbook of autism and pervasive developmental disorders.* New York: Wiley.

Cohen, J. A., & Mannarino, A. P. (2000). Predictors of treatment outcome in sexually abused children. *Child Abuse and Neglect, 24,* 983–994.

Cohen-Kettenis, P. T., & Van Goozen, S. H. M. (1997). Sex reassignment of adolescent transsexuals: A follow-up study. *Journal of the American Academy of Child and Adolescent Psychiatry, 36,* 263–271.

Colder, C. R., & Chassin, L. (1999). The psychosocial characteristics of alcohol users versus problem users: Data from a study of adolescents at risk. *Development and Psychopathology, 11,* 321–348.

Compton, S. N., Nelson, A. H., & March, J. S. (2000). Social phobia and separation anxiety symptoms in community and clinical samples of children and adolescents. *Journal of the American Academy of Child and Adolescent Psychiatry, 39,* 1040–1046.

Conners, C. K., Siltarenios, G., Parker, J. D. A., & Epstein, J. N. (1998a). The revised Conners Parent Rating Scale (CPRS-R): Factor structure, reliability, and criterion validity. *Journal of Abnormal Child Psychology, 26,* 257–268.

Conners, C. K., Siltarenios, G., Parker, J. D. A., & Epstein, J. N. (1998b). Revision and restandardization of the Conners Teacher Rating Scale (CTRS-R): Factor structure, reliability, and criterion validity. *Journal of Abnormal Child Psychology, 26,* 279–291.

Cormier, W. H., & Cormier, L. S. (1985). *Interviewing strategies for helpers* (2nd ed.). Monterey, CA: Brooks/Cole.

Cornell, D. G., Peterson, C. S., & Richards, H. (1999). Anger as a predictor of aggression among incarcerated adolescents. *Journal of Consulting and Clinical Psychology, 67,* 108–115.

Costello, E. J. (1989). Developments in child psychiatric epidemiology. *Journal of the American Academy of Child and Adolescent Psychiatry, 28,* 836–841.

Cox, A., Hopkinson, K., & Rutter, M. (1981). Psychiatric interviewing techniques: Pt. 2. Naturalistic study: Eliciting information. *British Journal of Psychiatry, 138,* 283–291.

Craske, M. G., Poulton, R., Tsao, J. C. I., & Plotkin, D. (2001). Paths to panic disorder/agoraphobia: An exploratory analysis from age 3 to 21 in an unselected birth cohort. *Journal of the American Academy of Child and Adolescent Psychiatry, 40,* 556–563.

Crick, N. R., & Grotpeter, J. K. (1995). Relational aggression, gender, and social-psychological adjustment. *Child Development, 66,* 710–722.

Cummings, J. G., Pepler, D. J., & Moore, T. E. (1999). Behavior problems in children exposed to wife abuse: Gender differences. *Journal of Family Violence, 14,* 133–156.

Dadds, M. R., Perrin, S., & Yule, W. (1998). Social desirability and self-reported anxiety in children: An analysis of the RCMAS Lie scale. *Journal of Abnormal Child Psychology, 26,* 311–317.

Deas-Nesmith, D., Brady, K. T., & Campbell, S. (1998). Comorbid substance use and anxiety disorders in adolescents. *Journal of Psychopathology and Behavioral Assessment, 20,* 139–148.

DeGangi, G. (2000). *Pediatric disorders of regulation in affect and behavior.* San Diego, CA: Academic Press.

Demers, S. T., & Fiorello, C. (1999). Legal and ethical issues in preschool assessment and screening. In E. V. Nuttall, I. Romero, & J. Kalesnik (Eds.), *Assessing and screening preschoolers: Psychological and educational dimensions* (2nd ed.). Boston: Allyn & Bacon.

DeWolfe, N. A., Byrne, J. M., & Bawden, H. N. (1999). Early clinical assessment of attention. *Clinical Neuropsychologist, 13,* 458–473.

Deykin, E. Y., & Buka, S. L. (1997). Prevalence and risk factors for posttraumatic stress disorder among chemically dependent adolescents. *American Journal of Psychiatry, 154,* 752–757.

Drotar, D. (1997). Relating parent and family functioning to the psychological adjustment of children with chronic health conditions: What have we learned? What do we need to know? *Journal of Pediatric Psychology, 22,* 149–165.

Dummit, E. S., III, Klein, R. G., Tancer, N. K., Asche, B., Martin, J., & Fairbanks, J. A. (1997). Systematic assessment of 50 children with selective mutism. *Journal of the American Academy of Child and Adolescent Psychiatry, 36,* 653–660.

Dunn, W. (1999). Assessment of sensorimotor and perceptual development. In E. V. Nuttall, I. Romero, & J. Kalesnik (Eds.), *Assessing and screening preschoolers: Psychological and educational dimensions* (2nd ed.). Boston: Allyn & Bacon.

DuPaul, G. J., Anastopoulos, A. D., Power, T. J., Reid, R., Ikeda, M. J., & McGoey, K. E. (1998). Parent ratings of attention-deficit/hyperactivity disorder symptoms: Factor structure and normative data. *Journal of Psychopathology and Behavioral Assessment, 20,* 83–102.

Durbrow, E. H. (1999). Cultural processes in child competence: How rural Caribbean parents evaluate their children. In A. S. Masten (Ed.), *Cultural processes in child development: The Minnesota Symposia on Child Psychology* (Vol. 29). Mahwah, NJ: Erlbaum.

Dykens, E. M. (2000). Psychopathology in children with intellectual disability [Annotation]. *Journal of Child Psychology, Psychiatry, and Allied Disciplines, 41,* 407–417.

Dykens, E. M., Sparrow, S. S., Cohen, D. J., Scahill, L., & Leckman, J. F. (1999). Peer acceptance and adaptive functioning. In J. F. Leckman & D. J. Cohen (Eds.), *Tourette's syndrome–Tics, obsessions, compulsions: Developmental psychopathology and clinical care.* New York: Wiley.

Edelbrock, C., Crnic, K., & Bohnert, A. (1999). Interviewing as communication: An alternative way of administering the Diagnostic Interview Schedule for Children. *Journal of Abnormal Child Psychology, 27,* 447–453.

Edelsoh, G. (1992). Self-reported depressive symptoms in first-grade children: Developmentally transient phenomena? *Journal of the American Academy of Child and Adolescent Psychiatry, 31,* 282–290.

Eisenberg, N., Wentzel, N. M., & Harris, J. D. (1998). The role of emotionality and regulation in empathy-related responding. *School Psychology Review, 27,* 506–521.

Ernst, M., Cookus, B. A., & Moravec, B. C. (2000). Pictorial Instrument for Children and Adolescents (PICA-III-R). *Journal of the American Academy of Child and Adolescent Psychiatry, 39,* 94–100.

Ewing-Cobbs, L., Kramer, L., Prasad, M., Canales, D. N., Louis, P. T., Fletcher, J. M., Vollero, H., Landry, S. H., & Cheung, K. (1998). Neuroimaging, physical, and developmental findings after inflicted and noninflicted traumatic brain injury in children. *Pediatrics, 102,* 300–307.

Fantuzzo, J. W., Coolahan, K., Mendez, J., McDermott, P., & Sutton-Smith, B. (1998a). Contextually relevant validation of peer play constructs with African American Head Start children. *Early Childhood Research Quarterly, 13,* 411–431.

Fantuzzo, J. W., DelGaudio, A., Atkins, M., Meyers, R., & Noone, M. (1998b). A contextually relevant assessment of the impact of child maltreatment on the social competencies of low-income urban children. *Journal of the American Academy of Child and Adolescent Psychiatry, 37,* 1201–1208.

Fantuzzo, J. W., Sutton-Smith, B., Coolahan, K. C., Manz, P. H., Canning, S., & Debnam, D. (1995). Assessment of preschool play interaction behaviors in young low-income children: Penn Interactive Peer Play Scale. *Early Childhood Research Quarterly, 10,* 105–120.

Faraone, S. V., Biederman, J., Mennin, D., Russell, R., & Tsuang, M. T. (1998). Familial subtypes of attention-deficit/hyperactivity disorder: A 4–year follow-up of children from antisocial-ADHD families. *Journal of Child Psychology, Psychiatry, and Allied Disciplines, 39,* 1045–1053.

Faraone, S. V., Biederman, J., Mennin, D., Wozniak, J., & Spencer, T. (1997). Attention-deficit/hyperactivity disorder with bipolar disorder: A familial subtype? *Journal of the American Academy of Child and Adolescent Psychiatry, 36,* 1378–1387.

Faust, D., Hart, K., & Guilmette, T. J. (1988). Pediatric malingering: The capacity of children to fake believable deficits on neuropsychological testing. *Journal of Counseling and Clinical Psychology, 56,* 578–582.

Faust, D., Hart, K., Guilmette, T. J., & Arkes, H. R. (1988). Neuropsychologists' capacity to detect adolescent malingerers. *Professional Psychology: Research and Practice, 19,* 508–515.

Federman, E. B., Costello, E. J., Angold, A., Farmer, E. M. Z., & Erkanli, A. (1997). Development of substance use and psychiatric comorbidity in an epidemiologic study of while and American Indian young adolescents: The Great Smoky Mountains study. *Drug and Alcohol Dependence, 44,* 69–78.

Feerick, M. M., & Haugaard, J. J. (1999). Long-term effects of witnessing marital violence for women: The contribution of childhood physical and sexual abuse. *Journal of Family Violence, 14,* 377–398.

Felice, M., Grant, J., Reynolds, B., Gold, S., Wyatt, M., & Heald, F. P. (1978). Follow-up observations of adolescent rape victims. *Clinical Pediatrics, 17,* 311–315.

Feng, H., & Cartledge, G. (1996). Social skill assessment of inner city Asian, African, and European American students. *School Psychology Review, 25,* 228–239.

Finch, A. J., Saylor, C. F., & Edwards, G. L. (1985). Children's Depression Inventory: Sex and grade norms for normal children. *Journal of Consulting and Clinical Psychology, 53,* 424–425.

Fisher, S. (1994). Identifying video game addiction in children and adolescents. *Addictive Behaviors, 19,* 545–553.

Fletcher, K. E. (1996). Childhood posttraumatic stress disorder. In E. J. Mash & R. A. Barkley (Eds.), *Child psychopathology.* New York: Guilford Press.

Flisher, A. J. (1999). Mood disorder in suicidal children and adolescents: Recent developments [Annotation]. *Journal of Child Psychology, Psychiatry, and Allied Disciplines, 40,* 315–324.

Flisher, A. J., Kramer, R. A., Hoven, C. W., King, R. A., Bird, H. R., Davies, M., Gould, M. S., Greenwald, S., Lahey, B. B., Regier, D. A., Schwab-Stone, M., & Shaffer, D. (2000). Risk behavior in a community sample of children and adolescents. *Journal of the American Academy of Child and Adolescent Psychiatry, 39,* 881–887.

Folstein, M. F., Folstein, S. E., & McHugh, P. R. (1975). "Mini-Mental State": A practical method for grading the cognitive state of patients for the clinician. *Journal of Psychiatric Research, 12,* 189–198.

Franzen, M., & Berg, R. (1989). *Screening children for brain impairment.* New York: Springer.

Frick, P. J., Kamphaus, R. W., Lahey, B. B., Loeber, R., Christ, M. A. G., Hart, E. L., & Tannenbaum, L. E. (1991). Academic underachievement and the disruptive behavior disorders. *Journal of Consulting and Clinical Psychology, 59,* 289–294.

Friedrich, W., Grambsch, P., Damon, L., Koverola, C., Wolfe, V., Hewitt, S., Lang, R., & Broughton, D. (1992). Child Sexual Behavior Inventory: Normative and clinical comparisons. *Psychological Assessment, 4,* 303–311.

Fritz, G. K., Fritsch, S., & Hagino, O. (1997). Somatoform disorders in children and adolescents: A review of the past 10 years. *Journal of the American Academy of Child and Adolescent Psychiatry, 36,* 1329–1338.

Fuller, C. G., & Sabatino, D. A. (1998). Diagnosis and treatment considerations with comorbid developmentally disabled populations. *Journal of Clinical Psychology, 54,* 1–10.

Garber, J., Van Slyke, D. A., & Walker, L. S. (1998). Concordance between mothers' and children's reports of somatic and emotional symptoms in patients with recurrent abdominal pain or emotional disorders. *Journal of Abnormal Child Psychology, 26,* 381–391.

Garralda, M. E. (1996). Somatization in children. *Journal of Child Psychology, Psychiatry, and Allied Disciplines, 37,* 13–33.

Geller, B., Craney, J. L., Bolhofner, K., BelBello, M. P., Williams, M., & Zimmerman, B. (2001). One-year recovery and relapse rates of children with a prepubertal and early adolescent bipolar disorder phenotype. *American Journal of Psychiatry, 158,* 303–305.

Geller, B., Williams, M., Zimmerman, B., Franzier, J., Beringer, L., & Warner, K. (1998). Prepubertal and early adolescent bipolarity differentiate from ADHD by manic symptoms, grandiose delusions, ultra-rapid or ultradian cycling. *Journal of Affective Disorders, 51,* 81–91.

Geller, B., Zimmerman, B., Williams, M., Bolhofner, K., Carney, J. L., DelBello, M. P., & Soutullo, C. A. (2000a). Diagnostic characteristics of 93 cases of prepubertal and early adolescent bipolar disorder phenotype by gender, puberty and comorbid attention-deficit/hyperactivity disorder. *Journal of Child and Adolescent Psychopharmacology, 10,* 157–164.

Geller, B., Zimmerman, B., Williams, M., Bolhofner, K., Carney, J. L., DelBello, M. P., & Soutullo, C. A. (2000b). Six-month stability and outcome of a prepubertal and early adolescent bipolar disorder phenotype. *Journal of Child and Adolescent Psychopharmacology, 10,* 165–173.

Giaconia, R. M., Reinherz, H. Z., Silverman, A. B., Pakiz, B., Frost, A. K., & Cohen, E. (1995). Traumas and posttraumatic stress disorder in a community population of older adolescents. *Journal of the American Academy of Child and Adolescent Psychiatry, 34,* 1369–1380.

Gil, E. (1993a). Age-appropriate sex play versus problematic sexual behaviors. In E. Gil & T. C. Johnson (Eds.), *Sexualized children*. Rockville, MD: Launch Press.

Gil, E. (1993b). Sexualized children. In E. Gil & T. C. Johnson (Eds.), *Sexualized children*. Rockville, MD: Launch Press.

Gold, M. A. (2000). Abortion. In S. M. Coupey (Ed.), *Primary care of adolescent girls*. Philadelphia: Hanley & Belfus.

Goldenring, J. M., & Cohen, E. H. (1988). Getting into an adolescent's heads. *Contemporary Pediatrics, 5,* 75–90.

Goldman, S., & Beardslee, W. (1999). Suicide in children and adolescents. In D. G. Jacobs (Ed.), *The Harvard Medical School guide to suicide assessment and intervention*. San Francisco: Jossey-Bass.

Goldman, S. J., D'Angelo, E. J., DeMaso, D. R., & Mezzacappa, E. (1992). Physical and sexual abuse histories among children with Borderline Personality Disorder. *American Journal of Psychiatry, 149,* 1723–1726.

Goodman, R. (1997). The Strengths and Difficulties Questionnaire: A research note. *Journal of Child Psychology, Psychiatry, and Allied Disciplines, 38,* 581–586.

Goodman, R., Meltzer, H., & Bailey, V. (1998). The Strengths and Difficulties Questionnaire: A pilot study of the validity of the self-report version. *European Child and Adolescent Psychiatry, 7,* 125–130.

Goodman, S. H., Schwab-Stone, M., Lahey, B. B., Shaffer, D., & Jensen, P. S. (2000). Major depression and dysthymia in children and adolescents: Discriminate validity and differential consequences in a community sample. *Journal of the American Academy of Child and Adolescent Psychiatry, 39,* 761–770.

Goodman, R., & Scott, S. (1999). Comparing the Strengths and Difficulties Questionnaire and the Child Behavior Checklist: Is small beautiful? *Journal of Abnormal Child Psychology, 27,* 17–24.

Goodwin, J. (1985). Post-traumatic symptoms in incest victims. In S. Eth & R. S. Pynoos (Eds.), *Post-traumatic stress disorder in children*. Washington, DC: American Psychiatric Press.

Gordon, M. (1983). *The Gordon Diagnostic System*. Boulder, CO: Clinical Diagnostic Systems.

Gottfried, A. W., Gottfried, A. E., Bathurst, K., & Guerin, D. W. (1994). *Gifted IQ, early developmental aspects: The Fullerton Longitudinal Study*. New York: Plenum Press.

Gould, M. S., King, R., Greenwald, S., Fisher, P., Schwab-Stone, M., Kramer, R., Flisher, A. J., Goodman, S., Canino, G., & Shaffer, D. (1998). Psychopathology associated with suicidal ideation and attempts among children and adolescents. *Journal of the American Academy of Child and Adolescent Psychiatry, 37,* 915–923.

Grant, B. F. (1998). The impact of a family history of alcoholism on the relationship between age of onset of alcohol use and DSM-IV Alcohol Dependence. *Alcohol Health and Research World, 22,* 144–147.

Green, M. L., Foster, M. A., Morris, M. K., Muir, J. J., & Morris, R. D. (1998). Parent assessment of psychological and behavioral functioning following pediatric acquired brain injury. *Journal of Pediatric Psychology, 23,* 289–299.

Greenbaum, P. E., Prange, M. E., Friedman, R. M., & Silver, S. E. (1991). Substance abuse prevention and comorbidity with other psychiatric disorders among adolescents with severe emotional disturbance. *Journal of the American Academy of Child and Adolescent Psychiatry, 30,* 575–583.

Greenspan, S. I., & Greenspan, N. T. (1991). *The clinical interview of the child.* Washington, DC: American Psychiatric Press.

Gresham, F. M., MacMillan, D. L., Bocian, K. M., Ward, S. L., & Forness, S. R. (1998). Comorbidity of hyperactivity–impulsivity–inattention and conduct problems: Risk factors in social, affective, and academic domains. *Journal of Abnormal Child Psychology, 26,* 393–406.

Griffiths, M. D. (1991). Amusement machine playing in childhood and adolescence: A comparative analysis of video games and fruit machines. *Journal of Adolescence, 14,* 53–73.

Grilo, C. M., Walker, M. L., Becker, D. F., Edell, W. S., & McGlashan, T. H. (1997). Personality disorders in adolescents with major depression, substance use disorders, and coexisting major depression and substance use disorders. *Journal of Consulting and Clinical Psychology, 65,* 328–332.

Grisso, T., Barnum, R., Fletcher, K. E., Cauffman, E., & Peuschold, D. (2001). Massachusetts Youth Screen Instrument for mental health needs of juvenile justice youths. *Journal of the American Academy of Child and Adolescent Psychiatry, 40,* 541–548.

Groholt, B., Ekeberg, O., Wichstrom, L., & Haldorsen, T. (2000). Young suicide attempters: A comparison between a clinical and an epidemiological sample. *Journal of the American Academy of Child and Adolescent Psychiatry, 39,* 868–875.

Grych, J. H., Jouriles, E. N., Swank, P. R., McDonald, R., & Norwood, W. D. (2000). Patterns of adjustment among children of battered women. *Journal of Consulting and Clinical Psychology, 68,* 84–94.

Gullone, E. (1999). The assessment of normal fear in children and adolescents. *Clinical Child and Family Psychology Review, 2,* 91–106.

Gupta, R., & Derevensky, J. L. (1996). The relationship between gambling and video-game playing behavior in children and adolescents. *Journal of Gambling Studies, 12,* 375–394.

Guyer, B. P. (2000). The adult who has ADHD: Finding success in the workplace or classroom. In B. P. Guyer (Ed.), *ADHD: Achieving success in school and in life.* Boston: Allyn & Bacon.

Guzder, J., Paris, J., Zelkowitz, P., & Feldman, R. (1999). Psychological risk factors for borderline pathology in school-age children. *Journal of the American Academy of Child and Adolescent Psychiatry, 38,* 206–212.

Guzder, J., Paris, J., Zelkowitz, P., & Marchessault, K. (1996). Risk factors for borderline pathology in children. *Journal of the American Academy of Child and Adolescent Psychiatry, 35,* 26–33.

Hahn, Y. S., & McLong, D. G. (1993). Risk factors in the outcome of children with minor head injury. *Pediatric Neurosurgery, 19,* 135–142.

Halperin, J. M., Matier, K., Bedi, G., Sharma, V., & Newcorn, J. H. (1992). Spec-

ificity of inattention, impulsivity, and hyperactivity to the diagnosis of at-
tention-deficit/hyperactivity disorder. *Journal of the American Academy of
Child and Adolescent Psychiatry, 31,* 190–196.

Hamby, S. L., & Finkelhor, D. (2000). The victimization of children: Recommendations for assessment and instrument development. *Journal of the
American Academy of Child and Adolescent Psychiatry, 39,* 829–840.

Handen, B. L., McAuliffe, S., Janosky, J., Feldman, H., & Breaus, A. M. (1998).
A playroom observational procedure to assess children with mental retardation and ADHD. *Journal of Abnormal Child Psychology, 26,* 269–277.

Handwerk, M. L., Larzelere, R. E., Friman, P. C., & Soper, S. H. (1999). Parent
and child discrepancies in reporting severity of problem behaviors in
three out-of-home settings. *Psychological Assessment, 11,* 14–23.

Harford, T. C., & Muthen, B. O. (2000). Adolescent and young adult antisocial
behavior and adult alcohol use disorders: A fourteen-year prospective follow-up in a national sample. *Journal of Studies on Alcohol, 61,* 524–528.

Hartung, C. M., & Widiger, T. A. (1998). Gender differences in the diagnosis of
mental disorders: Conclusions and controversies of the DSM-IV. *Psychological Bulletin, 123,* 260–278.

Harvey, A. G., & Bryant, R. A. (1998). The relationship between acute stress
disorder and posttraumatic stress disorder: A prospective evaluation of
motor vehicle accident survivors. *Journal of Consulting and Clinical Psychology, 66,* 507–512.

Hayward, C., Killen, J. D., Kraemer, H. C., Blair-Greiner, A., Strachowski, D.,
Cunning, D., & Taylor, B. (1997). Assessment and phenomenology of non-
clinical panic attacks in adolescent girls. *Journal of Anxiety Disorders, 11,*
17–32.

Hayward, C., Killen, J. D., Kraemer, H. C., & Taylor, C. B. (1998). Linking self-
reported childhood behavioral inhibition to adolescent social phobia.
*Journal of the American Academy of Child and Adolescent Psychiatry, 37,* 1308–
1316.

Heaton, R. K. (1981). *Wisconsin Card Sorting Test (WCST).* Odessa, FL: Psychological Assessment Resources.

Heber, R. (1959). A manual on terminology and classification in mental retardation (rev.). *American Journal of Mental Deficiency, 64*(Monograph Suppl.).

Heber, R. (1961). Modifications in the manual on terminology and classification
in mental retardation. *American Journal of Mental Deficiency, 65,* 499–500.

Hellgren, L., Gillberg, I. C., Bagenholm, A., & Gillberg, C. Children with deficits in attention, motor control, and perception (DAMP) almost grown up:
Psychiatric and personality disorders at age 16 years. *Journal of Child Psychology, Psychiatry, and Allied Disciplines, 35,* 1255–1271.

Henderson, H. A., & Fox, N. (1998). Inhibited and uninhibited children: Challenges in school settings. *School Psychology Review, 27,* 492–505.

Henderson, S. E., Barnett, A., & Henderson, L. (1994). Visuospatial difficulties
and clumsiness: On the interpretation of conjoint deficits. *Journal of Child
Psychology, Psychiatry, and Allied Disciplines, 35,* 961–969.

Henning-Stout, M. (1998). Assessing the behavior of girls: What we see and
what we miss. *Journal of School Psychology, 36,* 433–455.

Herzog, D. B., Dorer, D. J., Keel, P. K., Selwyn, S. E., Ekeblad, E. R., Flores, A. T., Greenwood, D. N., Burwell, R. A., & Keller, M. B. (1999). Recovery and relapse in anorexia and bulimia nervosa: A 7.5 year follow-up study. *Journal of the American Academy of Child and Adolescent Psychiatry, 38,* 829–837.

Hillier, L. M., & Morrongiello, B. A. (1998). Age and gender differences in school-age children's appraisals of injury risk. *Journal of Pediatric Psychology, 23,* 229–238.

Hinshaw, S., & Anderson, C. (1996). Conduct and oppositional defiant disorder. In E. J. Mash & R. A. Barkley (Eds.), *Child psychopathology.* New York: Guilford Press.

Hinshaw, S. P. (1992). Academic underachievement, attention deficits, and aggression: Comorbidity and implications for intervention. *Journal of Consulting and Clinical Psychology, 60,* 893–903.

Holmbeck, G. N., Belvedere, M. C., Christensen, M., Czerwinski, A. M., Hommeyer, J. S., Johnson, S. Z., & Kung, E. (1998). Assessment of adherence with multiple informants in pre-adolescents with Spina Bifida: Initial development of a multidimensional, multitask parent-report questionnaire. *Journal of Personality Assessment, 70,* 427–440.

Holmes, M. M. (1998). The clinical management of rape in adolescents. *Contemporary Pediatrics, 15,* 62–79.

Holmes, C. S., Respess, D., Greer, T., & Frentz, J. (1998). Behavior problems in children with diabetes: Disentangling possible scoring confounds on the Child Behavior Checklist. *Journal of Pediatric Psychology, 23,* 179–185.

Hooper, S. R., & Willis, W. G. (1989). *Learning disability subtyping: Neuropsychological foundations, conceptual models, and issues in clinical differentiation.* New York: Springer-Verlag.

Hopkinson, K., Cox, A., & Rutter, M. (1981). Psychiatric interviewing techniques: II. Naturalistic study: Eliciting feelings. *British Journal of Psychiatry, 138,* 406–415.

Horton, C. B., & Cruise, T. K. (2001). *Child abuse and neglect: The school's response.* New York: Guilford Press.

House, A. E. (1975). *An observational investigation of the relationship between mothers' visual tracking and the behavior of their children.* Unpublished doctoral dissertation, University of Tennessee, Knoxville.

House, A. E. (1999). *DSM-IV diagnosis in the schools.* New York: Guilford Press.

House, A. E., & Lewis, M. L. (1985). Wechsler Adult Intelligence Scale–Revised. In C. S. Newmark (Ed.), *Major psychological assessment instruments.* Boston: Allyn & Bacon.

House, A. E., & Stambaugh, E. E. (1979). Transfer of therapeutic effects from institution to home: Faith, hope, and behavior modification. *Family Process, 18,* 87–93.

Howe, M. J. A. (1999). *The psychology of high abilities.* New York: New York University Press.

Hudson, S. M., & Ward, T. (2001). Adolescent sexual offenders: Assessment and treatment. In C. R. Hollin (Ed.), *Handbook of offender assessment and treatment.* New York: Wiley.

Hughes, C., White, A., Sharpen, J., & Dunn, J. (2000). Antisocial, angry, and unsympathetic: "Hard-to-manage" preschoolers' peer problems and possible cognitive influences. *Journal of Child Psychology and Psychiatry, 41*, 169–179.

Hughes, J. N., & Baker, D. B. (1990). *The Clinical Child Interview*. New York: Guilford Press.

Isaac, G. (1991). Bipolar disorder in prepubertal children in a special education setting: Is it rare? *Journal of Clinical Psychiatry, 52*, 165–168.

Jacobs, D. G., Brewer, M., & Klein-Benheim, M. (1999). Suicide assessment: An overview and recommended protocol. In D. G. Jacobs (Ed.), *The Harvard Medical School guide to suicide assessment and intervention*. San Francisco: Jossey-Bass.

Jacobsen, L. K., & Rapoport, J. L. (1998). Research update: Childhood-onset schizophrenia: Implications of clinical and neurobiological research. *Journal of Child Psychology, Psychiatry, and Allied Disciplines, 39*, 101–113.

Jaffe, S.L. (1998). Adolescent substance abuse: Assessment and treatment. In A H. Esman, L. T. Flaherty, & H. A. Horowitz (Eds.), *Annals of the American Society for Adolescent Psychiatry: Vol. 23. Adolescent Psychiatry: Developmental and clinical studies*. Hillsdale, NJ: Analytic Press.

Jankowski, M. K., Leitenberg, H., Henning, K., & Coffey, P. (1999). Intergenerational transmission of dating aggression as a function of witnessing only same sex parents vs. opposite sex parents as perpetrators of domestic violence. *Journal of Family Violence, 14*, 267–279.

Jennett, B., & Bond, M. (1975). Assessment of outcome after severe brain damage: A practical scale. *Lancet, 2*, 480–484.

Johnson, J. G., Cohen, P., Skodol, A. E., Oldham, J. M., Kasen, S., & Brook, J. S. (1999). Personality disorders in adolescence and risk of major mental disorders and suicidality during adulthood. *Archives of General Psychiatry, 56*, 805–811.

Johnson, T. C. (1993a). Childhood sexuality. In Gil & Johnson (Eds.), Sexualized Children. Rockville, MD: Launch Press.

Johnson, T. C. (1993b). Preliminary findings. In E. Gil & T, C. Johnson (Eds.), *Sexualized children*. Rockville, MD: Launch Press.

Joiner, T. E., Rudd, M. D., Rouleau, M. R., & Wagner, K. D. (2000). Parameters of suicidal crises vary as a function of previous suicide attempts in youth inpatients. *Journal of the American Academy of Child and Adolescent Psychiatry, 39*, 876–880.

Kadesjo, B., & Gillberg, C. (2000). Tourette's disorder: Epidemiology and comorbidity in primary school children. *Journal of the American Academy of Child and Adolescent Psychiatry, 39*, 548–555.

Kamphaus, R. W. (1993). *Clinical assessment of children's intelligence*. Boston: Allyn & Bacon.

Kashani, J. H., Allan, W. D., Beck, J. C., Jr., Bledsoe, Y., & Reid, J. C. (1997). Dysthymic disorder in clinically referred preschool children. *Journal of the American Academy of Child and Adolescent Psychiatry, 36*, 1426–1433.

Kashani, J. H., & Carlson, G. A. (1987). Seriously depressed preschoolers. *American Journal of Psychiatry, 144*, 348–350.

Kashani, J. H., Holcomb, W. R., & Orvaschel, H. (1986). Depression and depressive symptoms in preschool children from the general population. *American Journal of Psychiatry, 143,* 1138–1143.

Kataoka, S. H., Zima, B. T., Dupre, D. A., Moreno, K. A., Yang, X., & McCracken, J. T. (2001). Mental health problems and service use among female juvenile offenders: Their relationship to criminal history. *Journal of the American Academy of Child and Adolescent Psychiatry, 40,* 549–555.

Katzman, D. K., & Davis, R. (2000). The female body image. In S. M. Coupey (Ed.), *Primary care of adolescent girls.* Philadelphia: Hanley & Belfus.

Kazdin, A. E. (1995). Conduct disorder. In F. C. Verhulst & H. M. Koot (Eds.), *The epidemiology of child and adolescent psychopathology.* New York: Oxford University Press.

Kearney, C. A., Albano, A. M., Eisen, A. R., Allan, W. D., & Barlow, D. H. (1997). The phenomenology of panic disorder in youngsters: An empirical study of a clinical sample. *Journal of Anxiety Disorders, 11,* 49–62.

Keel, P. K., Mitchell, J. E., Miller, K. B., Davis, T. L., & Crow, S. J. (2000). Predictive validity of bulimia nervosa as a diagnostic category. *American Journal of Psychiatry, 157,* 136–138.

Keenan, K., Loeber, R., & Green, S. (1999). Conduct disorders in girls: A review of the literature. *Clinical Child and Family Psychology Review, 2,* 3–19.

Kelly, G. A. (1955). *The psychology of personal constructs* (2 vols.). New York: Norton.

Kelly, J. B. (2000). Children's adjustment in conflicted marriage and divorce: A decade review of research. *Journal of the American Academy of Child and Adolescent Psychiatry, 39,* 963–973.

Kendziora, K. T., & O'Leary, S. G. (1998). Appraisals of child behavior by mothers of problem and nonproblem toddlers. *Journal of Abnormal Child Psychology, 26,* 247–255.

Kentgen, L. M., Klein, R. G., Mannuzza, S., & Davies, M. (1997). Test–retest reliability of maternal reports of lifetime mental disorders in their children. *Journal of Abnormal Child Psychology, 25,* 389–398.

Kernberg, P. F., Weiner, A. S., & Bardenstein, K. K. (2000). *Personality disorders in children and adolescents.* New York: Basic Books.

Kerwin, M. L. E., & Berkowitz, R. I. (1996). Feeding and eating disorders: Ingestive problems of infancy, childhood, and adolescence. *School Psychology Review, 25,* 316–328.

King, B. H., State, M. W., Shah, B., Davanzo, P., & Dykens, E. (1997). Mental retardation: A decade of progress: Part 1. *Journal of the American Academy of Child and Adolescent Psychiatry, 36,* 1656–1663.

Kinsella, G., Ong, B., Murtagh, D., Prior, M., & Sawyer, M. (1999). The role of the family for behavioral outcome in children and adolescents following traumatic brain injury. *Journal of Consulting and Clinical Psychology, 67,* 116–123.

Klinger, L. G., & Dawson, G., (1996). Autistic disorder. In E. J. Mash & R. A. Barkley (Eds.), *Child psychopathology.* New York: Guilford Press.

Kopp, S., & Gillberg, C. (1997). Selective mutism: A population based study. A research note. *Journal of Child Psychology, Psychiatry, and Allied Disciplines, 38,* 257–262.

Kovacs, M. (1992). *The Children's Depression Inventory*. Tonawanda, New York: Multi-Health Systems.

Kovacs, M., Gatsonis, C., Pollock, M., & Parrone, P. L. A. (1994). A controlled prospective study of DSM-III adjustment disorder in childhood. *Archives of General Psychiatry, 51*, 535–541.

Kresanov, K., Tuominen, J., Piha, J., & Almqvist, F. (1998). Validity of child psychiatric screening methods. *European Child and Adolescent Psychiatry, 7*, 85–95.

Kronenberger, W. C., & Meyer, R. G. (1996). *The child clinician's handbook*. Boston: Allyn & Bacon.

Krug, D. A., Arick, J., & Almond, P. (1980). Behavior checklist for identifying severely handicapped individuals with high levels of autistic behavior. *Journal of Child Psychology and Psychiatry, 21, 221–229.*

La Greca, A. M. (1999). The Social Anxiety Scales for children and adolescents. *Behavior Therapist, 22*, 133–136.

La Greca, A. M., & Lemanek, K. L. (1996). Editorial: Assessment as a process in pediatric psychology [Editorial]. *Journal of Pediatric Psychology, 21*, 137–151.

Lancaster, S. (1999). Being there: How parental mental illness can affect children. In V. Cowling (Ed.), *Children of parents with mental illness*. Melbourne, Victoria: Australian Council for Educational Research.

Lane, S. (1997). Assessment of sexually abusive youth. In G. Ryan & S. Lane (Eds.), *Juvenile sexual offending: Causes, consequences, and correction* (rev. ed.). San Francisco: Jossey-Bass.

Langer, L. M., & Tubman, J. G. (1997). Risky sexual behavior among substance-abusing adolescents: Psychosocial and contextual factors. *American Journal of Orthopsychiatry, 67*, 315–322.

Lavigne, J., Arend, R., Rosenbaum, D., Binns, H. J., Christoffel, K. K., & Gibbons, R. D. (1998a). Psychiatric disorders with onset in the preschool years: I. Stability of diagnoses. *Journal of the American Academy of Child and Adolescent Psychiatry, 37*, 1246–1254.

Lavigne, J., Arend, R., Rosenbaum, D., Binns, H. J., Christoffel, K. K., & Gibbons, R. D. (1998b). Psychiatric disorders with onset in the preschool years: II. Correlates and predictors of stable case status. *Journal of the American Academy of Child and Adolescent Psychiatry, 37*, 1255–1261.

Le Couteur, A., Rutter, M., Lord, C., Rios, P., Robertson, S., Holdgrafer, M., & McLennan, J. (1989). Autism Diagnostic Interview: A standardized investigator-based instrument. *Journal of Autism and Developmental Disorders, 19*, 363–387.

Lehmkuhl, G., Blanz, B., Lehmkuhl, U., & Braum-Scharm, H. (1989). Conversion disorder (DSM-III 300. 11): Symptomatology and course in childhood and adolescence. *European Archives of Psychiatry and Neurological Sciences, 238*, 155–160.

Leon, S. C., Lyons, J. S., & Uziel-Miller, N. D. (2000). Variations in the clinical presentations of children and adolescents at eight psychiatric hospitals. *Psychiatric Services, 51*, 786–790.

Leung, P. W. L., & Connolly, K. J. (1998). Do hyperactive children have motor organization and/or executive deficits? *Developmental Medicine and Child Neurology, 40,* 600–607.

Levy, H. B., Harper, C. R., & Weinberg, W. A. (1992). A practical approach to children failing in school. *Pediatric Clinics of North America, 39,* 895–928.

Lewinsohn, P. M., Rohde, P., & Seeley, J. R. (1995). Adolescent psychopathology: III. The clinical consequences of comorbidity. *Journal of the American Academy of Child and Adolescent Psychiatry, 34,* 510–519.

Lewinsohn, P. M., Rohde, P., & Seeley, J. R. (1998). Major depressive disorder in older adolescents: Prevalence, risk factors, and clinical implications. *Clinical Psychology Review, 18,* 765–794.

Lewinsohn, P. M., Zinbarg, R., Seeley, J. R., Lewinsohn, M., & Sack, W. H. (1997). Lifetime comorbidity among anxiety disorders and between anxiety disorders and other mental disorders in adolescents. *Journal of Anxiety Disorders, 11,* 377–394.

Lewis, D. O., Yeager, C. A., Cobham-Portorreal, C. S., Klein, N., Showalter, B. A., & Anthony, A. (1991). A follow-up of female delinquents: Maternal contributions to the perpetuation of deviance. *Journal of the American Academy of Child and Adolescent Psychiatry, 30,* 197–201.

Lezak, M. D. (1995). *Neuropsychological assessment* (3rd ed.). New York: Oxford University Press.

Li, C., Walton, J. R., & Nuttall, E. V. (1999). Preschool evaluation of culturally and linguistically diverse children. In E. V. Nuttall, I. Romero, & J. Kalesnik (Eds.), *Assessing and screening preschoolers: Psychological and educational dimensions* (2nd ed.). Boston: Allyn & Bacon.

Lifter, K. (1999). Descriptions of preschool children with disabilities or at-risk for developmental delay. In E. V. Nuttall, I. Romero, & J. Kalesnik (Eds.), *Assessing and screening preschoolers: Psychological and educational dimensions* (2nd ed.). Boston: Allyn & Bacon.

Lincoln, A. J., Bloom, D., Katz, M., & Boksenbaum, N. (1998). Neuropsychological and neurophysiological indices of auditory processing impairment in children with multiple complex developmental disorder. *Journal of the American Academy of Child and Adolescent Psychiatry, 37,* 100–112.

Lipschitz, D. S., Rasmusson, A. M., & Southwick, S. M. (1998). Childhood post-traumatic stress disorder: A review of neurobiologic sequelae. *Psychiatric Annals, 28,* 452–457.

Lish, J. D., Dime-Meenan, S., Whybrow, P. C., Price, R. A., & Hirschfeld, R. M. (1994). The National Depressive and Manic-Depressive Association (DMDA) survey of bipolar members. *Journal of Affective Disorders, 31,* 281–294.

Llorente, A. M., Ponton, M. O., Taussig, I. M., & Satz, P. (1999). Patterns of American immigration and their influence on the acquisition of neuropsychological norms for Hispanics. *Archives of Clinical Neuropsychology, 14,* 603–614.

Loeber, R., & Keenan, K. (1994). Interaction between conduct disorder and its comorbid conditions: Effects of age and gender. *Clinical Psychology Review, 14,* 497–523.

Logan, N. (1989). Diagnostic assessment of children. In R. J. Craig (Ed.), *Clinical and diagnostic interviewing.* Northvale, NJ: Aronson.

Looper, K., & Grizenko, N. (1999). Risk and protective factors scale: Reliability and validity in preadolescents. *Canadian Journal of Psychiatry, 44,* 138–143.

Lord, C., Rutter, M., Goode, S., Heemsbergen, J., Jordan, H., Mawhood, L., & Schopler, E. (1989). Autism Diagnostic Observation Schedule: A standardized observation of communicative and social behavior. *Journal of Autism and Developmental Disorders, 19,* 185–212.

Lord, C., Rutter, M., & Le Couteur, A. (1994). Autism Diagnostic Interview-Revised: A revised version of a diagnostic interview for caregivers of individuals with possible pervasive developmental disorders. *Journal of Autism and Developmental Disorders, 24,* 659–685.

Lothstein, L. M. (1992). Clinical management of gender dysphoria in young boys: Genital mutilation and DSM IV implications. *Journal of Psychology and Human Sexuality, 5,* 87–106.

Luckasson, R., Coulter, D., Polloway, E., Reiss, S., Schalock, R., Snell, M., Spitalnik, D., & Stark, J. (1992). *Mental retardation: Definitions, classification, and systems of support* (9th ed.). Washington, DC: American Association on Mental Retardation.

Lynskey, M. T., & Fergusson, D. M. (1995). Childhood conduct problems, attention deficit behavior, and adolescent alcohol, tobacco, and illicit drug use. *Journal of Abnormal Child Psychology, 23,* 281–302.

MacLeod, R. J., McNamee, J. E., Boyle, M. H., Offord, D. R., & Friedrich, M. (1999). Identification of childhood psychiatric disorder by informant: Comparisons of clinic and community samples. *Canadian Journal of Psychiatry, 44,* 144–150.

Majnemer, A., & Mazer, B. (1998). Neurologic evaluation of the newborn infant: Definition and psychometric properties. *Developmental Medicine and Child Neurology, 40,* 708–715.

March, J. S., & Leonard, H. L. (1996). Obsessive-Compulsive Disorder in children and adolescents: A review of the past 10 years. *Journal of the American Academy of Child and Adolescent Psychiatry, 35,* 1265–1273.

Marshall, R. D., Schneier, F. R., Lin, S.-H., Simpson, H. B., Vermes, D., & Liebowitz, M. (2000). Childhood trauma and dissociative symptoms in panic disorder. *American Journal of Psychiatry, 157,* 451–453.

Martin, C. S., & Winters, K. C. (1998). Diagnosis and assessment of alcohol use disorders among adolescents. *Alcohol Health and Research World, 22,* 95–105.

Matson, J. L., & Bamburg, J. W. (1998). Reliability of the Assessment of Dual Diagnosis (ADD). *Research in Developmental Disabilities, 19,* 89–95.

Matson, J. L., Gardner, W. I., Coe, D. A., & Sovner, R. (1991). A scale for evaluating emotional disorders in severely and profoundly mentally retarded persons. *British Journal of Psychiatry, 159,* 404–409.

Matson, J. L., & Smiroldo, B. B. (1997). Validity of the mania subscale of the Diagnostic Assessment of the Severely Handicapped–II (DASH-II). *Research in Developmental Disabilities, 18,* 1–5.

Matson, J. L., Smiroldo, B. B., & Hastings, T. L. (1998). Validity of the autism/pervasive developmental disorder subscale of the Diagnostic Assessment for the Severely Handicapped–II. *Journal of Autism and Developmental Disabilities, 28,* 77–81.

Max, J. E., Castillo, C. S., Lindgren, S. D., & Arndt, S. (1998a). The neuropsychiatric rating schedule: Reliability and validity. *Journal of the American Academy of Child and Adolescent Psychiatry, 37*, 297–304.

Max, J. E., & Dunisch, D. L. (1997). Traumatic brain injury in a child psychiatry outpatient clinic: A controlled study. *Journal of the American Academy of Child and Adolescent Psychiatry, 36*, 404–411.

Max, J. E., Koele, S. L., Castillo, C. C., Lindgren, S. E., Arndt, S., Bokura, H., Robin D. A., Smith, W. L., Jr., & Sato, Y. (2000). Personality change disorder in children and adolescents following traumatic brain injury. *Journal of the International Neuropsychological Society, 6*, 279–289.

Max, J. E., Koele, S. L., Smith, W. L., Sato, Y., Lindgren, S. D., Robin, D. A., & Arndt, S. (1998b). Psychiatric disorders in children and adolescents after severe traumatic brain injury: A controlled study. *Journal of the American Academy of Child and Adolescent Psychiatry, 37*, 832–840.

Max, J. E., Robin, D. A., Lindgren, S. D., Smith, W. L., Sato, Y., Mattheis, P. J., Stierwalt, J. A. G., & Castillo, C. S. (1997a). Traumatic brain injury in children and adolescents: Psychiatric disorders at two years. *Journal of the American Academy of Child and Adolescent Psychiatry, 36*, 1278–1285.

Max, J. E., Sharma, A., & Qurashi, M. I. (1997b). Traumatic brain injury in a child psychiatry inpatient population: A controlled study. *Journal of the American Academy of Child and Adolescent Psychiatry, 36*, 1595–1601.

Max, J. E., Smith, W. L., Sato, Y., Mattheis, P. J., Castillo, C. S., Lindgren, S. D., Robin, D. A., & Stierwalt, J. A. G. (1997c). Traumatic brain injury in children and adolescents: Psychiatric disorders in the first three months. *Journal of the American Academy of Child and Adolescent Psychiatry, 36*, 1278–1285.

Mazza, J. J. (2000). The relationship between posttraumatic stress symptomatology and suicidal behavior in school-based adolescents. *Suicide and Life-Threatening Behavior, 30*, 91–103.

Mazzocco, M. M. M., Pulsifer, M., Fiumara, A., Cocuzza, M., Nigro, F., Incorpora, G., & Barone, R. (1998). Autistic behaviors among children with Fragile X or Rett Syndrome: Implications for the classification of pervasive developmental disorder. *Journal of Autism and Developmental Disorders, 28*, 321–327.

McClellan, J. M., & Werry, J. S. (2000). Research Psychiatric Diagnostic Interviews For Children and Adolescents: Introduction. *Journal of the American Academy of Child and Adolescent Psychiatry, 39*, 19–27.

McClowry, S. G. (1998). The science and art of using temperament as the basis for intervention. *School Psychology Review, 27*, 551–563.

McGarvey, E. L., Canterbury, R. J., & Waite, D. (1996). Delinquency and family problems in incarcerated adolescents with and without a history of inhalant use. *Addictive Behaviors, 21*, 537–542.

McGrew, W. C. (1972). *An ethological study of children's behavior.* New York: Academic Press.

McKeown, R. E., Garrison, C. Z., Cuffe, S. P., Waller, J. L., Jackson, K. L., & Addy, C. L. (1998). Incidence and predictors of suicidal behaviors in a longitudinal sample of young adolescents. *Journal of the American Academy of Child and Adolescent Psychiatry, 37*, 612–619.

McLeod, J. D., & Nonnemaker, J. M. (2000). Poverty and child emotional and behavioral problems: Racial/ethnic differences in processes and effects. *Journal of Health and Social Behavior, 41,* 137–161.

McManus, M., Alessi, N. E., Grapentine, W. L., & Brickman, A. (1984). Psychiatric disturbance in serious delinquents. *Journal of the American Academy of Child and Adolescent Psychiatry, 23,* 602–615.

McNiel, D. E., Sandberg, D. A., & Binder, R. L. (1998). The relationship between confidence and accuracy in clinical assessment of psychiatric patients' potential for violence. *Law and Human Behavior, 22,* 655–669.

Meijer, M. (1995). *Borderline adolescents.* Amsterdam: Thesis.

Melchert, T. P. (1998). A review of instruments for assessing family history. *Clinical Psychology Review, 18,* 163–187.

Mesibov, G. B., Schopler, E., Schaffer, B., & Michal, N. (1989). Use of the Childhood Autism Rating Scale with autistic adolescents and adults. *Journal of the American Academy of Child and Adolescent Psychiatry, 28,* 538–541.

Miller, J. (2001). *One of the guys: Girls, gangs, and gender.* New York: Oxford University Press.

Miller, L. C., Barrett, C. L., & Hampe, E. (1974). Phobias of childhood in a prescientific era. In A. Davids (Ed.), *Child personality and psychopathology: Current topics* (Vol. 1). New York: Wiley.

Miller, W. H. (1975). *Systematic parent training: Procedures, cases, and issues.* Champaign, IL: Research Press.

Miller-Perrin, C. L., & Wurtele, S. K. (1990). Reactions to childhood sexual abuse: Implications for post-traumatic stress disorder. In C. L. Meek (Ed.), *Post-traumatic stress disorder: Assessment, differential diagnosis, and forensic assessment.* Sarasota, FL: Professional Resource Exchange.

Milne, J. M., Garrison, C. Z., Addy, C. L., McKeown, R. E., Jackson, K. L., Cuffe, S. P., & Waller, J. L. (1995). Frequency of phobic disorder in a community sample of young adolescents. *Journal of the American Academy of Child and Adolescent Psychiatry, 34,* 1202–1211.

Mitsis, E. M., McKay, K., Schulz, K. P., Newcorn, J. H., & Halperin, J. M. (2000). Parent–teacher concordance for DSM-IV attention-deficit/hyperactivity disorder in a clinic-referred sample. *Journal of the American Academy of Child and Adolescent Psychiatry, 39,* 308–313.

Moffit, T. E. (1993). The neuropsychology of conduct disorder. *Development and Psychopathology, 5,* 135–151.

Moolchan, E. T., Ernst, M., & Henningfield, J. E. (2000). A review of tobacco smoking in adolescents: Treatment implications. *Journal of the American Academy of Child and Adolescent Psychiatry, 39,* 682–693.

Moreau, D., & Weissman, M. M. (1992). Panic disorder in children and adolescents: A review. *American Journal of Psychiatry, 149,* 1306–1314.

Morenz, B., & Becker, J. (1995). The treatment of youthful sexual offenders. *Applied and Preventive Psychology, 4,* 247–256.

Morrison, J. A. (1993). *The first interview.* New York: Guilford Press.

Morrongiello, B. A., & Rennie, H. (1998). Why do boys engage in more risk taking than girls? The role of attributions, beliefs, and risk appraisals. *Journal of Pediatric Psychology, 23,* 33–43.

Moscicki, E. K. (1995) Suicide in childhood and adolescence. In F. C. Verhulst & H. M. Koot (Eds.), *The epidemiology of child and adolescent psychopathology.* New York: Oxford University Press.

Moscicki, E. K. (1999). Epidemiology of suicide. In D. G. Jacobs (Ed.), *The Harvard Medical School guide to suicide assessment and intervention.* San Francisco: Jossey-Bass.

Mota, V. L., & Schachar, R. J. (2000). Reformulating attention-deficit/hyperactivity disorder according to signal detection theory. *Journal of the American Academy of Child and Adolescent Psychiatry, 39,* 1144–1151.

Mouridsen, S. E., Rich, B., & Isager, T. (1999). Epilepsy in disintegrative psychosis and infantile autism: A long-term validation study. *Developmental Medicine and Child Neurology, 41,* 110–114.

Muris, P., Merckelbach, H., Mayer, B., & Prins, E. (2000). How serious are common childhood fears? *Behaviour Research and Therapy, 38,* 217–228.

Murphy, J. M., & Jellinek, M. S. (1988). Screening for psychosocial dysfunction in economically disadvantaged and minority group children: Further validation of the Pediatric Symptom Checklist. *American Journal of Orthopsychiatry, 58,* 450–456.

Murphy, J. M., Reede, J., Jellinek, M. S., & Bishop, S. J. (1992). Screening for psychosocial dysfunction in inner-city children: Further validation of the Pediatric Symptom Checklist. *Journal of the American Academy of Child and Adolescent Psychiatry, 31,* 1105–1111.

Nelson, V. S. (1992). Pediatric head injury. *Physical Medicine and Rehabilitation Clinics of North America, 3,* 461–474.

Newcomb, M. D., & Bentler, P. M. (1989). Substance use and abuse among children and teenagers. *American Psychologist, 44,* 242–248.

Newcorn, J. H., & Strain, J. (1992). Adjustment disorder in children and adolescents. *Journal of the American Academy of Child and Adolescent Psychiatry, 31,* 318–327.

Novins, D. K., Bechtold, D. W., Sack, W. H., Thompson, J., Carter, D. R., & Manson, S. M. (1997). The DSM-IV outline for cultural formulation: A critical demonstration with American Indian children. *Journal of the American Academy of Child and Adolescent Psychiatry, 36,* 1244–1251.

Ohayon, M. M., Guilleminault, C., & Priest, R. G. (1999). Night terrors, sleepwalking, and confusional arousals in the general population: Their frequency and relationship to other sleep and mental disorders. *Journal of Clinical Psychiatry, 60,* 268–276.

Olson, M. (1996). Tourette syndrome and tics. In Y. Frank (Ed.), *Pediatric behavioral neurology.* Boca Raton, FL: CRC Press.

O'Malley, P. M., Johnston, L. D., & Bachman, J. G. (1998). Alcohol use among adolescents. *Alcohol Health and Research World, 22,* 85–93.

Osman, A., Downs, W. R., Kopper, B. A., Barrios, F. X., Baker, M. T., Osman, J. R., Besett, T. M., & Linehan, M. M. (1998). The Reasons for Living Inventory for Adolescents (RFL-A): Development and psychometric properties. *Journal of Clinical Psychology, 54,* 1063–1078.

Othmer, I., & Othmer, S. C. (1994). *The clinical interview using DSM-IV: Vol. 1. Fundamentals.* Washington, DC: American Psychiatric Press.

Overmeyer, S., Taylor, E., Blanz, B., & Schmidt, M. H. (1999). Psychosocial adversities underestimated in hyperkinetic children. *Journal of Child Psychology, Psychiatry, and Allied Disciplines, 40,* 259–263.

Palla, B., & Litt, I. F. (1988). Medical complications of eating disorders in adolescents. *Pediatrics, 81,* 613–623.

Papolos, D., & Papolos, J. (1999). *The bipolar child.* New York: Broadway Books.

Parrot, A. (1989). Acquaintance rape among adolescents: Identifying risk groups and intervention strategies. *Journal of Social Work and Human Sexuality, 8,* 47–61.

Patterson, G. R. (1982). *Coercive family process.* Eugene, OR: Castalia.

Patterson, G. R., Reid, J. B., & Dishion, T. J. (1992). *Antisocial boys.* Eugene, OR: Castalia.

Perez, R. G., Ascaso, E., Massons, J. M. D., & de la Osa Chaparro, N. (1998). Characteristics of the subject and interview influencing the test–retest reliability of the Diagnostic Interview for Children and Adolescents–Revised. *Journal of Child Psychology, Psychiatry, and Allied Disciplines, 39,* 963–972.

Perez-Arce, P. (1999). The influence of culture on cognition. *Archives of Clinical Neuropsychology, 14,* 581–592.

Perkins, K., Ferrari, N., Rosas, A., Bessette, R., Williams, A., & Omar, H. (1997). You won't know unless you ask: The biopsychological interview for adolescents. *Clinical Pediatrics, 36,* 79–86.

Pfeffer, C. R. (1986). *The suicidal child.* New York: Guilford Press.

Pfefferbaum, B. (1997). Posttraumatic Stress Disorder in children: A review of the past 10 years. *Journal of the American Academy of Child and Adolescent Psychiatry, 36,* 1503–1511.

Phelps, L., Johnston, L. S., & Augustyniak, K. (1999). Prevention of eating disorders: Identification of predictor variables. *Eating Disorders, 7,* 99–108.

Phillips, K. A., Atala, K. D., & Albertini, R. S. (1995). Body dysmorphic disorder in adolescents. *Journal of the American Academy of Child and Adolescent Psychiatry, 34,* 1216–1220.

Pillow, D. R., Pelham, W. E., Hoza, B., Molina, B. S. G., & Stultz, C. H. (1998). Confirmatory factor analysis examining attention-deficit/hyperactivity disorder symptoms and other childhood disruptive behaviors. *Journal of Abnormal Child Psychology, 26,* 293–309.

Pilowsky, T., Yirmiya, N., Shulman, C., & Dover, R. (1998). The Autism Diagnostic Interview–Revised and the Childhood Autism Rating Scale: Differences between diagnostic systems and comparison between genders. *Journal of Autism and Developmental Disorders, 28,* 143–151.

Pliszka, S. R., Sherman, J. O., Barrow, M. V., & Irick, S. (2000). Affective disorder in juvenile offenders: A preliminary study. *American Journal of Psychiatry, 157,* 130–132.

Pollock, N. K., & Martin, C. S. (1999). Diagnostic orphans: Adolescents with alcohol symptoms who do not quality for DSM-IV abuse or dependence diagnoses. *American Journal of Psychiatry, 156,* 897–901.

Pollock, N. K., Martin, C. S., & Langenbucher, J. W. (2000). Diagnostic concordance of DSM-III, DSM-III-R, DSM-IV, and ICD-10 alcohol diagnoses in adolescents. *Journal of Studies of Alcohol, 61,* 439–446.

Ponton, M. O., & Ardila, A. (1999). The future of neuropsychology with Hispanic populations in the United States. *Archives of Clinical Neuropsychology, 14*, 565–580.

Power, T. J., Deherty, B. J., Panichelli-Mindel, S. M., Karustis, J. L., Eiraldi, R. B., Anastopoulos, A. D., & DuPaul, G. J. (1998). The predictive validity of parent and teacher reports of ADHD symptoms. *Journal of Psychopathology and Behavioral Assessment, 20*, 57–81.

Puura, K., Almqvist, F., Tamminen, T., Piha, J., Kumpulainen, K., Rasanen, E., et al. (1998). Children with symptoms of depression—What do adults see? *Journal of Child Psychology, Psychiatry, and Allied Disciplines, 39*, 577–585.

Ramirez, R. D. de, & Shipiro, E. S. (1998). Teacher ratings of attention-deficit/hyperactivity disorder symptoms in Hispanic children. *Journal of Psychopathology and Behavioral Assessment, 20*, 275–293.

Rapin, I. (1997). Classification and causal issues in autism. In D. J. Cohen & F. R. Volkmar (Eds.), *Handbook of autism and pervasive developmental disorders.* New York: Wiley.

Rapoport, J. L., & Ismond, D. R. (1996). *DSM-IV training guide for diagnosis of childhood disorders.* New York: Brunner/Mazel.

Reich, W. (2000). Diagnostic Interview for Children and Adolescents (DICA). *Journal of the American Academy of Child and Adolescent Psychiatry, 39*, 59–66.

Reid, R. (1995). Assessment of ADHD with culturally different groups: The use of behavioral rating scales. *School Psychology Review, 24*, 537–560.

Reid, R., DuPaul, G. J., Power, T. J., Anastopoulos, A. D., Rogers-Adkinson, D., Noll, M.-B., & Riccio, C. (1998). Assessing culturally different students for attention-deficit/hyperactivity disorder using behavior rating scales. *Journal of Abnormal Child Psychology, 26*, 187–198.

Reitan, R. M. (1984). *Aphasia and sensory-perceptual deficits in children.* Tucson, AZ: Neuropsychology Press.

Renaud, J., Brent, D. A., Birmaher, B., Chiappetta, L., & Bridge, J. (1999). Suicide in adolescents with disruptive disorders. *Journal of the American Academy of Child and Adolescent Psychiatry, 38*, 846–851.

Rey, G. J., Feldman, E., Rivas-Vazquez, R., Levin, B. E., & Benton, A. (1999). Neuropsychological test development and normative data on Hispanics. *Archives of Clinical Neuropsychology, 14*, 593–601.

Rey, J. M. (1993). Oppositional defiant disorder. *American Journal of Psychiatry, 150*, 1769–1778.

Reynolds, C. R., & Richmond, B. O. (1995). *Revised Children's Manifest Anxiety Scale.* Los Angeles: Western Psychological Services.

Riccio, C. A., Reynolds, C. R., & Lowe, P. A. (2001). *Clinical applications of continuous performance tests: Measuring attention and impulsive responding in children and adults.* New York: Wiley.

Ripple, C. H., & Luthar, S. S. (2000). Academic risk among inner-city adolescents: The role of personal attributes. *Journal of School Psychology, 38*, 277–298.

Risk Management Foundation of the Harvard Medical Institutions. (1999). Guidelines for identification, assessment, and treatment planning for suicidality. In D. G. Jacobs (Ed.), *The Harvard Medical School guide to suicide assessment and intervention.* San Francisco: Jossey-Bass.

Roberts, C., & Hindley, P. (1999). Practitioner review: The assessment and treatment of deaf children with psychiatric disorders. *Journal of Child Psychology, Psychiatry, and Allied Disciplines, 40,* 151–167.

Robertson, M. M., & Baron-Cohen, S. (1998). *Tourette syndrome: The facts* (2nd ed.). New York: Oxford University Press.

Robins, L. N. (1986). The consequences of conduct disorder in girls. In D. Olweus, J. Block, & M. Radke-Yarrow (Eds.), *The development of antisocial and prosocial behavior: Research, theories, and issues.* Orlando, FL: Academic Press.

Rosenfeld, W. D., & Coupey, S. M. (2000). Contraceptive counseling and prescription. In S. M. Coupey (Ed.), *Primary care of adolescent girls.* Philadelphia: Hanley & Belfus.

Rosenthal, S. L., Lewis, L. M., Succop, P. A., Burklow, K. A., Nelson, P. R., Shedd, K. D., Heyman, R. B., & Biro, F. O. (1999). Adolescents' views regarding sexual history taking. *Clinical Pediatrics, 38,* 227–233.

Rothbart, M. K., & Jones, L. B. (1998). Temperament, self-regulation, and education. *School Psychology Review, 27,* 479–491.

Rowe, K. J., & Rowe, K. S. (1992). The relationship between inattentiveness in the classroom and reading achievement (Part B): An explanatory study. *Journal of the American Academy of Child and Adolescent Psychiatry, 31,* 357–368.

Rubio-Stipec, M., Shrout, P. E., Canino, G., Bird, H. R., Jensen, P., Dulcan, M., & Schwab-Stone, M. (1996). Empirically defined symptom scales using the DISC 2.3. *Journal of Abnormal Child Psychology, 24,* 67–83.

Rutter, M., & Cox, A. (1981). Psychiatric interviewing techniques: 1. Methods and measures. *British Journal of Psychiatry, 138,* 273–282.

Ryan, C. C., & Futterman, D. (1998). *Lesbian and gay youth: Care and counseling.* New York: Columbia University Press.

Ryan, C. C., & Futterman, D. (2000). Lesbian adolescents. In S. M. Coupey (Ed.), *Primary care of adolescent girls.* Philadelphia: Hanley & Belfus.

Ryan, G. (1997a). Sexually abusive youth: Defining the population. In G. Ryan & S. Lane (Eds.), *Juvenile sexual offending: Causes, consequences, and correction* (rev. ed.). San Francisco: Jossey-Bass.

Ryan, G. (1997b). Incidence and prevalence of sexual offenses committed by juveniles. In G. Ryan & S. Lane (Eds.), *Juvenile sexual offending: Causes, consequences, and correction* (rev. ed.). San Francisco: Jossey-Bass.

Ryan, G. (1997c) Consequences for the victim of sexual abuse. In G. Ryan & S. Lane (Eds.), *Juvenile sexual offending: Causes, consequences, and correction* (rev. ed.). San Francisco: Jossey-Bass.

Ryan, G. (1997d). Consequences for the youth who has been abusive. In G. Ryan & S. Lane (Eds.), *Juvenile sexual offending: Causes, consequences, and correction* (rev. ed.). San Francisco: Jossey-Bass.

Ryan, G. (1997e). Perpetration prevention: Primary and secondary. In G. Ryan & S. Lane (Eds.), *Juvenile sexual offending: Causes, consequences, and correction* (rev. ed.). San Francisco: Jossey-Bass.

Ryan, G., & Lane, S. (1997a). Integrating theory and method. In G. Ryan & S.

Lane (Eds.), *Juvenile sexual offending: Causes, consequences, and correction* (rev. ed.). San Francisco: Jossey-Bass.

Ryan, G., & Lane, S. (1997b). Integrating theory and method. In G. Ryan & S. Lane (Eds.), *Juvenile sexual offending: Causes, consequences, and correction* (rev. ed.). San Francisco: Jossey-Bass.

Sachs, G. S., Baldassano, C. F., Truman, C. J., & Guille, C. (2000). Comorbidity of attention deficit hyperactivity disorder with early- and late-onset bipolar disorder. *American Journal of Psychiatry, 157*, 466–468.

Sandifer, M. G., Hordern, A., & Green, L. M. (1970). The psychiatric interview: The impact of the first three minutes. *American Journal of Psychiatry, 126*, 968–973.

Sands, R., Tricker, J., Sherman, C., Armatas, C., & Maschette, W. (1997). Disordered eating patterns, body image, self-esteem, and physical activity in preadolescent school children. *International Journal of Eating Disorders, 21*, 159–166.

Sarma, P. S. B. (1994). Physical and neurological examinations and laboratory studies. In K. S. Robson (Ed.), *Manual of clinical child and adolescent psychiatry*. Washington, DC: American Psychiatric Press.

Sattler, J. M. (1998). *Clinical and forensic interviewing of children and families: Guidelines for the mental health, education, pediatric, and child maltreatment fields*. San Diego: Author.

Saylor, C. F., Swenson, C. C., Reynolds, S. S., & Taylor, M. (1999). The Pediatric Emotional Distress Scale: A brief screening measure for young children exposed to traumatic events. *Journal of Clinical Child Psychology, 28*, 70–81.

Saywitz, K. J., & Snyder, L. (1996). Narrative elaboration: Test of a new procedure for interviewing children. *Journal of Consulting and Clinical Psychology, 64*, 1347–1357.

Scheeringa, M. S., Zeanah, C. H., Drell, M. J., & Larrieu, J. A. (1995). Two approaches to the diagnosis of posttraumatic stress disorder in infancy and early childhood. *Journal of the American Academy of Child and Adolescent Psychiatry, 34*, 191–200.

Schreier, H. A. (1999). Hallucinations in nonpsychotic children: More common than we think? *Journal of the American Academy of Child and Adolescent Psychiatry, 38*, 623–625.

Schteingart, J. S., Molnar, J., Klein, T. P., Lowe, C. B., & Hartmann, A. H. (1995). Homelessness and child functioning in the context of risk and protective factors moderating child outcomes. *Journal of Clinical Child Psychology, 24*, 320–331.

Screening test for bipolar disorder created. (2000). *Bipolar Disorder and Impulsive Spectrum Letter, 6*, 7–8.

Segal, B., Hobfoll, S. S., & F. Cromer (1984). Alcohol use by juvenile offenders. *International Journal of the Addictions, 19*, 541–549.

Shaffer, D., Fisher, P., Lucas, C. P., Dulcan, M. K., & Schwab-Stone, M. E. (2000). NIMH Diagnostic Interview Schedule for Children—Version IV (NIHM DISC-IV): Description, differences from previous versions, and reliability of some common diagnoses. *Journal of the American Academy of Child and Adolescent Psychiatry, 39*, 28–38.

Shaffer, D., Gould, M. S., Brasic, J., Ambrosini, P., Fisher, P., Bird, H., & Aluwahlia, S. (1983). A Children's Global Assessment Scale (CGAS). *Archives of General Psychiatry, 40,* 1228–1231.

Shaffer, H. J., LaBrie, R., Scanlan, K. M., & Cummings, T. N. (1994). Pathological gambling among adolescents: Massachusetts Gambling Screen (MAGS). *Journal of Gambling Studies, 10,* 339–362.

Shallice, T. (1982). Specific impairments of planning. *Philosophical Transactions of the Royal Society of London, 298,* 199–209.

Shapiro, E. G., & Rosenfeld, A. A. (1987). *The somatizing child: Diagnosis and treatment of conversion and somatization disorders.* New York: Springer-Verlag.

Shapiro, E. S. (1996). *Academic skills problems: Direct assessment and intervention* (2nd ed.). New York: Guilford Press.

Sheridan, S. M., Hungelmann, A., & Maughan, D. P. (1999). A contextualized framework for social skills assessment, intervention, and generalization. *School Psychology Review, 28,* 84–103.

Sherrill, J. T., & Kovacs, M. (2000). Interview Schedule for Children and Adolescents (ISCA). *Journal of the American Academy of Child and Adolescent Psychiatry, 39,* 67–75.

Shriver, M. D., Allen, K. D., & Mathews, J. R. (1999). Effective assessment of the shared and unique characteristics of children with autism. *School Psychology Review, 28,* 538–558.

Siegel, M., & Barthel, R. P. (1986). Conversion disorders on a child psychiatry consultation service. *Psychosomatics, 27,* 201–204.

Silberg, J., Pickles, A., Rutter, M., Hewitt, J., Simonoff, E., Maes, H., Carbonneau, R., Murrelle, L., Foley, D., & Eaves, L. (1999). The influence of genetic factors and life stress on depression among adolescent girls. *Archives of General Psychiatry, 56,* 225–232.

Silva, R. R., Alpert, M., Munoz, D. M., Singh, S., Matzner, F., & Dummit, S. (2000). Stress and vulnerability to posttraumatic stress disorder in children and adolescents. *American Journal of Psychiatry, 157,* 1229–1235.

Silverman, K. (2000). Sexual assault, rape, and sexual abuse. In S. M. Coupey (Ed.), *Primary care of adolescent girls.* Philadelphia: Hanley & Belfus.

Simmons, R. G., & Blyth, D. (1987). *Moving into adolescence: The impact of pubertal change and school context.* New York: Aldine De Gruyter.

Simpson, D., & Reilly, P. (1982). Pediatric coma scale. *Lancet, 2,* 450.

Skansgaard, E. P., & Burns, G. L. (1998). Comparison of DSM-IV ADHD combined and predominantly inattentive types: Correspondence between teacher ratings and direct observations of inattentive, hyperactivity/impulsivity, slow cognitive tempo, oppositional defiant, and overt conduct disorder symptoms. *Child and Family Behavior Therapy, 20,* 1–14.

Smart, D. W., & Smart, J. F. (1997). DSM-IV and culturally sensitive diagnosis: Some observations for counselors. *Journal of Counseling and Development, 75,* 392–398.

Sonuga-Barke, E., Minocha, K., Taylor, E., & Sandberg, S. (1993). Inter-ethnic bias in teachers' ratings of childhood hyperactivity. *British Journal of Developmental Psychology, 11,* 187–200.

Speltz, M. L., McClellan, J., DeKlyen, M., & Jones, K. (1999). Preschool boys with oppositional defiant disorder: Clinical presentation and diagnostic change. *Journal of the American Academy of Child and Adolescent Psychiatry, 38,* 838–845.

Spencer, S., Biederman, J., Harding, M., O'Donnel, D., Wilens, T., Faraone, S., Coffey, B., & Geller, D. (1998). Disentangling the overlap between Tourette's Disorder and ADHD. *Journal of Child Psychology, Psychiatry, and Allied Disciplines, 39,* 1037–1044.

Spreen, O., Risser, A. H., & Edgell, D. (1995). *Developmental neuropsychology.* New York: Oxford University Press.

Stahl, N. D., & Clarizio, H. F. (1999). Conduct disorder and comorbidity. *Psychology in the Schools, 36,* 41–50.

State, M. W., King, B. H., & Dykens, E. (1997). Mental retardation: A review of the past 10 years (Part 2). *Journal of the American Academy of Child and Adolescent Psychiatry, 36,* 1664–1671.

Steiner, H., & Lock, J. (1998). Anorexia nervosa and bulimia nervosa in children and adolescents: A review of the past 10 years. *Journal of the American Academy of Child and Adolescent Psychiatry, 37,* 352–359.

Steinhausen, H. C., & Juzi, C. (1996). Elective mutism: An analysis of 100 cases. *Journal of the American Academy of Child and Adolescent Psychiatry, 35,* 606–614.

Stevens, J., Quittner, A. L., & Abikoff, H. (1998). Factors influencing elementary school teachers' ratings of ADHD and ODD behaviors. *Journal of Clinical Child Psychology, 27,* 406–414.

Stevens, M. C., Fein, D. A., Dunn, M., Allen, D., Waterhouse, L. H., Feinstein, C., & Rapin, S. (2000). Subgroups of children with autism by cluster analysis: A longitudinal examination. *Journal of the American Academy of Child and Adolescent Psychiatry, 39,* 346–352.

Stone, W. L., Lee, E. B., Ashford, L., Brissie, J., Hepburn, S. L., Coonrod, E. E., & Weiss, B. H. (1999). Can autism be diagnosed accurately in children under 3 years? *Journal of Child Psychology, Psychiatry, and Allied Disciplines, 40,* 219–226.

Stormont, M., & Zentall, S. S. (1999). Assessment of setting in the behavioral ratings of preschoolers with and without high levels of activity. *Psychology in the Schools, 36,* 109–115.

Strub, R., & Black, F. W. (1988). *Neurobehavioral disorders: A clinical approach.* Philadelphia: Davis.

Strub, R., & Black, F. W. (1993). *The Mental Status Examination in neurology* (3rd ed.). Philadelphia: Davis.

Swedo, S. E., Leonard, H. L., Mittleman, B. B., Allen, A. J., Rapoport, J. L., Dow, S. P., Kanter, M. E., Chapman, F., & Zabriskie, J. (1997). Identification of children with pediatric autoimmune neuropsychiatric disorders associated with streptococcal infections by a marker associated with rheumatic fever. *American Journal of Psychiatry, 154,* 110–112.

Szymanski, L. S. (1994). Mental retardation and mental health: Concepts, aetiology and incidence. In N. Bouras (Ed.), *Mental health in mental retardation.* London: Cambridge University Press.

Taylor, H. G., Yeates, K. O., Wade, S. L., Drotar, D., Klein, S. K., & Stancin, T. (1999). Influences on first-year recovery from traumatic brain injury in children. *Neuropsychology, 13*, 76–89.

Teasdale, G., & Jennett, B. (1974). Assessment of coma and impaired consciousness: A practical scale. *Lancet, 2*, 81–84.

Teeter, P. A., & Semrud-Clikeman, M. (1997). *Child neuropsychology: Assessment and interventions for neurodevelopmental disorders.* Boston: Allyn & Bacon.

Teglasi, H. (1998a). Introduction to the mini-series: Implications of temperament for the practice of school psychology. *School Psychology Review, 27,* 475–478.

Teglasi, H. (1998b). Temperament constructs and measures. *School Psychology Review, 27,* 564–585.

Teglasi, H., & Epstein, S. (1998) Temperament and personality theory: The perspective of cognitive-experiential self-theory. *School Psychology Review, 27,* 534–550.

Thomas, A., & Chess, S. (1977). *Temperament and behavior disorders in children.* New York: University Press.

Thomas, J. M., & Clark, R. (1998). Disruptive behavior in the very young child: Diagnostic classification: 0–3 guides identification of risk factors and relational interventions. *Infant Mental Health Journal, 19,* 229–244.

Thompson, R. J., Jr., & Gustafson, K. E. (1996). *Adaptation to chronic medical illness.* Washington, DC: American Psychological Association.

Thornton, C., & Russell, J. (1997). Obsessive compulsive comorbidity in the dieting disorders. *International Journal of Eating Disorders, 21,* 83–87.

Tofler, I. R., Knapp, P. K., & Drell, M. J. (1999). The "achievement by proxy" spectrum: Recognition and clinical response to pressured and high-achieving children and adolescents. *Journal of the American Academy of Child and Adolescent Psychiatry, 38,* 213–216.

Towbin, K. E., Dykens, E. M., Pearson, G. S., & Cohen, D. J. (1993). Conceptualizing "borderline syndrome of childhood" and "childhood schizophrenia" as a developmental disorder. *Journal of the American Academy of Child and Adolescent Psychiatry, 32,* 775–782.

Tracey, S. A., Chorpita, B. F., Douban, J., & Barlow, D. H. (1997). Empirical evaluation of DSM-IV generalized anxiety disorder criteria in children and adolescents. *Journal of Clinical Child Psychology, 26,* 404–414.

U.S. Department of Education. (1997). *To assure the free appropriate public education of all children with disabilities.* Washington, DC: U.S. Government Printing Office.

Valla, J., Bergeron, L., & Smolla, N. (2000). The Dominic-R: A Pictorial Interview for 6- to 11-year-old children. *Journal of the American Academy of Child and Adolescent Psychiatry, 39,* 85–93.

Van der Gaag, R. J., Buitelaar, J., Van den Ban, E., Bezemer, M., Nijo, L., & Van Engeland, H. (1995). A controlled multivariate chart review of multiple complex developmental disorder. *Journal of the American Academy of Child and Adolescent Psychiatry, 34,* 1096–1106.

Vela, R. M., Gottlieb, E. H., & Gottlieb, H. P. (1983). Borderline syndromes in childhood: A critical review. In K. S. Robson (Ed.), *The borderline child: Approaches to etiology, diagnosis, and treatment.* New York: McGraw-Hill.

Viswanathan, V., Bridges, S. J., Whitehouse, W., & Newton, R. W. (1998). Childhood headaches: Discrete entities or continuum? *Developmental Medicine and Child Neurology, 40,* 544–550.

Vitaro, F., Gendreau, P. L., Tremblay, R. E., & Oligny, P. (1998). Reactive and proactive aggression differentially predict later conduct problems. *Journal of Child Psychiatry, Psychology, and Allied Disciplines, 39,* 377–385.

Volkmar, F. R., & Cohen, D. J. (1996). Nonautistic pervasive developmental disorders. In R. Michaels (Ed.), *Psychiatry* (Vol. 2). Baltimore: Lippincott Williams & Wilkins.

Volkmar, F. R., Klin, A., Marans, W. D., & McDougle, C. J. (1996). Autistic disorder. In F. R. Volkmar (Ed.), *Psychoses and pervasive developmental disorders in childhood and adolescence.* Washington, DC: American Psychiatric Press.

Volkmar, F. R., Klin, A., & Pauls, D. (1998). Nosological and genetic aspects of Asperger syndrome. *Journal of Autism and Developmental Disorders, 28,* 457–463.

Vygotsky, L. S. (1962). *Thought and language.* Cambridge, MA: MIT Press.

Vygotsky, L. S. (1978). *Mind in society.* Cambridge, MA: Harvard University Press.

Wahler, R. G., House, A. E., & Stambaugh, E. E., II. (1976). *Ecological assessment of child problem behavior.* New York: Pergamon Press.

Walter, A. L., & Carter, A. S. (1997). Gilles de la Tourette's syndrome in childhood: A guide for school professionals. *School Psychology Review, 26,* 28–46.

Walton, J. W., Johnson, S. B., & Algina, J. (1999). Mother and child perceptions of child anxiety: Effects of race, health, and stress. *Journal of Pediatric Psychology, 24,* 29–39.

Waschbusch, D. A., Daleiden, E., & Drabman, R. S. (2000). Are parents accurate reporters of their child's cognitive abilities? *Journal of Psychopathology and Behavioral Assessment, 22,* 61–77.

Webb, J. T. (2000, August). *Misdiagnosis and dual diagnosis of gifted children: Gifted and LD, ADHD, OCD, oppositional defiant disorder.* Paper presented at the annual convention of the American Psychological Association, Washington, DC. Available at http://www.sengifted.org in July 2001.

Webster-Stratton, C. (1996). Early-onset conduct disorder: Does gender make a difference? *Journal of Consulting and Clinical Psychology, 64,* 540–551.

Webster-Stratton, C., & Lindsay, D. W. (1999). Social competence and conduct problems in young children: Issues in assessment. *Journal of Clinical Child Psychology, 28,* 25–43.

Weinberg, N. Z., Rahdert, E., Colliver, J. D., & Glantz, M. D. (1998). Adolescent substance abuse: A review of the past 10 years. *Journal of the American Academy of Child and Adolescent Psychiatry, 37,* 252–261

Weiner, D. A., Abraham, M. E., & Lyons, J. (2001). Clinical characteristics of youths with substance use problems and implications for residential treatment. *Psychiatric Services, 52,* 793–799.

Wekerle, C., & Wolfe, D. A. (1996). Child maltreatment. In E. J. Mash & R. A. Barkley (Eds.), *Child psychopathology*. New York: Guilford Press.

Weller, E. B., Weller, R. A., Fristad, M. A., Rooney, M. T., & Schecter, J. (2000). Children's Interview for Psychiatric Symptoms (ChIPS). *Journal of the American Academy of Child and Adolescent Psychiatry, 39,* 76–84.

Wenar, C., & Kerig, P. (2000). *Developmental psychopathology* (4th ed.). Boston: McGraw-Hill.

Werry, J. S. (1996). Childhood schizophrenia. In F. R. Volkmar (Ed.), *Psychoses and pervasive developmental disorders in childhood and adolescence.* Washington, DC: American Psychiatric Press.

Wicks-Nelson, R., & Israel, A. C. (2000). *Behavior disorders in childhood* (4th ed.). Upper Saddle River, NJ: Prentice-Hall.

Widom, C. S. (1999). Posttraumatic stress disorder in abused and neglected children grown up. *American Journal of Psychiatry, 156,* 1223–1229.

Wiederman, M. W., & Pryor, T. (1996). Substance use and impulsive behaviors among adolescents with eating disorders. *Addictive Behavior, 21,* 269–272.

Wiers, R. W., Gunning W. B., & Sergeant, J. A. (1998). Is a mild deficit in executive functions in boys related to childhood ADHD or to parental multigenerational alcoholism? *Journal of Abnormal Child Psychology, 26,* 415–430.

Wilkinson-Ryan, T., & Westen, D. (2000). Identity disturbance in borderline personality disorder: An empirical investigation. *American Journal of Psychiatry, 157,* 528–541.

Willemsen-Swinkels, S. H. N., Buitelaar, J. K., Dekker, M., & van Engeland, H. (1989). Subtyping stereotypic behavior in children: The association between stereotypic behavior, mood, and heart rate. *Journal of Autism and Developmental Disorders, 28,* 547–557.

Wills, T. A., & Cleary, S. D. (1999). Peer and adolescent substance use among 6th–9th graders: Latent growth analyses of influence versus selection mechanisms. *Health Psychology, 18,* 453–463.

Wilson, G. T., Heffernan, K., & Black, C. M. D. (1996). Eating Disorders. In E. J. Mash & R. A. Barkley (Eds.), *Child psychopathology*. New York: Guilford Press.

Wing, L. (1997). Syndromes of autism and atypical development. In D. J. Cohen & F. R. Volkmar (Eds.), *Handbook of autism and pervasive developmental disorders.* New York: Wiley.

Wintgens, A., Lepine, S., Lefebvre, F., Glorieux, J., Gauthier, Y., & Robaey, P. (1998). Attachment, self-esteem, and psychomotor development in extremely premature children at preschool age. *Infant Mental Health Journal, 19,* 394–408.

Wise, A. J., & Spengler, P. M. (1997). Suicide in children younger than age fourteen: Clinical judgment and assessment issues. *Journal of Mental Health Counseling, 19,* 318–335.

Woodward, L. J., & Fergusson, D. M. (2000). Childhood peer relationship problems and later risks of educational underachievement and unemployment. *Journal of Child Psychology, Psychiatry, and Allied Disciplines, 41,* 191–201.

World Health Organization. (1992). *International classification of disease* (10th ed.). Geneva: Author.

Yates, A. (1987). Psychological damage associated with extreme eroticism in young children. *Psychiatric Annals, 17,* 257–261.

Yeates, K. O. (2000). Closed-head injury. In K. O. Yeates, M. D. Ris, & H. G. Taylor (Eds.), *Pediatric neuropsychology: Research, theory, and practice.* New York: Guilford Press.

Ychuda, R. (1999). Biological factors associated with susceptibility to posttraumatic stress disorder. *Canadian Journal of Psychiatry, 44,* 34–39.

Zahn-Waxler, C. (1993). Warriors and worriers: Gender and psychopathology. *Development and Psychopathology, 5,* 79–89.

Zalsman, G., Netanel, R., Fischel, T., Freudenstein, O., Landau, E., Orbach, I., Weizman, A., Pfeffer, C. R., & Apter, A. (2000). Human figure drawings in the evaluation of severe adolescent suicidal behavior. *Journal of the American Academy of Child and Adolescent Psychiatry, 39,* 1024–1031.

Zappella, M., Gillberg, C., & Ehlers, S. (1998). The preserved speech variant: A subgroup of the Rett complex: A clinical report of 30 cases. *Journal of Autism and Developmental Disorders, 28,* 519–526.

Zarek, D., Hawkins, D., & Rogers, P. D. (1987). Risk factors for adolescent substance abuse: Implications for pediatric practice. *Pediatric Clinics of North America, 34,* 481–493.

Zero to Three/National Center for Clinical Infant Programs. (1994). *Diagnostic classification of mental health and developmental disorders of infancy and early childhood.* Arlington, VA: National Center for Clinical Infant Programs.

Zoccolillo, M. (1993). Gender and the development of conduct disorder. *Development and Psychopathology, 5,* 65–78.

Zoccolillo, M., Meyers, J., & Assiter, S. (1997). Conduct disorder, substance dependence, and adolescent motherhood. *American Journal of Orthopsychiatry, 67,* 152–157.

# Index